T0340697

**Diabetes and
Kidney Disease**

Diabetes and
Kidney Disease

EDITED BY

Gunter Wolf MD, MHBA

Professor and Chairman
Department of Internal Medicine III
University of Jena
University Hospital
Jena, Germany

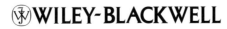

A John Wiley & Sons, Ltd., Publication

This edition first published 2013 © 2013 by John Wiley & Sons, Ltd.

Wiley-Blackwell is an imprint of John Wiley & Sons, formed by the merger of Wiley's global Scientific, Technical and Medical business with Blackwell Publishing.

Registered office: John Wiley & Sons, Ltd, The Atrium, Southern Gate, Chichester, West Sussex, PO19 8SQ, UK

Editorial offices: 9600 Garsington Road, Oxford, OX4 2DQ, UK
The Atrium, Southern Gate, Chichester, West Sussex, PO19 8SQ, UK
111 River Street, Hoboken, NJ 07030-5774, USA

For details of our global editorial offices, for customer services and for information about how to apply for permission to reuse the copyright material in this book please see our website at www.wiley.com/wiley-blackwell

The right of the author to be identified as the author of this work has been asserted in accordance with the UK Copyright, Designs and Patents Act 1988.

Library of Congress Cataloging-in-Publication Data
Diabetes and kidney disease / edited by Gunter Wolf.
    p. ; cm.
Includes bibliographical references and index.
ISBN 978-0-470-67502-1 (hardback : alk. paper)
I. Wolf, Gunter, 1961–
[DNLM: 1. Diabetic Nephropathies. WK 835]
LC Classification not assigned
616.4'62–dc23
                              2012036995

A catalogue record for this book is available from the British Library.

Wiley also publishes its books in a variety of electronic formats. Some content that appears in print may not be available in electronic books.

Cover image: Courtesy of Hermann J. Kissler, Christiane Rüster, Utz Settmacher
Cover design by Garth Stewart

Set in 8/12 pt Stone Serif by Toppan Best-set Premedia Limited
Printed and bound in Singapore by Markono Print Media Pte Ltd

1   2013

Contributors, vii

Kerstin Amann MD
Professor of Nephropathology
Department of Pathology
Universität Erlangen-Nürnberg
Erlangen, Germany

Carsten A. Böger MD
Department of Internal Medicine II
Nephrology
University Medical Center Regensburg
Regensburg, Germany

Martin Busch MD
Consultant, Nephrologist and Lecturer
Department of Internal Medicine III
Jena University Hospital, Jena, Germany

Christoph Daniel PhD
Nephropathology, Department of Pathology
Universität Erlangen-Nürnberg
Erlangen, Germany

Jörg Dötsch MD
Professor of Pediatrics
University Hospital of Cologne
Department of Pediatric and Adolescent
Medicine
Cologne, Germany

Muriel A. Ghosn MD
Medical Chief Resident
Department of Internal Medicine
American University of Beirut
Beirut, Lebanon

Hans-Peter Hammes MD
Section Head, Endocrinology
5th Medical Department
UMM – University of Heidelberg
Mannheim, Germany

Anita Hansen MD
Medical Faculty
Department of Nephrology
Heinrich-Heine University Düsseldorf
Düsseldorf, Germany

Christoph Hasslacher
Professor of Internal Medicine
Diabetesinstitut Heidelberg
St. Josefskrankenhaus
Heidelberg, Germany

Andrea Icks MD DPH MBA
Institute of Biometrics and Epidemiology
German Diabetes Center;
Senior Lecturer
Department of Public Health
Faculty of Medicine
Heinrich-Heine University
Düsseldorf, Germany

Bethany Karl DO
Nephrology Fellow
Center for Renal Translational Medicine
University of California
CA, USA

Hermann J. Kissler MD
Visceral Surgery Fellow
Department of General, Visceral and
Vascular Surgery
Jena University Hospital
Jena, Germany

Helmut Kleinwechter MD
Specialist in Diabetology
Diabetologikum Kiel
Diabetes Center and Diabetes Education
Center
Kiel, Germany

Michael Koch MD
Head
Center of Nephrology Mettmann, Germany;
Clinic of Urology and Nephrology
Niederberg Hospital Velbert, Germany

Gabriele Lehmann MD
Department of Internal Medicine III
Jena University Hospital
Jena, Germany

Ivonne Loeffler PhD
Postdoctoral Research Fellow
Department of Internal Medicine III
Jena University Hospital
Jena, Germany

Peter R. Mertens MD
Professor of Medicine
Director
Department of Nephrology and
Hypertension, Diabetes and Endocrinology
Otto-von-Guericke University Magdeburg
Magdeburg, Germany

Ulrich A. Müller MD MSc
Department of Medicine III
Jena University Hospital
Jena, Germany

Thomas Neumann MD
Consultant Rheumatologist
Department of Internal Medicine III
Jena University Hospital
Jena, Germany

Kai D. Nüsken MD
Division of Pediatric Nephrology
Department of Pediatric and Adolescent
Medicine
University Hospital of Cologne
Cologne, Germany

Ivo Quack MD
Medical Faculty
Department of Nephrology
Heinrich-Heine University Düsseldorf
Düsseldorf, Germany,

Eberhard Ritz MD
Professor of Nephrology
Department Internal Medicine
Division of Nephrology
Nierenzentrum
Carola Ruperto University Hospital
Heidelberg, Germany

Lars Christian Rump MD
Professor of Medicine
Department of Nephrology
Heinrich-Heine University Düsseldorf
Düsseldorf, Germany

Christiane Rüster MD
Attending Physician, Nephrologist
Department of Internal Medicine III
Jena University Hospital
Jena, Germany

Alexander Sämann MD
Department of Medicine III
Jena University Hospital
Jena, Germany

Ute Schäfer-Graf MD, PhD
Specialist in Perinatology and Diabetology
Berlin Diabetes and Pregnancy Center
Department of Gynecology and Obstetrics
St. Joseph Hospital
Berlin, Germany

Utz Settmacher MD
Professor of Surgery
Chairman
Department of General, Visceral and
Vascular Surgery
Jena University Hospital
Jena, Germany

Kumar Sharma MD FAHA
Director
Center for Renal Translational Medicine
Professor of Medicine
University of California
CA, USA

Christoph Wanner MD
Professor of Medicine
Department of Medicine
Division of Nephrology
University of Würzburg
Würzburg, Germany

Fuad N. Ziyadeh MD FASN FACP
Professor of Medicine and Biochemistry
Chairman, Department of Internal Medicine
American University of Beirut
Beirut, Lebanon

In 1801 the English physician Erasmus Darwin (1731–1802) recognized some patient with diabetes whose urine could be coagulated by heat, indicating proteinuria, and associated this finding with dropsy and general swelling. In 1936, the seminal discovery by Kimmelstiel and Wilson showed the morphologic changes by the description of glomerular lesions in diabetics with nephropathy. Today, diabetic renal disease is now worldwide the major cause of end-stage renal failure. Besides the uncountable individual suffering of patients with diabetic nephropathy, there is an increasing economical burden for such patients. Patients with diabetic renal disease have a very high cardiovascular morbidity and mortality. The spectrum of patients with diabetes and renal disease has completely been changed: 25 year ago diabetic nephropathy was a feature of patients with type 1 diabetes, type 2 diabetes was considered a relatively rare even a "normal" process of aging. Now, the increasing pandemic of patients with type 2 diabetes makes this group the largest suffering from diabetic nephropathy, albeit the incidence of patients with type 1 diabetes has also increased in recent years. The current book provides an up-to-date review of many aspects, not only of diabetic nephropathy but of the more complex relationship between the kidney and diabetes. All the contributors to this book are experts in their fields. It covers a wide range of topics from epidemiology, pathophysiology and genetics to concrete treatment recommendations and algorithms for the practicing physician. Furthermore, the reader will also find chapters on topics normally not found in standard books on diabetic nephropathy, such as diabetic nephropathy in children, the relationship between retinal and renal diabetic complications and diabetes, bone, and the kidney. Therefore, the book is not only for the expert nephrologists and diabetologists, but also for general internists and primary care physicians. The authors have put an enormous amount of work into this book. They would be happy if this contribution could help to better care for patients with diabetes and renal affections. Many thanks to Wiley-Blackwell (especially Jennifer Seward) for agreeing to start this ambiguous projects and for the continuous help while carrying it out.

Professor Dr. Gunter Wolf MD, MHBA
Department of Internal Medicine III
University of Jena
Jena, Germany

Part I

Introduction and Pathophysiology

History of diabetic nephropathy: a personal account

Eberhard Ritz

Carola Ruperto University Hospital, Heidelberg, Germany

Type 2 diabetes and diabetes-associated nephropathy have currently become worldwide epidemics, but they are by no means completely novel diseases. No unequivocal description of diabetes mellitus is found in the *Corpus Hippocraticum* or in the subsequent European medical literature; in Europe it was centuries before the sweet taste of urine in subjects with diabetes was described by Thomas Willis in 1674, and for sugar as the responsible chemical compound to be identified in the urine by Matthew Dobson in 1776.

In contrast, an impressive body of evidence documents the common presence of diabetes, presumably the result of genetics and lifestyle, in ancient India and China, and later in Arabia and Iran, pointing to the diagnostic acumen of the physicians of these countries in the distant past.

The characteristic "sweet urine" in diabetes was mentioned in the Indian Sanskrit literature covering medicine and presumably written between 300 BC and AD 600 [1]. These ancient physicians mentioned "sugar cane urine" (*Iksumeha*) or "honey urine" (*Madhumeha* and *Hastimeha*) as well as "urine flow like elephant in heat". They noted that ants and insects would rush to such honey urine—strongly suggesting that this observation was the consequence of glycosuria and diabetes. This condition was correctly ascribed to excessive food intake and insufficient exercise; the authors also mentioned the cardinal symptoms: polyphagia, polyuria, and polydipsia; even the secondary sequelae of diabetes, such as abscess formation, carbuncles, lassitude, and floppiness, were reported. Proposed interventions included the very rational advice of active physical exercise and long marches. In China, the oldest description of diabetes as "Xiao-ke" (wasting thirst or emaciation and thirst) syndrome can be traced back more than 2000 years to the *Yellow Emperor's Classic of Internal Medicine*. Ancient Chinese physicians had

Diabetes and Kidney Disease, First Edition. Edited by Gunter Wolf.
© 2013 John Wiley & Sons, Ltd. Published 2013 by John Wiley & Sons, Ltd.

noted that "sweet" urine was a manifestation of a disease characterized by hunger and poly-phagia, by thirst and polydipsia as well as by polyuria. In addition, Chinese literature has described the characteristic complications of skin abscesses, infections, blindness, turbid urine, and edema. The pathogenesis of this condition was ascribed to improper fatty, sweet, and excessively rich diet. Interventions with diet therapy, exercise, herbal medicine, and acupuncture were proposed.

In Arabian (and Persian) literature diabetes, called "Aldulab" (water wheel), as a disease char-acterized by polydipsia, polyuria, and marasm was described by the scholar Abū Alī al-Husain ibn Abdullāh ibn Sīnā (Avicenna AD 980–1037) [2]. It is also of interest that Maimonides, a Jewish physician who emigrated from Toledo to Egypt commented on a disease in Egypt of fat, elderly men characterized by polyuria and rapid physical decay; he stated that he had never seen this condition in his native Toledo, illustrating the apparent rarity of diabetes in Europe at that time. Subsequently, in medieval Europe diabetes definitely existed, at least in the upper class, as suggested by the available descriptions of the terminal diseases of Henry VIII of England, Louis XIV of France, August der Starke of Saxony, and others. However, it was centuries before the sweet taste of urine in diabetes was described by Thomas Willis (in 1674) and before sugar in the urine was identified as a distinct chemical substance by Matthew Dobson (in 1776).

Nevertheless some key observations had been made very early. Domenico Cotugno (*De Ischiade Nervosa*, Commentarius Gräffer, Vienna, 1770) described what in retrospect presumably was proteinuria in a nephrotic patient with coagulable urine; later proteinu-ria was described in diabetic patients on many occasions.

In the 19th century, with increasing wealth and an increasing prevalence of obesity, a pro-gressive increase in the frequency of type 2 diabetes was noted. In type 2 diabetes, pro-teinuria was repeatedly described in the 19th century, but end-stage renal disease (ESRD) was apparently uncommon in type 2 diabetic patients, presumably because most patients died from cardiovascular events or other (mostly infectious) complications before the manifestations of advanced kidney disease appeared. The failure to recognize renal disease as a sequela of diabetes is illustrated by the fact that Friedrich Theodor von Frerichs had written a brilliant description on the pathophysiology underlying proteinuria and kidney disease [3]; yet, disappointingly, in his encyclopedic book on diabetes (*Über den Diabetes*, Berlin, 1884, Verlag August Hirschwald), the standard book on diabetes in the German literature, he mentioned only tubular and interstitial lesions of the kidney, and did not mention the glomeruli at all. Surprisingly, he states that the kidneys of diabetic patients are usually small and that interstitial tissue is increased.

Later, Armanni described vacuolization in proximal tubular epithelial cells with subnu-clear deposits of glycogen and fat in the kidneys of diabetic patients (Armanni–Ebstein lesion) [4].

It was Griesinger who first provided a systematic analysis of kidney morphology [5] describing, 64 autopsies of diabetic individu-als. This analysis was based on the available literature and included seven of his own patients whom he had treated up to this point in Tübingen, reflecting the relative rarity of diabetes at that time. Fifty-eight per cent of the patients were between 20 and 40 years, and he stated that diabetes was rare elderly people. He stated,

the opinion that the kidneys are infrequently affected in this disease and changes of the kidneys, if any, would consist only in true hypertrophy is wrong. In any case, these dis-eases of the kidneys complicate diabetes in a remarkable fashion and are the trigger for a series of pathological processes in many advanced cases. The frequency of these renal lesions is in line with the frequent finding that many diabetic patients have protein in their urine, mostly not constantly, but often at times copiously. . . . there are, however, cases where – with the onset of albuminuria – sugar disappears from the urine. In these cases usually morbus Brightii takes its known course with generalized hydrops etc. In the majority of cases, moderate albuminuria coexists with glycosuria . . . .

Another description of kidney lesions was provided by Abeille [6], who stated,

most frequently one finds only simple hypertrophy of the kidney at autopsy . . . in some cases these organs were the seat of Bright's disease, i.e. albuminuria associated with glucosuria . . . it has been stated that albuminuria documents regression of the disease . . . to the contrary it is the result of functional trouble or evidence of structural lesions as a result of Bright's disease.

What had been widely known in the 19th century was the high prevalence of albuminuria in diabetes; characteristic is the observation of Schmitz, who stated that in 1200 diabetics he found different amounts of urinary protein in 824 cases; he stated "I never saw uremia to occur in an albuminuric diabetic patient, presumably because they died beforehand from cardiovascular causes" [7]. Naunyn [8] had an interest in diabetes, and the pancreatic secretion of a glycemia-lowering substance had been discovered by Mehring and Minkowski at his clinic in Strasburg. Naunyn found albuminuria in 34 of 134 young diabetic patients, of whom six patients excreted >1 g of albumin per day. He also confirmed the above-mentioned observation that glycosuria disappeared when proteinuria increased. The same observation was also made by van Noorden [9].

At this time, a key finding for the understanding of diabetic nephropathy was the discovery by Etienne Lancereaux in 1880 that there are two types of diabetes, i.e. type 1 (diabete maigre) and type 2 (diabetes obese).

It is of interest that in the 19th century and even in the first decades of the 20th century, chronic kidney disease in diabete patients is not mentioned at all in major textbooks on kidney disease, e.g., by Volhard or Fishberg. Franz Volhard in his ground-breaking description of kidney disease [10] completely ignored diabetes as a cause of kidney disease in this seminal work. Even later in Fishberg's book [11], the reference to diabetes is limited to diabetic coma and to prerenal azotemia; he stated "nephritis is extremely rare in diabetes and if it occurs, it is not the result of excessive 'work' of the kidney, but is caused by accompanying problems, e.g., tuberculosis, cardiac disease, arteriosclerosis." In summary, apart from recognizing diabetes as a cause of proteinuria, diabetes was not on the radar of most physicians with an interest in nephrology. Even among diabetologists, nephropathy was not at the forefront of interest until approximately 20 years after the introduction of insulin treatment—the latency until severe renal problems arise.

Étienne Lancereaux (1829–1910) in his paper "Le diabete maigre: ses symptomes, son evolution, son prognostie et son traitement" had introduced the concept of "diabète maigre" and "diabète obese" in 1880. In retrospect, it is of interest to note that the breakthroughs achieved by the early descriptions of Kimmelstiel [12] and of Allen [13] almost all concerned patients with type 2 diabetes with a relatively long duration of the disease, presumably because type 1 diabetic patients had often succumbed before they had time to develop glomerulosclerosis. After insulin became available, it usually took up to two decades for terminal kidney disease to develop. Subsequently, however, in the 1960s and 1970s, the focus of attention in clinical and anatomical studies on diabetic nephropathy was on type 1 diabetic patients who had at this point in time lived long enough to develop advanced diabetic nephropathy, which takes more than 10 to 20 years to develop.

All this started with the brilliant description of intercapillary lesions in diabetic patients by Paul Kimmelstiel and Clifford Wilson in 1936 [12]. Kimmelstiel was born to a Jewish merchant family in Hamburg and was associate professor at the Department of Pathology in Hamburg–Eppendorf. In 1933 he emigrated to the USA and worked at the Harvard Institute of Pathology, where he met Clifford Wilson with whom he described the intercapillary changes of the glomerulus in diabetes mellitus in a landmark publication. He studied the kidneys of eight patients who had presented with massive edema (out of proportion to existing cardiac failure) with hypertension of the "benign" type and with a history of long-standing diabetes. The glomeruli were regularly hyalinized (staining for fat, but only exceptionally yielding double refraction) and the number of capillaries was reduced. Often a ring of open capillaries surrounded central hyaline masses. A very high degree of "arteriosclerosis" with fatty degeneration was seen in the arterioles. Although the basement membrane of the capillaries was preserved for a long time, it eventually changed and the capillary walls thickened homogeneously near the central hyaline masses; the capillaries collapsed and finally merged with the central hyaline. There was no definite proof of an inflammatory process. He gave a very detailed account of the differences between this novel lesion and intercapillary glomerulonephritis as described by Fahr, an extracapillary glomerulonephritis emphasizing the striking hyaline thickening of the intercapillary connective tissue of the glomerulus. The non-inflammatory degenerative nature of the lesion suggested to him that both arteriosclerosis and

diabetes were involved in its causation, and prompted him to coin the novel term "intercapillary glomerulosclerosis". Interestingly, in 1934, MacCallum had described glomerular lesions resembling Kimmelstiel–Wilson lesions; however, he failed to make the connection to diabetes and ascribed this to "the ageing process of the glomerulus".

Kimmelstiel's concept of a diabetes-specific glomerular disease was confirmed and more firmly identified as a sequela of diabetes by Allen in New York [13]. He popularized the concept of a specific glomerular lesion caused by diabetes, based on autopsies of a much larger cohort of 105 diabetic patients, 34% of whom showed this specific lesion. He noted that it was virtually specific for diabetes (which is no longer absolutely true today, e.g., it may be seen in κ-light chain nephropathy etc.).

In the early 1970s, more and more diabetic patients were started on hemodialysis; these were initially almost exclusively young patients with type 1 diabetes (interestingly the first type 1 diabetic patient who started hemodialysis in Downstate Medical Center Brooklyn as a compassionate case was the husband of a dialysis nurse). The initial outcomes were most unsatisfactory [14], and in these days it was stated "Diabetic nephropathy is irreversible in humans; no case of recovery or cure has been reported in the literature; once the clinical signs of nephropathy have become manifest, the natural course is inexorable progressive to death" [15]. The helpless situation of the physician at this time was illustrated by the statement ". . . the renal failure will progress in spite of all forms of therapy. In the terminal stage the physician's role will mostly be of psychological nature, attempting to maintain a reasonable degree of optimism in the patient . . ." [16]. It was only later on that the major proportion of patients with advanced diabetic nephropathy developing terminal renal failure suffered from type 2 diabetes. In retrospect it is amusing that we [17] had great difficulty to get our paper published which indicated a "similar risks of nephropathy in patients with type 1 or 2 diabetes mellitus"—this statement was based on the finding that the cumulative risk of proteinuria after 25 years of diabetes mellitus was 57% in type 2 diabetes and 46% in type 1 diabetes. Obviously it was felt that renal complications were mostly restricted to patients with type 1 diabetes. In the early 1970s, when diabetics first started on dialysis, it was mainly relatively young type 1 diabetic patients. Today this has become a small minority (2.2% of diabetic patients on hemodialysis in Germany [18] while type 1 plus type 2 diabetes currently accounts for 49.6% of all hemodialysis patients in Germany [18].

The progress in understanding the underlying pathophysiology of diabetic nephropathy, the introduction of treatments to prevent, stop, or at least retard progression of diabetic nephropathy, and the progressively better outcomes of the treatment of end-stage diabetic nephropathy by dialysis or transplantation has been an impressive success story in recent decades. For reasons of space we focus on interventions that interfere with the progression of diabetic nephropathy.

A major initial step forward was the introduction of quantitative morphology by Osterby in Aarhus. She showed that in the early stage of diabetes the basement membranes were normal (thus excluding the then popular hypothesis of a pre-existing capillary defect predisposing to diabetic nephropathy). She concluded that such changes of the capillary membrane were the consequence of hyperglycemia—thus opening the window to prevention by achieving near-normal glycemia [19]

In those days, the notion prevailed that diabetic nephropathy was a unidirectional process with continuous downhill deterioration. The observation of Fioretto [20] provided evidence that the lesions of diabetic nephropathy are potentially reversible after pancreas transplantation. Using quantitative methods to evaluate

glomerular morphology, she studied at baseline and after 5 and 10 years eight microalbuminuric type 1 diabetic patients who had received a pancreas transplant. Before transplantation median albuminuria was 103 mg/day; it had decreased to 20 mg/day 10 years after pancreas transplantation. Although 5 years after pancreas transplantation the thickness of the glomerular and tubular basement membranes had not changed, after 10 years the thickness of the glomerular basement membrane had significantly decreased from 570 ± 64 nm to 404 ± 38 nm; the mesangial fractional volume had decreased as well (baseline 0.33 ± 0.007; at 10 years 0.27 ± 0.02 $p = 0.05$), thus documenting that in principle the lesions of diabetic nephropathy are even reversible with longstanding normoglycemia.

In an important later study on the morphology underlying progression, Osterby showed that the onset of proteinuria is associated with widespread disconnection of the junction between the proximal tubuli and the associated glomerulus, leading to atubular glomeruli and loss of glomerular function [21]. She also showed that in type 2 diabetes, the lesions are more heterogeneous and resemble the typical histological pattern of type 1 diabetic lesions only in a minority of cases [22].

In the clinical arena, the door for early diagnosis of glomerulopathy was opened with the availability of an immunoassay for urinary albumin in low concentrations [23]. The establishment of this novel methodology permitted Keen's collaborator Giancarlo Viberti [24] to examine 87 patients with insulin-dependent diabetes mellitus in whom the urinary albumin excretion rate (AER) was measured in 1966/67; at follow-up after 15 years, 63 of the original cohort were alive and were restudied; the others had died in between. The development of albustix-positive proteinuria was related to past AER values in 1966/67: the advanced stage of proteinuria had developed in only two of 55 patients with an initial AER <30 mg/min, but in seven of eight patients with AER 30–140 mg/min—illustrating the power of "microalbuminuria" to predict the evolution of clinical diabetic nephropathy. With foresight he postulated that such levels of AER are potentially reversible, pointing to the possibility of the prevention of diabetic kidney disease. This key observation was quickly confirmed by other authors, specifically Mogensen [25] and Parving [26].

Furthermore, Mogensen [27] provided the evidence that in type 2 diabetic patients microalbuminuria was predictive of renal and cardiovascular risk and stated that "screening for microalbuminuria in such population will identify high risk patients with abnormalities that are potentially treatable." Today, monitoring of urine albumin excretion is part and parcel of the standard of care for diabetes and has done much to increase awareness of the renal (and cardiovascular) complications of diabetes.

The potential significance of albuminuria soon broadened beyond the issue of kidney disease with the proposal of the "Steno hypothesis" that "albuminuria in type 1 diabetes is not only an indication of renal disease, but a new independent risk marker of proliferative retinopathy and macroangiopathy as a result of a generalized abnormality ("leakiness") of vascular beds [28].

It has recently been argued that the concept of "micro"-albuminuria should be abandoned and that urine albumin concentration should be treated as a continuous variable which reflects the progressive increase in both renal and cardiovascular risks in patients with progressively higher concentrations of urinary albumin [29], but because of the inertia of medical nomenclature the term microalbuminuria persists to this day.

Despite the early documentation of Mogensen that microalbuminuria predicts clinical proteinuria and early mortality, the common view was that the risk of developing nephropathy

and uremia was very high in type 1 diabetes, but substantially less elevated in type 2 diabetes. Since in those days type 2 diabetes occurred mostly in elderly individuals with limited life expectancy and high cardiovascular mortality, the true renal risk in type 2 diabetes had been underestimated, because most patients did not survive to experience advanced renal complications. The study of Hasslacher [17] addressed this issue by evaluating all patients with type 2 and type 1 diabetes without severe secondary disease who were followed in the university hospital in Heidelberg between 1970 and 1985. After 25 years it was found that the cumulative risk of proteinuria was virtually identical, i.e., 57% in type 2 and 47% in type 1 diabetes; the cumulative risk of renal failure 5 years after the onset of proteinuria was 63% and 59% respectively. This finding documented that in patients with type 2 and type 1 diabetes the renal risk is similar.

Apart from progress in the understanding of the diagnostic value of albuminuria and of the underlying renal pathology, enormous progress had also been made in the prevention and treatment of diabetic nephropathy. One major step concerned glycemic control. This was first evaluated in type 1 diabetes by the landmark prospective controlled Diabetes Control and Complications study [30, 31] and by the subsequent observational Epidemiology of Diabetes Interventions and Complications follow-up study [32]. Young type 1 diabetic patients with no or mild retinopathy had been randomized to conventional or intensified glycemic control (insulin pump or three daily injections). The study clearly documented the benefit of intensive control: the onset of albuminuria >40 mg/day was lower by 39% and onset of proteinuria by 54% [22]. The detailed analysis of the progression of diabetic nephropathy showed that the beneficial effect on albuminuria was independent of blood pressure, age, diabetes duration, baseline glycosylated hemoglobin (HbA1c), and retinopathy [33]. The controlled trial was followed by an observational follow-up in which glycemic control was no longer significantly different between the two arms of the study population. Nevertheless, 22 years after the start of the study a glomerular filtration rate (GFR) <60 mL/min/1.73 m² was observed in 24 patients in the group with initially intensified versus 46 patients with initially standard treatment [32]. Indeed today, given better glycemic control and more efficient blood pressure-lowering agents including renin–angiotensin system (RAS) blockade, type 1 diabetic patients in most countries have become a small minority of the total number of diabetic patients requiring treatment for end-stage kidney disease.

A second quantum leap forward was the introduction of antihypertensive treatment. In the past it was thought that blood pressure elevation was necessary to guarantee adequate renal perfusion. I couldn't find a reference to this in the literature, but I learned from Carl Erik Mogensen that as a young physician he tried to lower blood pressure in a type 1 diabetic patient with the newly introduced beta-blockers, although this had been strictly forbidden by the chief of department—obviously because of the then frequent side effects. Against the advice of the authorities, he gave antihypertensive treatment and some years later he could show that this had reduced the progressive loss of GFR in type 1 diabetic patients. This prompted him to carry out a short-term study and a long-term study [34, 35] in six young male diabetic patients with intermittent albustix-positive proteinuria and in 10 young male diabetics with constant proteinuria—a ridiculously small group compared with today's mega trials; he measured glomerular filtration and plasma flow as well as urinary albumin excretion using exact techniques. In the patients without constant proteinuria, no deterioration in renal function was noted during a mean control period of 32 months. In contrast, in patients with constant proteinu-

ria, the decrease in GFR and renal plasma flow (RPF) was 0.91 mL/min/month ± 0.68 and 4.38 mL/min/month ± 3.23 respectively. A positive correlation was found between the rate of decrease in GFR on the one hand and diastolic pressure and albuminuria on the other. After this pioneer study, Mogensen performed an interventional uncontrolled study [35] in six insulin-dependent, juvenile-onset diabetic patients. Blood pressure was lowered from an average of 162/103 mmHg to a mean level of 144/95 mmHg for 73 months. The diastolic pressure was lowered to 95 mmHg, the GFR loss was 1.23 mL/min/month in the run-in period and reduced to 0.49 mL/min/month on antihypertensive treatment; finally a dramatic 95% decrease in albuminuria was seen. This led Mogensen to firmly conclude that antihypertensive treatment slows the decline in renal function in diabetic nephropathy. Based on this finding, which was also reported by Parving [26, 36] at the same time, antihypertensive treatment has become a bedrock of today's management of diabetic nephropathy.

The third advance in the management of diabetic nephropathy was the introduction of RAS blockade. With the availability of captopril and subsequently of alternative angiotensin-converting enzyme (ACE) inhibitors, in a number of studies different investigators documented the beneficial acute and intermediate-term effect of RAS blockade on lowering albuminuria/proteinuria over and above what was seen with alternative antihypertensive agents [37–42] in relatively small cohorts.

A sufficiently large prospective study on nephropathy of type 1 diabetes was performed by a collaborative study group. The effect of captopril was compared with placebo in 409 patients with proteinuria >500 mg/day and serum creatinine >2.5 mg/dL. Doubling of s-creatinine was significantly less frequent in patients on captopril ($n = 25$) versus placebo ($n = 43$); furthermore, a small but significant difference in the rate of decline in creatinine clearance was found: $11 \pm 21\%$ per year in the captopril versus $17 \pm 20\%$ in the placebo group, thus documenting that captopril protects against deterioration in renal function in insulin-dependent diabetes with nephropathy significantly more effectively than blood pressure control alone. An impressive 50% reduction in the combined end point of death, dialysis, and transplantation was noted on captopril [43]. Remission of nephrotic-range proteinuria was more frequent in the nephrotic probands of the captopril group (7/42 versus 1/66 in the placebo group; in parallel, GFR by iothalamate clearance declined significantly only in the group which had not achieved remission, thus documenting that captopril protects against deterioration in renal function in insulin-dependent diabetic nephropathy significantly more effectively than blood pressure control alone [31]. A further follow-up study compared two levels of target blood pressure [mean arterial pressure (MAP) 92 mmHg versus 100–107 mmHg]; there was no difference in the GFR loss, but proteinuria was significantly less (535 mg/24 hour) in the captopril than in the placebo group [44], which led the authors to suggest that in this population the target MAP should be 92 mmHg.

Because type 2 diabetes is much more frequent than type 1, a major challenge was to document the effect of RAS blockade on nephropathy in type 2 diabetes. In the meantime, angiotensin receptor blockers had become available. The study of Barnett [45] in type 2 diabetic patients at relatively early stages of diabetic nephropathy documented that both ACE inhibitors (enalapril) and angiotensin receptor blockers (irbesartan) were equally effective to achieve a stable plateau of GFR after approximately 4 years following the start of treatment. In type 2 diabetic patients at more advanced stages of diabetic nephropathy, two contemporaneous controlled studies were performed: one with Losartan [46] and the other with Irbesartan [47]. Both came to the

same conclusion, i.e., apart from reducing proteinuria, the composite end point of doubling of baseline serum creatinine, development of ESRD or death from any cause was reached in a smaller proportion of patients.

The fourth recent advance was by the Steno Memorial Hospital group in Copenhagen in a controlled study of patients with type 2 diabetes and microalbuminuria. The study provided the proof that intensified multifactorial intervention is more effective than standard treatment according to guidelines (i.e. those valid at the time the study was started). In this study 151 patients were randomly assigned to a group according to the (then) guidelines of the Danish society or to intensified treatment, which consisted of reduction of saturated fat, light to moderate exercise, no smoking (advise which was futile), captopril (irrespective of blood pressure), vitamin C, etc. An effort was made to achieve glycosylated hemoglobin (HbA1c) <6.5%. After a 3.8-year follow-up progression to overt nephropathy was already less (OR 0.27) as was progression of retinopathy (OR 0.45) or autonomic neuropathy (OR 0.32) [48]. After a follow-up of 7.8 years, 47 patients achieved remission to normoalbuminuria. This was associated with less decline in GFR (Δ –2.3 $\pm$ 0.4 mL/min/year) compared with patients who progressed to overt nephropathy (GFR Δ $\pm$ 0.5 mL/min/year). The start of antihypertensive treatment was also associated with remission to normoalbuminuria (OR 2.32) as was a 1% decrease in HbA1c [49]. In this cohort, the hazard ratio (HR) of a cardiovascular (CV) event was lowered to 0.47, of nephropathy 0.39, and of retinopathy 0.42—globally, approximately 50% risk reduction. The study was followed by an observational follow-up. After no less than 13.3 years a significant effect was also seen on cardiovascular mortality and ESRD: 24 patients in the intensive treatment versus 40 in the conventional treatment group had died (hazard ratio 0.54); both CV death (HR 0.43) and CV events (HR 0.41) were lower in the intensive treatment group. Only one patient in the intensive versus six patients in the conventional treatment group had developed end-stage kidney disease, suggesting an effect of metabolic memory.

Obviously, compared with the sad state of treatment of diabetic nephropathy 40 years ago [14], the prognosis of diabetic nephropathy has been improved dramatically. But the number of patients, mostly with type 2 diabetes, currently entering end-stage kidney disease, continues to be a challenge and will require novel approaches in the future.

1. Frank LL. Diabetes mellitus in the texts of old Hindu medicine (Charaka, Susruta, Vagbhata). *Am J Gastroenterol* 1957;**27**:76–95.
2. Mujais SK, Nephrologic beginnings: the kidney in the age of Ibn Sina (980–1037 AD). *Am J Nephrol* 1987;**7**:133–6.
3. Schwarz U, Ritz E. Glomerulonephritis and progression–Friedrich Theodor von Frerichs, a forgotten pioneer. *Nephrol Dial Transplant* 1997;**12**:2776–8.
4. Giordano C, De Santo NG, Lamendola MG, Capodicasa G. The genesis of the Armanni-Ebstein lesion in diabetic nephropathy. *J Diabet Complications* 1987;**1**:2–3.
5. Griesinger W. Studien über Diabetes. *Archiv Physiologie Heilkunde* 1859; **3**:1–75.
6. Abeille J. *Traité des maladies a urines albumineuses et sucrées*. Paris: J.-B. Baillère, 1865, p. 6.48
7. Schmitz R. *Ueber die prognostische Bedeutung und die Aetiologie der Albuminurie bei Diabetes. Berliner Klinische Wochenschrift* 1891;**28**: 373–7.
8. Naunyn B. *Der Diabetes Mellitus*, 2nd edn. Vienna: Alfred Hölder, 1906.
9. Van Noorden C. *Die Zuckerkrankheiten— ihre Bedeutung*, 6th edn Berlin: A. Hirschfeld, 1912.
10. Volhard F, Fahr T. *Die Brightsche Nierenkrankeit*. Berlin: Springer, 1914.
11. Fishberg AM. *Hypertension and nephritis*, 4th edn. Philadelphia, PA: Lea and Febiger, 1939.
12. Kimmelstiel P, Wilson C. Intercapillary lesions in the glomeruli of the kidney. *Am J Pathol* 1936;**12**:83–98.7.
13. Allen AC. So called intercapillary glomerulosclerosis—a lesion associated with diabetes. *Arch Pathol* 1941;**32**:33–51.
14. Ghavamian M, Gutch CF, Kopp KF, Kolff WJ. The sad truth about hemodialysis in diabetic nephropathy. *JAMA* 1972;**222**:1386–9.
15. Kussman MJ, Goldstein H, Gleason RE. *The clinical course of diabetic nephropathy. JAMA* 1976;**236**:1861–3.
16. Thomsen AChr. *The kidney in diabetes mellitus*. Copenhagen: Munksgaard, 1965.
17. Hasslacher C, Ritz E, Wahl P, Michael C. Similar risks of nephropathy in patients with type I or type II diabetes mellitus. *Nephrol Dial Transplant* 1989;**4**:859–63.
18. Icks A, Haastert B, Genz J, *et al*. Incidence of renal replacement therapy (RRT) in the diabetic compared with the non-diabetic population in a German region, 2002–08. *Nephrol Dial Transplant* **26**:264–9.
19. Østerby R. Morphometric studies of the peripheral glomerular basement membrane in early juvenile diabetes. I. Development of initial basement membrane thickening. *Diabetologia* 1972;**8**(2):84–92.
20. Fioretto P, Steffes MW, Sutherland DE, *et al*. Reversal of lesions of diabetic nephropathy after pancreas transplantation. *N Engl J Med* 1998;**339**:69–75.
21. Najafian B, Kim Y, Crosson JT, Mauer M. Atubular glomeruli and glomerulotubular

junction abnormalities in diabetic nephropathy. *J Am Soc Nephrol* 2003;**14**:908–17.

22. Fioretto P,Caramori ML, Mauer M. The kidney in diabetes: dynamic pathways of injury and repair. The Camillo Golgi Lecture 2007. *Diabetologia* 2008;**51**:1347–55.

23. Keen H, Chlouverakis C. An immunoassay method for urinary albumin at low concentrations. *Lancet* 1963;**2**:913–4.

24. Viberti GC, Hill RD, Jarrett RJ, *et al.* Microalbuminuria as a predictor of clinical nephropathy in insulin-dependent diabetes mellitus. *Lancet* 1982;**1**:1430–2.

25. Mogensen CE. Long-term antihypertensive treatment inhibiting progression of diabetic nephropathy. *BMJ* 1982;**285**:685–8.

26. Parving HH, Andersen AR, Smidt UM, Svendsen PA. Early aggressive antihypertensive treatment reduces rate of decline in kidney function in diabetic nephropathy. *Lancet* 1983;**1**:1175–9.

27. Mogensen CE. Microalbuminuria predicts clinical proteinuria and early mortality in maturity-onset diabetes. *N Engl J Med* 1984;**310**:356–60.

28. Deckert T, Feldt-Rasmussen B, Borch-Johnsen K, *et al.* Albuminuria reflects widespread vascular damage. The Steno hypothesis. *Diabetologia* 1989;**32**:219–26.

29. Ruggenenti P, Remuzzi G. Time to abandon microalbuminuria? *Kidney Int* 2006;**70**:1214–22.

30. The Diabetes Control and Complications Trial Research Group. The effect of intensive treatment of diabetes on the development and progression of long-term complications in insulin-dependent diabetes mellitus. *N Engl J Med* 1993;**329**:977–86.

31. Hebert LA, Bain RP, Verme D, *et al.* Remission of nephrotic range proteinuria in type I diabetes. Collaborative Study Group. *Kidney Int* 1994;**46**:1688–93.

32. de Boer IH, Sun W, Cleary PA, *et al.* Intensive diabetes therapy and glomerular filtration rate in type 1 diabetes. *N Engl J Med* **365**:2366–76.

33. The Diabetes Control and Complications (DCCT) Research Group. Effect of intensive therapy on the development and progression of diabetic nephropathy in the Diabetes Control and Complications Trial. *Kidney Int* 1995;**47**:1703–20.

34. Mogensen CE. Progression of nephropathy in long-term diabetics with proteinuria and effect of initial anti-hypertensive treatment. *Scand J Clin Lab Invest* 1976;**36**:383–8.

35. Mogensen CE. Renal function changes in diabetes. Diabetes 1976;**25**(Suppl): 872–9.

36. Parving HH, Andersen AR, Smidt UM, *et al.* Reduced albuminuria during early and aggressive antihypertensive treatment of insulin-dependent diabetic patients with diabetic nephropathy. *Diabetes Care* 1981;**4**:459–63.

37. Björck S, Herlitz H, Nyberg G, *et al.* Effect of captopril on renal hemodynamics in the treatment of resistant renal hypertension. *Hypertension* 1983;**5**:III152–3.

38. Björck S, Mulec H, Johnsen SA, *et al.* Contrasting effects of enalapril and metoprolol on proteinuria in diabetic nephropathy. *BMJ* 1990;**300**:904–7.

39. Bjorck S, Mulec H, Johnsen SA, *et al.* Renal protective effect of enalapril in diabetic nephropathy. *BMJ*, 1992;**304**:339–43.

40. Passa P, LeBlanc H, Marre M. *Effects of enalapril in insulin-dependent diabetic subjects with mild to moderate*

uncomplicated hypertension. *Diabetes Care*, 1987;**10**:200–4.

41. Mimran A, Insua A, Ribstein J, *et al.* Contrasting effects of captopril and nifedipine in normotensive patients with incipient diabetic nephropathy. *J Hypertens* 1988;**6**:919–23.

42. Parving HH, Hommel E, Smidt UM. Protection of kidney function and decrease in albuminuria by captopril in insulin dependent diabetics with nephropathy. *BMJ* 1988;**297**: 1086–91.

43. Lewis EJ, Hunsicker LG, Bain RP, Rohde RD. The effect of angiotensin-converting-enzyme inhibition on diabetic nephropathy. The Collaborative Study Group. N Engl J Med 1993;**329**:1456–62.

44. Lewis JB, Berl T, Bain RP, *et al.* Effect of intensive blood pressure control on the course of type 1 diabetic nephropathy. Collaborative Study Group. *Am J Kidney Dis* 1999;**34**:809–17.

45. Barnett AH, Bain SC, Bouter P, *et al.* Angiotensin-receptor blockade versus converting-enzyme inhibition in type 2 diabetes and nephropathy. *N Engl J Med* 2004;**351**:1952–61.

46. Brenner BM, Cooper ME, de Zeeuw D, *et al.* Effects of losartan on renal and cardiovascular outcomes in patients with type 2 diabetes and nephropathy. *N Engl J Med* 2001;**345**:861–9.

47. Lewis EJ, Hunsicker LG, Clarke WR, *et al.* Renoprotective effect of the angiotensin-receptor antagonist irbesartan in patients with nephropathy due to type 2 diabetes. *N Engl J Med* 2001;**345**:851–60.

48. Gaede P, Vedel P, Parving HH, Pedersen O. Intensified multifactorial intervention in patients with type 2 diabetes mellitus and microalbuminuria: the Steno type 2 randomised study. *Lancet* 1999;**353**:617–22.

49. Gaede P, Tarnow L, Vedel P, Parving HH, *et al.* Remission to normoalbuminuria during multifactorial treatment preserves kidney function in patients with type 2 diabetes and microalbuminuria. *Nephrol Dial Transplant* 2004;**19**:2784–8.

Chapter 2

Epidemiology of chronic kidney disease in diabetes

Andrea Icks[1,2] and Michael Koch[2,3]

¹German Diabetes Center, Institute for Biometry and Epidemiology, Düsseldorf, Germany
²Faculty of Medicine, Heinrich-Heine University Düsseldorf, Düsseldorf, Germany
³Center of Nephrology, Mettmann, Düsseldorf, Germany

Key points

- Valid epidemiological data regarding diabetes and chronic kidney disease are scarce.
- Diabetes-related kidney disease is the leading cause of renal replacement therapy.
- The risk of developing chronic kidney disease in people with diabetes seems to be declining. Nevertheless, with an aging population and the increasing prevalence of diabetes, the number of affected persons remains high.

- The risk of developing diabetes-related chronic kidney disease and, in particular, renal replacement therapy differs with age, sex, ethnic background, and region.
- Epidemiological studies with standardized methods addressing the diabetic population are warranted to get a more valid insight in the incidence and prevalence and the progression of chronic kidney disease in diabetes, its trends and its differences between regions and subgroups.

Introduction

This chapter gives an overview of the epidemiology of chronic kidney disease (CKD) in diabetes. We will focus on (1) incidences of CKD in different stages and of end-stage renal disease (ESRD) requiring renal replacement therapy, namely maintenance dialysis or transplantation, i.e., new cases in a disease-free defined population during a defined period of observation, and (2) prevalences of these endpoints, i.e., the total number of affected persons in a defined period (often at an index date or within 1 year) in a defined population.

Epidemiological measures and pitfalls

This is not an easy task. Some figures are often reported in review articles or overviews regarding renal disease in diabetes [see, for example, 1–4]. In individuals with in either type 1 or type 2 diabetes, it has been reported that 25–40%

Diabetes and Kidney Disease, First Edition. Edited by Gunter Wolf.
© 2013 John Wiley & Sons, Ltd. Published 2013 by John Wiley & Sons, Ltd.

will develop diabetic nephropathy in a 25-year period. Diabetes is considered to be the leading cause for ESRD: The proportion of diabetes-related ESRD among all cases of ESRD is reported to be about 25–55%. There are some hints that the incidences of CKD and ESRD are declining in both type 1 and type 2 diabetes. There are large differences between regions and ethnic groups; however, the data are controversial. Knowledge remains uncertain, mainly because of methodological issues.

• *The numerator* (cases): The definition of CKD in general and diabetes-related CKD differs. Several studies have investigated albuminuria or proteinuria using several definitions. Others have analyzed renal impairment, which, however, has been defined in different ways, frequently using different formulae to estimate the glomerular filtration rate (eGFR). Diabetes-related ESRD is poorly defined: it may be ESRD in individuals with diabetes, or in individuals when diabetes is the main cause of ESRD, or just ESRD due to diabetic nephropathy. Furthermore, most data stem from ESRD registers. Even when registers are complete, the incidence of ESRD depends on access to or acceptance of ESRD, so that the proportion of individuals classified with ESRD probably differs between regions and time periods.

• *The denominator* (the population at risk): Incidence and prevalence of diabetes-related CKD or ESRD may be estimated in the general population (diabetic as well as non-diabetic), in the estimated diabetic population, or in selected samples, e.g. clinic-based patient cohorts or participants in clinical trials. Incidence and prevalence in the general population are difficult to interpret, since the figures depend largely on the prevalence of diabetes in the population, which differs by region and with time trends because of changing incidences, survival, and detection rates. Studies using clinic-based or primary care-based populations or clinical trials will probably overestimate incidence and prevalence, since participants differ from the general diabetic population, e.g., the selection may be of individuals with more severe illness. Thus, whenever possible we will focus on epidemiological studies within population-based diabetic samples. Even then, several problems occur, in particular in type 2 diabetes. It is well known that a high number of individuals with type 2 diabetes are undiagnosed [5]. It is considered that this proportion has declined during previous years because of higher awareness concerning undetected diabetes and improved screening initiatives. Hence, the population of individuals with diabetes might have increased due to a higher detection of previously unknown cases. These individuals may differ from the previously diagnosed population and may be suffering from milder forms of diabetes. A further point is that the definition of diabetes differs with calendar year and region. Foe example, several Scientific Diabetes Associations have lowered the threshold of fasting glucose from 140 to 126 mg/dL [6].

• *The study design*: Study populations differ with respect to age, gender, ethnic background, and demographic variables, which are all considered to influence CKD. Studies differed with respect to their observation period and epidemiological measures. Prevalence may be assessed as "point prevalence" or period prevalence, e.g., 1 year or even life time prevalence. The same is true for incidence: incidence may be estimated as incidence rates per defined person times, or as cumulative incidences for different observation periods. An important issue is the database. Using data from routine statistics, e.g., social insurance data, will largely underestimate CKD, since only diagnosed cases can be identified, and it is well known that a large proportion of CKD is undiagnosed [7].

When looking for epidemiological data in the following, one has to keep in mind these points, which contribute to problems in interpreting results (Box 2.1).

Box 2.1 **Epidemiological factors contributing to variation in the recorded incidence and prevalences of end-stage renal disease (ESRD) in diabetes**

Bias
Ascertainment bias (expanding access to ESRD treatment)
Classification bias (insulin-requiring type 2 diabetes coded as type 1 disease; diagnostic preference when more than one cause of ESRD is present
Lead-time/length bias (resulting from starting treatment at an earlier stage of disease)

Changing demography
Aging of the population
Immigration of persons at high risk for diabetes

Rising incidence of diabetes

Longer survival of persons with diabetes

Changing medical management of diabetes
Fewer diabetic patients developing nephropathy
Slower progression of diabetic nephropathy

Longer survival of persons with ESRD

Chronic kidney disease without end-stage renal disease

Incidence of chronic kidney disease in individuals with diabetes

The population-based incidence of CKD in type 1 diabetes, as defined by persistent microalbuminuria, has been declining for several years. Based on data from a population-based incidence register in Sweden, the cumulative incidence of persistent microalbuminuria after 25 years of diabetes decreased from 30% among patients in whom diabetes developed between 1961 and 1965 to 8.9% among those in whom it developed from 1966 to 1970 [8]. After 20 years of diabetes, the cumulative incidence decreased from 28.0% among the patients in whom diabetes developed from 1961 to 1965 to 5.8% among those in whom it developed from 1971 to 1975. Up to the end of the observation time in 1991, persistent microalbuminuria had not developed in any patient in whom diabetes was diagnosed in the period 1976–1980. The mean glycosylated hemoglobin (HbA1c) was significantly higher in patients with than those without persistent albuminuria [8].

More recent data have been reported by the Epidemiology of Diabetes Interventions and Complications Study, the follow-up to the Diabetes Control and Complications Trial (DCCT) study [see, for example, 9, 10]. However, participants in the DCCT were a selected population with a diabetes duration of 1–5 years; hence, the data are difficult to compare with population-based data.

Data describing the incidence of CKD in type 2 diabetes are not available from population-based samples but from clinic-based studies or clinical trials. The UK Prospective Diabetes Study included individuals with newly diagnosed type 2 diabetes for a randomized study which aimed to evaluate intensive diabetes care. Of 5102 participants, prospective analyses were undertaken in those without albuminuria ($n = 4031$) or with normal plasma creatinine ($n = 5032$) at diagnosis. Development of albuminuria (microalbuminuria or macroalbuminuria) or renal impairment

(Cockroft–Gault estimated creatinine clearance <60 mL/min or doubling of plasma creatinine) was estimated. After 15 years of follow-up, 38% had developed albuminuria, 29% renal impairment, and 14% both conditions. Of the people who had developed renal impairment, 51% did not have preceding albuminuria. Men had an increased risk of developing micro- or macroalbuminuria compared with women (18% and 47% increase), but a 45% lower risk of developing renal insufficiency. People with Indian Asian ethnicity had an about twofold higher risk for both conditions than white Caucasians, whereas the risk in Afro-Caribbeans was not significantly higher. Risk factors for both conditions were baseline systolic blood pressure, urinary albumin, and plasma creatinine. Distinct sets of further risk factors were associated with the two outcomes, consistent with the concept that they are not linked inexorably in type 2 diabetes [11].

In a hospital-based study in Italy, 1449 patients with type 2 diabetes without CKD at baseline were followed up for 5 years. The 5-year cumulative incidence of CKD, defined as persistent macroalbuminuria [albumin-to-creatinine ratio (ACR) ≥30 mg/mmol in at least two of three samples] or modification of diet in renal disease (MDRD) eGFR <60 mL/min/1.73 m² was 13.4%. Age, sex, body mass index, hypertension, smoking history, diabetes duration, lipids, current use of medication, and baseline albuminuria were significantly associated [12].

Prevalence of chronic kidney disease in individuals with diabetes

The prevalence of CKD in type 1 diabetes was estimated in a population-based sample of 648 adult patients with type 1 diabetes in Germany [13]. Nephropathy, defined as at least microalbuminuria or elevated serum creatinine, was observed in 30% of the patients. The probability of having at least macroalbuminuria was 3.5-fold higher in patients in the lowest socioeconomic group than those in the highest socioeconomic group [13]. In a more recent study, 25.2% of type 1 diabetic individuals had MDRD eGFR <60 mL/min/1.73 m² [14].

The prevalence of CKD in general or type 2 diabetes has been estimated in several countries in general, or in primary care-based populations with diabetes (Table 2.1). In Hong Kong the prevalence of renal impairment (defined as MDRD eGFR below 60 mL/min/1.73 m²) was 11.9% [15]. In a population-based study in Taiwan, using the same definition, the prevalence was 15.1%. The prevalence of proteinuria was 29.4% [16]. In a population-based sample in Shanghai, 32.8% of type 2 diabetic patients had CKD stage 3–5, based on the Cockcroft Gault equation [17]. In Australia, the prevalence of proteinuria (ACR >2.5 or 3.5 mg/mmol in men and women) in a primary care-based study was 34.6%, and the prevalence of renal impairment, using MDRD-based eGFR, was 23.1% [18]. Only a subgroup of patients had both abnormal eGFR and abnormal proteinuria. In another study from Australia, the prevalence of CKD was assessed in individuals with screen-detected diabetes, using an oral glucose tolerance test. The prevalence of proteinuria (protein to creatinine ratio ≥0.2 mg/mg) was 8.7%, fourfold higher than in those without diabetes, which was 1.9%, and the prevalence of Cockcroft–Gault estimated GFR <60 mL/min was 27.6%, threefold higher than in individuals without diabetes, which was 9.8% [19]. Thus, the prevalence of at least proteinuria in the study of Chabdan was much lower than the study of Thomas, probably due to the different diabetic populations (population of individuals with screen-detected diabetes compared with patients with diagnosed diabetes in primary care, a higher proportion of people from Asia and Aborigines or Pacific Islanders in the population of Thomas).

In the USA, based on National Health and Nutrition Examination Survey (NHANES) data,

Table 2.1 Prevalence of CKD in general or type 2 diabetes

Study	Population	Definitions	Proteinuria prevalence	Renal impairment prevalence	CKD prevalence
Lin 2007, Taiwan 1999–2001	Random sample of individuals aged 30+; diabetic population identified by OGTT	Proteinuria: urine protein to creatinine ratio ≥0.2 mg/mg Renal impairment: MDRD estimated GFR	29.4%; higher in females than males (33.6% vs 24.0%; increasing with increasing age	15.2%; higher in females than in males (20.8% vs 8.1%) and increasing with increasing age	31.5%
Lu 2008 China 2004	Random sample of diabetic patients 30+	Proteiuria: Microalbuminuria: ACR 30–299 mg/g, Macroalbuminuria: ACR ≥300 mg/g Renal impairment: Cockcroft–Gault estimated GFR	Microalbuminuria: 41.7%, macroalbuminuria: 7.7%	32.8% (type 2)	63.9% male patients had a higher percentage of CKD Stages 3–5 and female patients had a higher percentage of CKD stages 1–2. Increased risk associated with duration of diabetes (OR 1.026) and older age (OR 1.066) and duration
So 2006, China 1995–2000	All newly referred type 2 diabetic patients without a history of macrovascular disease or ESRD to a hospital in Hong Kong	Proteinuria Microalbuminuria: ACR 3.5–25 mg/mmol, Macroalbuminuria: >25 mg/mmol Renal impairment: MDRD estimated GFR	Microalbuminuria: 26.3% Macroalbuminuria: 12.7%	11.9% (eGFR 15–60) Higher proportions of patients with stages 2–4 renal function were male and smokers	41.6% (CKD 1–4)
Chabdan 2003, Australia 1999–2000	Random sample of individuals aged 25+, 92.8% Caucasian, diabetic population identified by OGTT	Proteinuria: urine protein to creatinine ratio ≥0.2 mg/ mg; renal impairment: Cockcroft–Gault estimated GFR	8.7% Similar in men and women; increasing with increasing age	27.6% Higher in women than in men; increasing with increasing age	Not reported for diabetic population

Study	Population	Definitions	Albuminuria/proteinuria findings	Renal impairment	Other
Thomas 2006, Australia 2005	Randomly selected GPs each recruiting 10–15 diabetic patients	Proteinuria Microalbuminuria: ACR 3.5–35 mg/mmol (women) or 2.5–25 mg/mmol (men) Macroalbuminuria: ACR >35 mg/mmol (women) or >25 mg/mmol (men) Renal impairment: MDRD estimated GFR	Microalbuminuria: 27.3% Macroalbuminuria: 7.3% Statistically similar in men and women, no association between age and duration of diabetes Higher proportion of Indigenous Australians or Pacific Islanders with eGFR <60 had an abnormal ACR compared with patients of European Ancestry.	23.1% Higher in female than in male (OR 2.27), older age (OR per 10-year difference 2.21)	47.1 % had at least one of the symptoms microalbuminuria, macroalbuminuria or renal impairment
Middleton 2006, UK 2004	All adults with diabetes in primary and secondary care (96.1% Caucasian)	Renal impairment: MDRD estimated GFR		27.5% Higher in female than in male (OR 2.11), older age (OR per year 1.09)	
Wolf 2006 Germany 2000–2004	Individuals insured with Dt. BKK	Proteinuria Albuminuria: ≥20 mg/L or self-rated as "positive" Renal impairment: MDRD estimated GFR	18%	25.2% (type 1) 35.7% (type 2) (eGFR 30–59)	CKD stages 2–5: 75.6% (type 1) 88% (type 2)
Hallan 2006 Norway 1995–1997	Random sample of diabetic patients 20+	Renal impairment: MDRD estimated GFR		14.4%	
Süleymanlar 2011 Turkey	Random sample of diabetic patients 18+	Proteinuria Microalbuminuria: ACR 30–299 mg/g, Macroalbuminuria: ACR ≥300 mg/g Renal impairment: MDRD estimated GFR	Microalbuminuria: 19.7% Macroalbuminuria: 5.3%	11.1%	32.4%

ACR, albumin-to-creatinine ratio; CKD, chronic kidney disease; GFR, glomerular filtration rate; MDRD, modification of diet in renal disease; OGTT, oral glucose tolerance test.

the prevalence of CKD as defined by albuminuria and MDRD eGFR in the diabetic population has remained relatively stable since 1999, between 40.5% in 2001–2002 and 35.87% in 2007–2008 [20].

The prevalence of renal impairment (defined as MDRD eGFR below 60 mL/min/1.73 m^2) in a primary care-based study in the UK was 22.5% [21]. In Germany, in a sample of health insurance, 18% had proteinuria, and 35.7% of type 2 diabetic individuals had MDRD eGFR <60 mL/min/1.73 m^2 [14]. In Norway, in a random sample of diabetic patients aged 20 years or above, the prevalence of renal impairment, defined as MDRD eGFR <60 mL/min/1.73 m^2 was 14.4% [22]. In Turkey, it was 11.1% [23]. In this study, also proteinuria was assessed (defined as ACR 30–299 mg/g or ≥300 mg/g). The prevalences of micro- and macroalbuminuria were 19.7% and 5.3%, respectively. In total, 32.4% of the individuals with diabetes had CKD [23]. Thus, the figures vary in the different studies (Table 2.1). The differences may be due to regional differences and different study designs and definitions of CKD and diabetes. Differences were observed for sex, age, and ethnic background (Table 2.1).

Anothaisintawee et al. [24] included four of the above-mentioned studies [15, 16, 18, 21] in a systematic review and meta-analysis for CKD stage 3 or higher (defined as MDRD eGFR below 60 mL/min/1.73 m^2). The pooled prevalence was 18.2%, almost twofold higher than in the general population, where it was 10.6%.

As mentioned above, the presence of type 2 diabetes is often unknown. Furthermore, an obviously high number of individuals have subthreshold elevated blood glucose values, namely impaired fasting glucose or impaired glucose tolerance, often called "prediabetes" (International Diabetes Federation). Plantinga et al. [25] analyzed the prevalence of CKD in individuals with previously undetected diabetes and those with prediabetes. They used NHANES data and included 8188 indi-

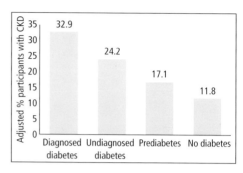

Figure 2.1 National Health and Nutrition Examination Survey 1999–2006: Participants with CKD by diabetes status (Platinga 2010). CKD, chronic kidney disease.

viduals with data for fasting glucose, serum creatinine, and urinary albumin–creatinine ratio. CKD was defined as MDRD-based eGFR <60 mL/min/1.73 m^2 or albumin–creatinine ratio ≥30 mg/g. The age and sex-adjusted prevalence of CKD in individuals with diagnosed diabetes, undiagnosed diabetes, prediabetes, and without diabetes were 32.9%, 24.2%, 17.1%, and 11.8%, respectively (Figure 2.1).

Renal replacement therapy

Before we address ESRD requiring renal replacement therapy in association with diabetes, we will have a look on ESRD in general.

Worldwide, there are large differences regarding incidence and prevalence of ESRD (Figure 2.2). The highest incidences are found in Morelos (Mexico) [597 per million population (pmp)], Jalisco (Mexico) (419 pmp), the USA (371 pmp), and Taiwan (347 pmp), lowest incidences in Russia (35 pmp) and Bangladesh (13 pmp) [20]. Note that these incidences are not adjusted for age and sex, and that large differences exist particularly regarding the age distribution within the different countries. Figure 2.2 also presents age-specific incidences. Also, within one country differences are large, not only in the USA but also, for example, in Spain and in Europe: Canary Islands (172 pmp), Catalonia (143 pmp),

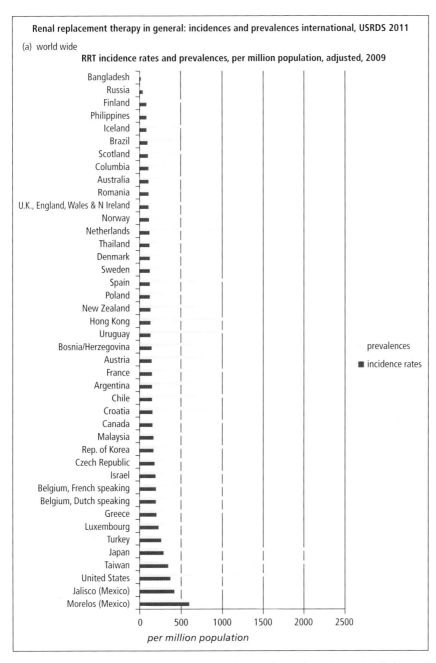

Renal replacement therapy in general: incidences and prevalences international, USRDS 2011

(a) world wide

RRT incidence rates and prevalences, per million population, adjusted, 2009

Renal replacement therapy in general: incidence and prevalence international: (a) worldwide; (b) European regions. U.S. Renal Data System, USRDS 2011 Annual Data Report: Atlas of End-Stage Renal Disease in the United States, National Institutes of Health, National Institute of Diabetes and Digestive and Kidney Diseases, Bethesda, MD, 2011. RRT, renal replacement therapy.

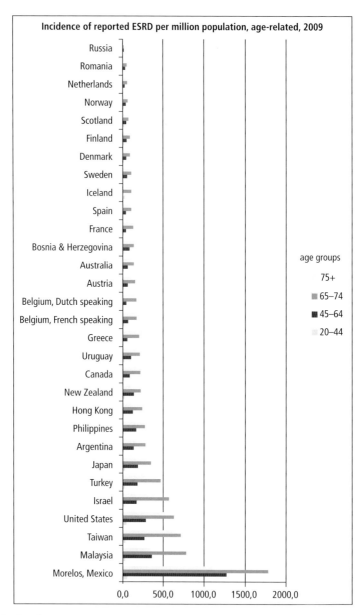

Figure 2.2 (Continued)

Basque country (129 pmp) Extremadura (108 pmp), Castile-La Mancha (94 pmp); age- and sex-adjusted rates were, respectively, 193.0 pmp, 142.3 pmp, 117.5 pmp, 100.4 pmp, 93.1 pmp) [26] (Figure 2.2b).

There are large differences between sub-groups. For the US data, as expected, the inci-dence of ESRD increases with increasing age (2011 incidence rates in people aged 0–19, 20–44, 45–64, 65–74, and 75+ years are 16, 131,

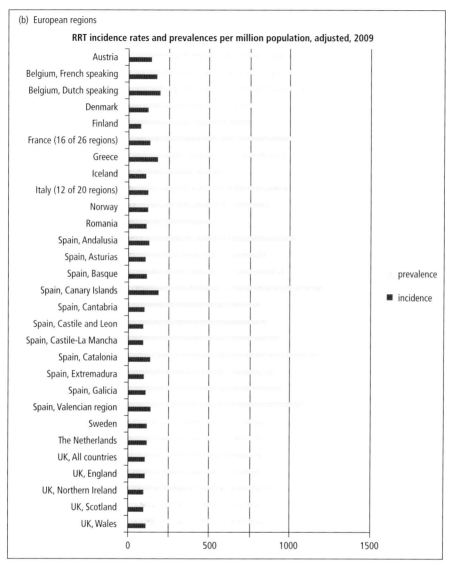

(b) European regions

RRT incidence rates and prevalences per million population, adjusted, 2009

prevalence

■ incidence

(Continued)

610, 1407, and 1762 pmp, respectively; rates are adjusted for race and gender) [20]. In men, the incidence is higher than in women (452 and 282 pmp, adjusted for race and age). Incidence rates are highest in African Americans, followed by Native American and Asian/Pacific Islander (incidence rates 976, 523 and 403 pmp, respectively). The lowest incidence rates are observed in White Americans (277 pmp). Incidence rates for Hispanics are higher than those for non-Hispanics: 501 versus 345 pmp (all rates adjusted for age and gender) [20].

Incidence of renal replacement therapy in diabetes

Most data regarding the incidence of ESRD are obtained from ESRD registers. In most countries, the underlying cause of ESRD is reported, so that diabetes-related ESRD can be identified. However, most countries present only data of the general population, not of their diabetic populations.

When the incidence of ESRD is reported, it must be kept in mind that case definitions may differ: ESRD in the diabetic population may be all cases of ESRD independent of the cause of ESRD or only diabetes-related ESRD—the most frequent figure in incidence estimates based on ESRD registers—and specific diabetic nephropathy. Furthermore, in type 1 diabetes populations, those including children and adolescents may differ from those including young adults. It must also be kept in mind that studies which are based on diabetes incidence registers follow patients from diabetes onset, whereas clinic-based studies may include patients with a longer diabetes duration. Incidence data from ESRD registers assess new cases in the general population, i.e., the duration of diabetes is distributed between new onset and long duration.

As the incidence of CKD declines, so the incidence of ESRD in type 1 diabetes is considered to decline. Results have been reported by Nishimura *et al.*, who assessed the long-term incidence and temporal trends of ESRD in childhood-onset diabetes using a population-based cohort of 1075 type 1 diabetes patients from Allegheny County, USA [27]. The 20-year cumulative incidence of ESRD fell from 9.1% in patients with diabetes onset from 1965 to 1969 to 3.6% in those diagnosed from 1975 to 1979. On the basis of data from population-based incidence registers, a study from Finland reported an incidence of ESRD of 2.2% and 7.8% at 20 and 30 years, respectively. The incidence has continuously declined between 1965 and 1990. The risk of ESRD did not differ between sexes, and was lowest in patients who were diagnosed at an age younger than 5 years [28]. In Sweden, the cumulative incidence of ESRD after 30 years was even lower, with a higher incidence in male (4.1%) than in female patients (2.5%) [29]. In both male and female patients, diabetes onset before the age of 10 years was associated with the lowest risk of ESRD. The highest risk for ESRD was found in male patients with diabetes onset at age 20–34 years (threefold increase compared with male subjects with diabetes onset at age 0–9 years). In female patients, the highest risk was observed for those with diabetes onset at age 10–19 years (2.8-fold increased compared with those with onset at age 0–9 years) [29].

For the general diabetic population, data for diabetes-related ESRD from the USA suggest that also in type 2 diabetes the incidence of ESRD has been declining in recent years: up to 1990, the incidence (age and sex adjusted to the 2005 population) was found to have increased to 355 per 100 000 diabetic population in 1995, and to have declined thereafter to 254 in 2009 [20, 30] (Figure 2.3). In the diabetic population, the incidence of ESRD was highest in Black or African American individuals (4264 pmp), followed by the American Indian or Alaska Native population (3504 pmp) and Asian population (2635 pmp). The lowest incidence rates were found in the white population (2040 pmp). Kidney failure rates were higher in diabetic men (2633 pmp) than in diabetic women (2207 pmp) [20]. However, it must be considered that the diabetic population changed during the observed period, with higher detection of previously unknown diabetes and probably higher survival, as well as changed definitions of diabetes (see above).

Estimates of the incidence of ESRD in the diabetic population are also available for Spain and for Germany. In Spain there are large variations between regions: Lorenzo and colleagues found the incidence to be between 21 and

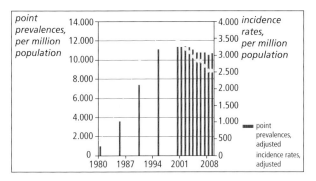

Trend of incidence and prevalence of diabetes-related end-stage renal disease. U.S. Renal Data System, USRDS 2011 Annual Data Report: Atlas of End-Stage Renal Disease in the United States, National Institutes of Health, National Institute of Diabetes and Digestive and Kidney Diseases, Bethesda, MD, 2011.

148 per 100 000 diabetic population [31]. In Germany, all ESRD cases in the diabetic population have been estimated to be about 160 per 100 000 diabetic population. Although the number of cases should be higher than in the USA and the Spanish diabetic populations since not only diabetes-related ESRD was included, the incidence was lower than in the US population; however, it was higher than in Spain [32, 33]. Thus, the pattern is the same picture regarding the incidence of all ESRD cases (above): the highest incidences are seen in Taiwan and the USA; Germany and Spain are in the middle area, with lower incidences in Spain [26].

In a population-based study from Italy [34], type 2 diabetes was addressed. A total of 1408 patients with type 2 diabetes were followed up after an average of 6.7 years. The incidence ESRD was 1.04 per 1000 person-years. However, no actual data or trend analyses are available.

Prevalence of renal replacement therapy in diabetes

The USRDS database shows point prevalences of ESRD in the diabetic population. The prevalence (age and sex adjusted to the 2005 population) increased to about 1150 per 100 000

population and remained relatively stable, reaching a prevalence of 1070 per 100 000 population in 2009 (UDRDS 2011) (Figure 2.3).

Summary and perspectives

Valid epidemiological data regarding diabetes and chronic kidney disease are scarce. Different study designs make it difficult to compare results from different regions or time periods. However, the available data suggest that the risk of developing chronic kidney disease, in particular renal replacement therapy, is declining in type 1 and, for few years at least in the USA, in type 2 diabetes. For most countries, the incidence of diabetes-related ESRD is only estimated in the general population. Using these data, the ESRD Incidence Study Group has analyzed the mean annual change in incidence of treated ESRD, by type of diabetes, in Europeans from eight countries or regions, non-indigenous Canadians, and non-indigenous Australians, aged 30–44 or 45–64 years, for the period 1998–2002 [35]. They found a 5–20% decline in the incidence of diabetes-related ESRD in type 1 diabetes in the study period, but not in type 2 diabetes. Perhaps 2002 was too early to see a decline in the incidence of type 2 diabetes-related ESRD in the study regions. Also in the

USA, the decline in the incidence of ESRD in the diabetic population has been seen only since 1996 [20]. Controversial findings regarding a decreasing incidence of ESRD in type 1 diabetes in recent years come from a clinic-based cohort in the USA. In the Joslin Clinic, the incidence rates of ESRD within 6 years of follow-up in cohorts enrolled in 1991–1995, 1996–2000, and 2001–2004 were 5.3, 5.5, and 6.8 per 100 000 person-years, respectively [36]. However, the data are difficult to compare with register- and population-based estimates, since in the Joslin clinic, patients may have been selected and they were not followed from the onset of diabetes. Nevertheless, incidence and prevalence are high and may further increase due to the aging population and, perhaps, an improvement in the survival of patients with diabetes.

Large differences are observed for incidence and prevalence of ESRD independent of diabetes, not only between countries, but also between regions within single countries. Corresponding data are scarce in the diabetic population, but the incidence of diabetes-related ESRD in the USA, Germany, and Spain suggest that large differences also exist in the diabetic population,. For the prevalence of CKD in the diabetic population, there seem to be large differences. The reasons are not clear; however, it has to be taken into account that data are difficult to compare due to different study designs, as outlined above.

An interesting question is whether progression from CKD before ESRD to ESRD differs between regions and time periods. Only one study has analyzed the first part of the question, mainly in the general population. Hallan and colleagues compared Norwegian and US data with respect to prevalence data for CKD stages (population survey in Norway, NHANES data in the USA, with data for albuminuria as well as GFR) and ESRD incidences derived from ESRD registers. They found that the prevalence of CKD is similar in the USA and European countries; however, the transition rates to ESRD are two to three times higher in the USA than in Norway [22]. In non-diabetic individuals, patients in stages 3 or 4 have a twofold higher risk in the USA of reaching ESRD than in Norway. In diabetic individuals, the risk was 2.8 times higher.

In conclusion, epidemiological studies with standardized methods addressing the diabetic population are warranted to gain a more valid insight for incidence and prevalence and the progression of CKD in diabetes, its trends and its differences between regions and subgroups.

References

1. Williams ME, Stanton RC. Diabetic kidney disease: current challenges. In: Himmelfarb J, Sayegh MH (eds) *Chronic kidney disease, dialysis, and transplantation*, 3rd edn. Boston, MA: Elsevier, 2010, pp. 39–56.

2. Rossing P. Diabetic nephropathy: worldwide epidemic and effects of current treatment on natural history. *Curr Diab Rep* 2006;**6**:479–83.

3. Harvey JN. Trends in the prevalence of diabetic nephropathy in type 1 and type 2 diabetes. *Curr Opin Nephrol Hypertens* 2003;**12**:317–22.

4. Jones CA, Krolewski AS, Rogus J, et al. Epidemic of end-stage renal disease in people with diabetes in the United States population: do we know the cause? *Kidney Int* 2005; **67**:1684–91.

5. International Diabetes Federation (IDF). *Diabetes atlas*, 4th edn. Brussels: International Diabetes Federation, 2009.

6. The Expert Committee on the Diagnosis and Classification of Diabetes Mellitus: Report of the Expert Committee on the Diagnosis and Classification of Diabetes Mellitus. *Diabetes Care* 1997;**20**:1183–97.

7. Coresh J, Byrd-Holt D, Astor BC, et al. Chronic kidney disease awareness,

prevalence, and trends among US adults, 1999 to 2000. *J Am Soc Nephrol* 2005;**16**:180–8.

8. Bojestig M, Arnqvist HJ, Hermansson G, *et al.* Declining incidence of nephropathy in insulin-dependent diabetes mellitus. *N Engl J Med* 1994;**330**:15–18.

9. Mollitch ME, Steffes M, Sun W *et al.*, for the EDIC Study Group. Development and progression of renal insufficiency with and without albuminuria in adults with type 1 diabetes in the Diabetes Control and Complications Trial and the Epidemiology of Diabetes Interventions and Complications Study. *Diabetes Care* 2010;**33**:1536–43.

10. De Boer IH, Rue TC, Cleary PA, *et al.*, for the DCCT/EDIC Study Research Group. Long-term outcomes of patients with type 1 diabetes mellitus and microalbuminuria. *Arch Intern Med* 2011;**171**:412–20.

11. Retnakaran R, Cull CA, Thorne KT, *et al.*, for the UKPDS Study Group. Risk factors for renal dysfunction in type 2 diabetes. U.K. Prospective Diabetes Study 74. *Diabetes* 2006;**55**:1832–9.

12. Zoppini G, Targher G, Chonchol M, *et al.* Serum uric acid levels and incident chronic kidney disease in patients with type 2 diabetes and preserved kidney function. *Diabetes Care* 2012;**35**:99–104.

13. Mühlhauser I, Overmann H, Bender R, *et al.* Social status and quality of care for adult people with type 1 diabetes mellitus—a population-based study. *Diabetologia* 1998;**41**:1139–50.

14. Wolf G, Müller N, Tschauner T, *et al.* Prevalence of chronic kidney disease in the Diabetes TÜV of the German Companies' Health Insurance 2000–2004 [in German]. *Medizinische Klinik* 2006;**101**:441–7.

15. So WY, Kong APS, Ma RCW, *et al.* Glomerular filtration rate, cardiorenal endpoints, and all-cause mortality in type 2 diabetic patients. *Diabetes Care* 2006;**29**:2046–52.

16. Lin CH, Yang WC, Tsai ST, *et al.* A community-based study of chronic kidney disease among type diabetics in Kinnen, Taiwan. *Diabetes Res Clin Practice* 2007;**75**:306–12.

17. Lu B, Song X, Dong X, *et al.* High prevalence of chronic kidney disease in population-based patients diagnosed with type 2 diabetes in downtown Shanghai. *J Diabetes Complications* 2008;**22**:96–103.

18. Thomas MC, Weekes AJ, Broadley OJ, *et al.* The burden of chronic kidney disease in Australian patients with type 2 diabetes (the NEFRON study). *Med J Aust* 2006;**185**:140–4.

19. Chadban SJ, Briganti EM, Kerr PG, *et al.* Prevalence of kidney damage in Australian adults: The AusDiab Kidney Study. *J Am Soc Nephrol* 2003;**14**:S131–8.

20. U.S. Renal Data System (USRDS). *Annual Data report: atlas of end-stage renal disease in the United States.* Bethesda, MD: National Institutes of Health, National Institute of Diabetes and Digestive and Kidney Diseases, 2011.

21. Middleton RJ, Foley RN, Hegarty J, *et al.* The unrecognized prevalence of chronic kidney disease in diabetes. *Nephrol Dial Transplant* 2006;**21**:88–92.

22. Hallan SI, Coresh J, Astor BC, *et al.* International comparison of the relationship of chronic kidney disease prevalence and ESRD risk. *J Am Soc Nephrol* 2006;**17**:2275–84.

23. Süleymanlar G, Utas C, Arinsoy T, *et al.* A population-based survey of Chronic REnal Diease I Turkey—the CREDIT study. *Nephrol Dial Transplant* 2011;**26**: 1862–71.

24. Anothaisintawee T, Rattanasiri S, Ingsathit A, *et al.* Prevalence of chronic kidney disease: a systematic review and

meta-analysis. *Clin Nephrol* 2008;**71**: 244–54.

25. Plantinga LC, Crews DC, Coresh J, *et al.* Prevalence of chronic kidney disease in US adults with undiagnosed diabetes or prediabetes. *Clin J Am Soc Nephrol* 2010;**5**:673–82.

26. ERA-EDTA. *Annual Report 2009*. http:// www.era-edta-reg.org/files/annualreports/ pdf/AnnRep2009.pdf.

27. Nishimura R, Dorman JS, Bosnyak Z, *et al.* Incidence of ESRD and survival after renal replacement therapy in patients with type 1 diabetes: a report from the Alleghen County Registry. *Am J Kidney Dis* 2003;**42**:117–24.

28. Finne P, Reunanen A, Stenman S, *et al.* Incidence of end-stage renal disease in patients with type 1 diabetes. *JAMA* 2005;**294**:1782–7.

29. Möllsten A, Svensson M, Waernbaum I, *et al.*, for the Swedish Childhood Diabetes Study Group. Cumulative risk, age at onset, and sex-specific differences for developing end-stage renal disease in young patients with type 1 diabetes. *Diabetes* 2010;**59**:1803–8.

30. Burrows NR, Li Y, Geiss LS. Incidence of treatment for end-stage renal disease among individuals with diabetes in the US continues to decline. *Diabetes Care* 2010;**33**:73–7.

31. Lorenzo V, Boronat M, Saavedra P, *et al.* Disproportional high incidence of diabetes-related end-stage renal disease in the Canary Islands. An analysis based on estimated population at risk. *Nephrol Dial Transplant* 2010;**25**:2282–8.

32. Icks A, Haastert B, Genz J, *et al.* Incidence of renal replacement therapy (ESRD) in the diabetic compared to the non-diabetic population in a German region, 2002–2008. *Nephrol Dial Transplant* 2011;**26**:264–9.

33. Hoffmann F, Haastert B, Koch M, *et al.* The effect of diabetes on incidence and mortality in end-stage renal disease in Germany. *Nephrol Dial Transplant* 2011;**26**:1634–40.

34. Bruno G, Biggeri A, Merletti F, *et al.* Low incidence of end-stage renal disease and chronic renal failure in type 2 diabetes. *Diabetes Care* 2003;**26**: 2353–8.

35. The ESRD Incidence Study Group. Divergent trends in the incidence of end-stage renal disease due to Type 1 and Type 2 diabetes in Europe, Canada and Australia during 1998–2002. Diabet Med 2006;**23**:1364–9.

36. Rosolowsky ET, Skupien J, Smiles AM, *et al.* Risk for ESRD in type 1 diabetes remains high despite renoprotection. *J Am Soc Nephrol* 2011;**22**:545–53.

Genetic risk factors for diabetic nephropathy

Carsten A. Böger[1] and Peter R. Mertens[2]

[1]University Medical Center Regensburg, Regensburg, Germany
[2]Otto-von Guericke University Magdeburg, Magdeburg, Germany

Key points

- Only approximately 30% of patients with diabetes eventually develop nephropathy.
- First evidence linking diabetic nephropathy with genetic variants was collected from family studies.
- Separating the interaction of genes from non-genetic factors (cardiovascular risk factors, social and economic factors, nutrition and physical activity, epigenetics) remains difficult.
- Therefore, genetic studies need to account for non-genetic factors affecting diabetic nephropathy risk to exclude spurious findings due to confounding.
- A key to successful genetic analyses is phenotype definition, which has recently become standardized.
- Cohort size and composition is a critical challenge in genetic analysis of diabetic nephropathy because of bias with smaller cohorts.

- There are different methods for genetic analyses (linkage analysis, candidate gene approach, or genome-wide studies).
- In particular, results of candidate genes are often difficult to replicate because of small cohort size. The gold standard is genome-wide analysis with large cohorts.
- Probably the most convincing finding obtained in family-based studies is the association of a genetic region at 18q22.3.
- Genes associated with diabetic nephropathy have not yet altered diagnostic or treatment algorithms of this disease.

Diabetic nephropathy (DN) is a microangiopathic manifestation of diabetes occurring in about 30% of patients [1] and is associated with high risk for cardiovascular morbidity and mortality and end-stage renal disease (ESRD). Numbers vary strongly between ethnicities (e.g., higher prevalence in Pima Indians [2]). Major questions relating to DN are still unanswered: What drives the onset and progression

Diabetes and Kidney Disease, First Edition. Edited by Gunter Wolf.
© 2013 John Wiley & Sons, Ltd. Published 2013 by John Wiley & Sons, Ltd.

of DN? How may one estimate the risk for DN? What is the relative contribution of genetic background (ethnicity), individual genetic risk profile, glycemic control, and environmental factors. This chapter summarizes methods of genetic research and evidence linking genetic variants with the overall risk for DN, embedded in a conceptual overview and an outlook on translation of genetic research into clinical practice.

The first evidence linking DN with genetic variants was collected from family studies and incidence models. In the Wisconsin epidemiologic study, Klein *et al.* [3] observed that metabolic control was equal in those with and without nephropathy. Familial clustering of diabetic nephropathy independent of metabolic control was observed in a landmark study in patients with type 1 diabetes performed by Seaquist *et al.* [4] The fourfold higher risk for siblings of patients with type 1 diabetes indicates strong genetic effects on outcome in this study. Additional family studies displayed familial aggregation of diabetic nephropathy in both type 1 and type 2 diabetes [2, 5]. For type 2 diabetes patients with first-degree family members known to have DN, the relative risk for developing DN ranges from twofold in Caucasian-Americans to 9.2-fold in African Americans, Mexican Americans, Asian Indians, and Nauruans. Such large differences due to ethnicity were reported by Freedman *et al.* in 1993 [6]: for relatives of African American patients with type 2 diabetes the relative risk for renal replacement treatment is fivefold compared with European-Americans, even after adjusting for socioeconomic factors. Indirect evidence for an important role of genetic variation in DN risk comes from epidemiological studies which showed that the incidence rate of diabetic nephropathy peaks at a duration of diabetes of about 15 years [7] with an incidence rate of 2–3% per year, in contrast to an incidence rate of 0.5–1% after 20 years of dia-

betes duration [7, 8]. A time-dependent peak in diabetes complication incidence rates beyond which, for example, poor glycemic control does not contribute profoundly to risk is a strong indicator that other factors such as genetic variation contribute to overall risk. Moreover, the Diabetes Control and Complications Trial (DCCT, $n = 1441$; mean therapy duration 6.5 years) and the subsequent Epidemiology of Diabetes Interventions and Complications cohort study (EPIC trial, $n = 1375$, median follow-up 22 years) indicate that intensive antihyperglycemic therapy over a prolonged period of 6.5 years could reduce some but not all of the risk for estimated glomerular filtration rate (eGFR) below 60 mL/min/1.73 m² [9], again indicating further risk factors at play. About 25% of diabetics will not develop DN independent of the quality of glycemic control (summarized in Rich [10]), thus supporting the concept of protective factors. Dissecting the interaction of genes with non-genetic factors (cardiovascular risk factors, social and economic factors, nutrition and physical activity, epigenetics) is key to approaching these questions (Figure 3.1).

Pharmacological treatment of traditional cardiovascular risk factors (diabetes, hypertension, smoking, and dyslipoproteinemia) has significantly improved outcomes in diabetes. However, in spite of improved blood pressure and glucose control renal events such as microalbuminuria [11] and doubling of serum creatinine or ESRD [12] are only partially averted. Recently, *heritability* for the two main measures of kidney function, GFR and albuminuria, were estimated at 36–75% and 16–49%, respectively, not only in studies with diagnosed type 2 diabetes but also in the general population [13, 14]. Non-genetic risk factors confound the search for genetic variants associated with DN, with cardiovascular risk factors, predominantly diabetes, hypertension, and smoking, determining a significant

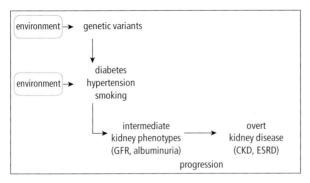

Proposed model of interaction of genes, environment and chronic kidney disease (CKD) risk factors in the development of diabetic nephropathy. ESRD, end-stage renal disease; GFR, glomerular filtration rate.

portion of non-genetic risk (Figure 3.1). As discussed above, the risk for diabetic nephropathy is time dependent with reduced risk with prolonged diabetes duration over 15 years [7, 8], and improved glycemic control retards the onset of diabetic nephropathy [9, 15–17]. Similar evidence exists for the control of hypertension in diabetes [18, 19]. Thus, genetic studies need to account for non-genetic factors affecting DN risk to exclude spurious findings due to confounding.

What is diabetic nephropathy?

Key to successful genetic analyses is a definitive phenotype definition. In contrast to kidney diseases where diagnosis is based on a kidney biopsy (e.g., immunoglobulin (Ig)A nephropathy, membranous nephropathy, Alport's syndrome) or imaging studies (e.g. autosomal dominant polycystic kidney disease), the diagnosis of diabetic nephropathy is almost always made clinically and not by histology. Given risk of bleeding during kidney biopsy, the procedure is only performed if it promises to have an impact on clinical decision making. Thus, it is usually performed to exclude non-

diabetic kidney diseases, and not to confirm suspected DN.

The clinical diagnosis takes into account the typical course of DN: after many years of diabetes duration with normal GFR and absent albuminuria, DN onset is marked by mildly elevated albuminuria (albumin excretion rate ≥30 mg per day, also termed microalbuminuria) with or without hyperfiltration and increased GFR. Subsequently, DN is characterized by mostly overlapping stages of declining GFR and progressive proteinuria that may reach the nephrotic range [20]. In the early stages, regression to normalbuminuria is frequently observed [21]. Further, macroalbuminuria is not a condition *sine qua non* for profound kidney damage. Indeed, studies indicate that chronic kidney disease in diabetes may evolve in the absence of considerable proteinuria and progress to end-stage renal disease [22].

Unfortunately, there is no uniform definition of DN across published genetic studies, which are mostly (cross-sectional) case–control studies. Since microalbuminuria can be transient and not always due to DN (e.g., transient microalbuminuria due to physical exercise or by fever), diabetic nephropathy cases are usually defined as those with high levels of albuminuria (defined mostly as ≥300 mg/day, macroalbuminuria) and/or ESRD in the absence of other causes of ESRD [23–25]. The presence of macroalbuminuria over a certain time prior to or at diagnosis of ESRD is not always used as a criterion for the DN diagnosis since this information is frequently not available in cross-sectional studies, especially in type 2 diabetes. The presence of diabetic retinopathy is used in some studies to make the diagnosis of diabetic nephropathy more likely [26]. Controls are mostly defined as those with long-standing diabetes (>15 years) and normal range albuminuria (<30 mg/day). A GFR ≥60 mL/min/1.73 m^2 is not always taken as a criterion to define controls without DN.

Diagnosing DN clinically and without histology leads to several issues that are important to consider when reviewing results of genetic analyses.

1. Histological alterations observed with DN are not uniform [27, 28]. Pathognomonic thickening of basal membranes is often accompanied by diverse other histological features. These may include nodular matrix accumulation (termed Kimmelstiel–Wilson nephritis [29]) or recruitment of inflammatory cells into the tubulointerstitium with prominent inflammatory reaction [28]. Phenotypic alterations observed in DN have recently been summarized [27]. A generally accepted classification will be of paramount relevance for future studies, when comparative designs are sought and therapeutic interventions are eventually planned. Overall, these issues raise the question whether DN constitutes a single diagnosis or rather an umbrella term for diverse glomerular and tubulointerstitial subentities [27]. Any type of disease misclassification reduces statistical power and may explain inconsistent findings between genetic studies.

2. In cases with *overt proteinuria* and absence of nephritic sediment, misclassification of diabetic nephropathy may occur due to clinical mimicry of other kidney disease. Approximately 30% of such patients have non-diabetic kidney diseases [30]. In a recent study with 576 con-secutive biopsies, the diagnoses of those without non-diabetic kidney disease were mostly immune complex glomerulonephritis and secondary focal glomerulosclerosis [30]. Such misclassification reduces the statistical power for genetic analyses, potentially leading to false-negative results for the phenotype of DN, but not to false-positive results (i.e., associations with undiagnosed glomerulopathy).

3. In patients with diabetes who have *reduced eGFR but normal albuminuria*, underlying hypertensive nephropathy (so-called benign nephrosclerosis) is a likely diagnosis given the high prevalence of hypertension in diabetes patients. This is supported by data from diabetic patients, where a substantial proportion develops decreased eGFR without concurrent or prior elevated albuminuria [31, 32]. One of the most challenging tasks is dissection of the intertwined diagnoses of DN and hypertension-related nephrosclerosis. Hypertension may be the primary driving force of kidney disease or, conversely, a co-factor developing with kidney disease progression. In the majority of diabetic patients, even without metabolic syndrome, such as type 1 diabetics, hypertension evolves. At the time of enrolment in the DCCT/EPIC trial none of the type 1 diabetes patients was diagnosed hypertensive, 22 years later more than 50% of patients were hypertensive [9].

4. Two different measures of kidney function are used to define the DN phenotype: albuminuria and GFR. Recently, it has been challenged that these two traits have the same genetic background [13], which is supported by recent data from genome-wide association studies of eGFR and albuminuria in general population studies [33–35]. This may be a cause of false-negative results.

What is the optimal study design?

Cohort size and composition is a critical challenge in genetic analysis of DN. As a cohort's sample size decreases to smaller than $n = 1000$, the more prone it is to bias due to sampling strategy, to false-positive or -negative results in genetic analyses, and to low power especially for low-frequency variants. Ideally, cohorts for the study of DN have long-term prospective follow-up, a large sample size, and provide a representative sample of the general population with type 2 diabetes mellitus. The higher effort necessary for performing a prospective study compared with a cross-sectional study is well invested since misclassification of type 2 diabetes mellitus complications is reduced by prospective study design: for example, a patient in a cross-sectional study with a one-time normal urinalysis and short diabetes duration is misclassified as "control" without diabetic nephropathy if macroalbuminuria and reduced eGFR occur after this single cross-sectional examination. Longitudinal studies allow the analysis of the full spectrum of kidney disease in type 2 diabetes mellitus: incident microalbuminuria or eGFR $<60\,mL/min/1.73\,m^2$, preclinical kidney function decline, progression of CKD, and incident ESRD. Recruiting a representative sample of the general population with type 2 diabetes mellitus is particularly challenging since very healthy or very ill type 2 diabetes mellitus patients are underrepresented in most observational studies. Further sources of bias are the level of care and complexity of comorbidities in recruiting outpatient departments. For example, patients recruited only in a university center tend to have more comorbidities and severe type 2 diabetes mellitus manifestations than patients recruited in a general practitioner's office, and differences in intensity of care may affect the outcomes too. Thus, documentation of the mode of ascertainment or recruiting is imperative to allow for the statistical adjustment for this type of bias.

In addition to assessing a patient's ethnicity (e.g., Caucasian versus African American), an important design issue is population substructure, i.e., undetected differences in genetic background even within the same ethnicity [36–38]. Population substructure can be detected and controlled for in genetic studies by principal component analysis or by the method of "genomic control" [39].

In summary, any epidemiological or genetic epidemiological analysis of a cohort requires careful consideration of cohort design, sample size, ethnicity and phenotype definition.

Methods for genetic studies

Linkage analyses are classical genetic mapping approaches performed in families with index patients affected by a rare disease. Success in discovering mutations causing diseases with a Mendelian mode of inheritance and mostly a pathognomonic clinical phenotype linked to a single gene is often reported [40]. This method systematically examines the whole genome, and thus has no prior candidate gene. In diseases with a clear Mendelian mode of inheritance, variants discovered typically have large effects explaining essentially all of the disease risk (Figure 3.2) [41].

The so-called *candidate gene approach* investigates the association between common genetic variants in candidate genes for disease phenotypes such as DN based on *a priori* biological hypotheses. Confirmatory replication is rarely achieved due to a multitude of study design issues, such as inadequate power, low significance threshold, and differences in phenotype definition between studies. Despite limitations, this method has been widely used (reviewed in Maeda [42], McKnight *et al.* [43]) until the first genome-wide association studies were published in 2005. Since then candidate gene studies have become an accepted method to confirm loci identified by GWAS or other genome-wide genetic methods [44, 45].

Genome-wide association studies (GWAS) have been catalyzed by the publication of the human genome in 2001 by technological advances in the high-throughput detection of

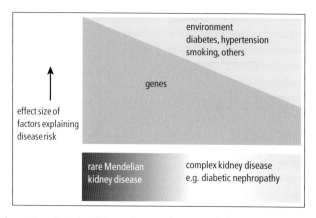

Figure 3.2 Role of genetic variants in etiology of rare and common kidney diseases.

genome sequence variation and the unraveling of the genetic architecture in humans of different ethnic origin in the HapMap project [46]. Commercial sources offer the necessary high throughput genotyping technologies for rapidly genotyping more than 10^6 single nucleotide polymorphisms (SNPs) across the whole genome per person in a single analytical process. In contrast to candidate gene studies, GWAS have the advantage of being unbiased by biological hypotheses since a SNP panel is analyzed that captures most of an individual's genetic variation.

Linear (for continuous traits, e.g. eGFR) and logistic (for dichotomous traits, e.g. DN or ESRD) regression models are used to calculate the degree of association of the risk allele with a certain phenotype, such as DN, for each of the SNPs genotyped. By using the information on human genetic variation in the HapMap data set, these large data sets may be further enhanced by the imputation of the further several million SNPs that lie between the genotyped SNPs [47, 48]. This extension of the SNP number studied increases the coverage of genomic variation within the genome, making the pooling of data from different studies for joint GWAS meta-analysis possible even if the studies were genotyped on different genotyping platforms. The advantage of GWAS meta-analyses is that the higher sample size increases the power to detect the small effects associated with each SNP typically observed for common diseases such as DN (Figure 3.2) [41].

To exclude false-positive results when performing several million statistical tests, it is necessary to correct for multiple testing. Applying the method described by Bonferroni to GWAS with 1 million genome-wide independent SNPs, a SNP association is deemed genome-wide significant if the p-value is less than 5×10^{-8}. This "Bonferroni penalty" reduces power, thus requiring very large sample sizes. To confirm results of this first stage of locus discovery, confirmation in independent individuals is mandatory in a second stage of genetic testing of the SNPs identified in stage 1 GWAS [41].

While the current HapMap-imputed SNP data set provides reliable data on SNPs with a *minor allele frequency* above 10%, there is considerable uncertainty about the quality of information on SNPs with a minor allele frequency less than 10% [49]. This problem is further aggravated by the fact that most studies are underpowered to adequately analyze SNPs with such low minor allele frequency. However, imputation of >7 million SNPs with improved coverage of such low-frequency variants is now possible with the availability of the sequence information of several hundred individuals of European origin in the 1000 Genomes data set [47, 49]. These data sets will be used in the near future and are hoped to close the gap between common variant approaches (GWAS) and rare mutation approaches (linkage analysis).

Important caveats regarding interpretation of genetic analyses include (1) publication bias, whereby non-significant findings may not be published and thus be underrepresented, (2) between-study heterogeneity in design, phenotype definition, population stratification [36], and ethnicity, potentially leading to random effects, and (3) the SNPs identified through GWAS are rarely the causal variants, but rather identify genetic loci for further functional study. The SNP identified could tag any functional entity. Depending on genetic architecture at that locus, several genes and their regulatory regions may be included.

In summary, when reviewing results of genetic analyses of DN, it is important to consider the caveats regarding phenotype defini-

tion, study design and methods of genetic analyses raised above.

Family-based linkage analyses

Family-based linkage studies have identified several genetic regions associated with DN (reviewed in Freedman *et al.* [50]), but the small effect size and borderline significance level do not allow the conclusion that these loci are unequivocally related to DN risk. Methodological issues obscuring clear findings include non-uniform study designs and phenotype definitions, and inadequate statistical power (Table 3.1). Probably the most convincing finding obtained in family-based studies is the association of a genetic region at 18q22.3 with advanced DN, which was confirmed in Pima Indians in the same study [51]. Subsequent genetic and functional studies by the same group in Mannheim identified genetic variants in the Carnosinase 1 (*CNDP1*) gene to explain this genetic signal [52], confirmed by several other studies [53].

Overview of genome-wide association studies (GWAS) and family based linkage studies for diabetic nephropathy

Locus (gene name)	Lowest p-value in SNP-GWAS	Highest LOD-score in linkage analysis	Ethnicity	Phenotype	References
3p13	NA	2.76	AA	Albuminuria in DM1 or DM2	[75]
3q13	NA	4.55	AA	ESRD/proteinuria in DM2	[76]
3q21.3	NA	2.67	Fi	ESRD/proteinuria in DM1	[77]
3q25.1	NA	3.1	EA	ESRD/proteinuria in DM1	[78]
6p24.3	NA	3.09	EA	ESRD/proteinuria in DM1 or DM2	[75]

(*Continued*)

Table 3.1 (Continued)

Locus (gene name)	Lowest p-value in SNP-GWAS	Highest LOD-score in linkage analysis	Ethnicity	Phenotype	References
7p14.1 (ELMO1)	NA	8×10^{-6}	Ja, EA, AA, PI	ESRD/proteinuria in DM1 or DM2	[26, 56, 57, 79, 80]
7p21.3	NA	2.81	AI	ESRD/proteinuria in DM1 or DM2	[75]
7q21.2	NA	2.96	EA	Albuminuria in DM1 or DM2	[75]
7q21.1/ 7q21.3	NA	$p = 6 \times 10^{-4}$/ 6×10^{-5}	EA/AA	Albuminuria/ESRD/ proteinuria in DM1 or DM2	[81]
7q36.2	NA	3.1	>90% EA	Albuminuria in DM2	[82]
8q24 (PVT1)	2×10^{-5}	NA	PI, EA	Albuminuria/ESRD in DM1 and DM2	[58], [59]
9q21.32 (FRMD3)	5×10^{-7}	NA	EA	ESRD/proteinuria in DM1	[23]
10q22.3 (ZMIZ1)	NA	8.1×10^{-5}	EA	ESRD/proteinuria in DM1	[56]
10q23.31	3.1	NA	>90% EA	eGFR in DM2	[83]
11p15.5 (CARS)	3.1×10^{-6}	NA	EA	ESRD/proteinuria in DM1	[23]
12p13.2 (KLRA1)	6×10^{-4}	NA	EA	ESRD/proteinuria in DM1	[56]
TMPO (12q22)	5×10^{-4}	NA	EA	ESRD/proteinuria in DM1	[56]
12q24.11 (ACACB)	1.4×10^{-6}	NA	Ja	ESRD/proteinuria in DM2	[84]
13q34 (IRS2)	1×10^{-4}	NA	EA	ESRD/proteinuria in DM1	[56]
13q34 (rs1411766)	NA	1.8×10^{-6}	EA, Ja	ESRD/proteinuria in DM1 or DM2	[23], [85]
16q13 (SLC12A3)	8.7×10^{-5}	NA	Ja	ESRD/proteinuria in DM2	[54]
18q22.3 (CNDP1)	6.1	2×10^{-4}	Tu, AA, EA, AI	ESRD/proteinuria in DM2	[51, 76, 81, 86, 87]

AA, African-Americans; AI, American-Indians; EA, European-Americans; MA, Mexican-Americans; Fi, Finnish; Ja, Japanese; Tu, Turkish; ACR, albumin-to-creatinine ratio; DM1, type 1 diabetes mellitus; DM2, type 1 diabetes mellitus.

Genome-wide association studies

The first GWAS of DN was performed in Japanese patients with type 1 diabetes. SNPs in SLC12A3, the gene encoding the thiazide-sensitive sodium chloride cotransporter and mutated in Gitelman's syndrome, were signifi-cantly associated with DN [54]. An analysis of a larger number of SNPs in the same subjects revealed ELMO1 (engulfment and cell motility 1) and ACACB (acetyl coenzyme A carboxylase beta) as potential loci for DN. Both have been validated by functional studies. The protein expressed by ELMO1 is a mammalian homologue of the *Caenorhabditis elegans ced-12* gene product, which is required for engulfment of dying cells and for cell migration. A known link to kidney disease has not been published [55]. Further genetic evidence supports the notion of *ELMO1* as an interesting candidate for DN, since it showed nominally significant association in another GWAS in type 1 diabetics of European descent [56], in a fine-mapping study in African Americans with type 2 diabetes [57], and in Pima Indians. However, the SNPs identified differ between studies, are not completely correlated, and did not reach genome-wide significance. Further, correlated alleles do not consistently show either a protective or damaging effect. Thus, further work is required to elucidate the mechanisms by which genetic variants at the *ELMO1* locus affect DN risk.

Plasmacytoma variant 1 (*PVT1*) has been identified by genome-wide analysis of over 100 000 SNPs in Pima Indians, in a study analyzing genetic risk for ESRD due to diabetes type 2 [58]; results were confirmed in Caucasians with ESRD attributed to diabetes type 1 [59].

Further, *FRMD3* and *CARS* were associated with diabetic nephropathy in a large GWAS of patients with type 1 diabetes from the GoKinD collection [23]. Though none of the reported SNPs reached genome-wide significance, these findings were confirmed by an independent, prospective study of type 1 diabetes patients (DCCT/EDIC), and by expression in human kidney.

However, none of the GWAS performed for DN have identified SNPs with genome-wide significance. Since analyses of dichotomous traits such as DN require large sample sizes to attain adequate statistical power, the GWAS of DN published so far are notoriously underpowered. Pooling of GWAS from several GWAS by meta-analysis is currently under way in the FIND (diabetes mellitus type 2, [60]) and GENIE consortia (diabetes mellitus type 1), although sample size ($n < 10 000$) is not yet

comparable with recently published GWAS meta-analyses of eGFR and albuminuria in general population cohorts (sample size >65 000 [33, 34, 61–63]).

Thus, in contrast to the exciting discovery of the *MYH9/APOL1* locus associated with non-diabetic ESRD in African Americans, the search for genetic variants associated with ESRD due to DN in African Americans has not been as successful [38, 64, 65]. A recent GWAS of ESRD in African Americans with type 2 diabetes found no SNPs with genome-wide significance, but several loci were named [66]. The formally significant association of variants in *MYH9* with DN in a candidate gene study may be attributed to underlying non-diabetic kidney disease since biopsies were not performed [67]. Recent genetic analyses indicate that there are genetic variants associated with incident CKD and progressive kidney disease irrespective of underlying primary insults [43, 68–70], but GWAS have not been published for this clinically important phenotype.

The future of genetic analyses

The effect sizes of the SNPs identified in GWAS are very small, and account only for a fraction of the heritability observed in family studies [13, 41]. For example, the 16 SNPs associated with eGFR in GWAS meta-analysis of over 67 000 individuals in the general population account for only 1.4% of the interindividual variation of eGFR in this sample [33], while heritability of eGFR lies at 36–75% [13]. This gap has been termed "missing heritability" [41], with several potential explanations: (1) There may be further frequent variants [minor allele frequency (MAF) 10–50%] with smaller effect size. GWAS or GWAS meta-analyses with higher sample sizes should detect these; (2) less frequent variants (MAF 1–10%) may account for larger effects, which may be detected by using a set of SNPs that provides more reliable genetic information at low MAF than current

SNP panels do [47], or by performing whole-genome sequencing thus covering the total individual genomic variation; (3) gene–gene and gene–environment interactions may dilute the main variant effect. Larger GWAS accounting for such interactions could detect SNPs involved in networks. However, cohorts with adequate sample sizes and detailed environmental phenotyping in sufficient quality are not (yet) available. The multitude of gene–gene interactions to be searched would involve an enormous number of tests. Another approach with recent success is to integrate data on genetic variants with databases obtained by genome-wide analysis of gene expression, or information on body fluid metabolites or peptides [71, 72].

Translation into animal models

In an optimal setting, genetic findings from GWAS or association studies with candidate genes will allow to directly link genetic aberration with a single gene or a limited number of genes whose function may be unraveled by *in vitro* and experimental studies. What are the advantages and merits of such an approach? Experimental models performed in animals with gene deletion(s) (at times several genes may be knocked out at the same time, even conditionally after birth) allow the relative contribution of genetic effects on diabetic nephropathy to be assessed. Under such circumstances targeted therapy may be devised and tested. There are however some important aspects to consider before one may envision translational approaches towards animal studies. Rodents exhibit a completely different genetic background, some mouse strains are susceptible to nephropathy, others are resistant. A recent study analyzed the dependency of albuminuria in aging mice on genetic background, in respect of loci for human diabetic nephropathy on mouse chromosome 8. By haplotype association mapping the authors compared the haplotypes of relatively closely related mouse inbred strains regarding their renal phenotype (albumin-to-creatinine ratio) at age 12, 18, and 24 months. Two of the identified nine susceptibility loci were significantly associated with DN loci in human type 1 diabetes patients [73]. The results underscore common underlying genes that predispose to kidney disease in mice and humans. Conversely, they emphasize the relevance of gene–gene interactions.

Furthermore, typical histopathologic findings for DN are not common in rodents with prolonged diabetes alone. In rats, only the combination of hypertension and diabetic metabolism results in a renal phenotype.

Translation into clinical use

Once genetic variants have been identified, there is still a long way to go before patients will benefit in day-to-day care. Bioinformatic tools and systems biology approaches are key to the analysis of large-scale and multidimensional data and will further aid in clarifying whether a genetic variant is "harmful" to the organism [74]. In principle, such findings need not necessarily identify only a single protein but may also identify complex pathways. The aim is to utilize the information to design successful interventions. Alternatively, the development of highly predictive marker proteins will ensure that they are utilized to identify those patients at highest risk for DN.

Glossary

Minor allele frequency (MAF): the presence of two or more alleles at a specific chromosomal position defines a polymorphic site in the genome, e.g., a single nucleotide polymorphism. The minor allele frequency gives the frequency that the rarer of the alleles occurs in a genotyped population.

Heritability: The extent to which a trait manifestation is determined by heritable factors which are assumed to be genetically determined. The degree of heritability is determined in pedigree analysis of family studies.

1. Adler AI, Stevens RJ, Manley SE, *et al.* Development and progression of nephropathy in type 2 diabetes: the United Kingdom Prospective Diabetes Study (UKPDS 64). *Kidney Int* 2003;**63**:225–32.

2. Pettitt DJ, Saad MF, Bennett PH, *et al.* Familial predisposition to renal disease in two generations of Pima Indians with type 2 (non-insulin-dependent) diabetes mellitus. *Diabetologia* 1990;**33**: 438–43.

3. Klein R, Klein BE, Moss SE, *et al.* The Wisconsin epidemiologic study of diabetic retinopathy. IV. Diabetic macular edema. *Ophthalmology* 1984;**91**: 1464–74.

4. Seaquist ER, Goetz FC, Rich S, Barbosa J. Familial clustering of diabetic kidney disease. Evidence for genetic susceptibility to diabetic nephropathy. *N Engl J Med* 1989;**320**:1161–5.

5. Quinn M, Angelico MC, Warram JH, Krolewski AS. Familial factors determine the development of diabetic nephropathy in patients with IDDM. *Diabetologia* 1996;**39**:940–5.

6. Freedman BI, Spray BJ, Tuttle AB, Buckalew VM, Jr. The familial risk of end-stage renal disease in African Americans. *Am J Kidney Dis* 1993;**21**: 387–93.

7. Krolewski AS, Warram JH, Rand LI, Kahn CR. Epidemiologic approach to the etiology of type I diabetes mellitus and its complications. *N Engl J Med* 1987;**317**:1390–8.

8. Forsblom CM, Groop PH, Ekstrand A, Groop LC. Predictive value of microalbuminuria in patients with insulin-dependent diabetes of long duration. *BMJ* 1992;**305**:1051–3.

9. de Boer IH, Sun W, Cleary PA, Lachin JM, Molitch ME, Steffes MW, *et al.* Intensive diabetes therapy and glomerular filtration rate in type 1 diabetes. *N Engl J Med* 2011;**365**:2366–76.

10. Rich SS. Genetics of diabetes and its complications. *J Am Soc Nephrol* 2006;**17**:353–60.

11. Agrawal L, Azad N, Emanuele NV, *et al.* Observation on renal outcomes in the Veterans Affairs Diabetes Trial. *Diabetes Care* 2011;**34**:2090–4.

12. Keane WF, Brenner BM, de Zeeuw D, *et al.* The risk of developing end-stage renal disease in patients with type 2 diabetes and nephropathy: the RENAAL study. *Kidney Int* 2003;**63**:1499–507.

13. Placha G, Canani LH, Warram JH, Krolewski AS. Evidence for different susceptibility genes for proteinuria and ESRD in type 2 diabetes. *Adv Chronic Kidney Dis* 2005;**12**:155–69.

14. O'Seaghdha CM, Fox CS. Genetics of chronic kidney disease. *Nephron Clin Pract* 2011;**118**:c55–63.

15. Krolewski AS, Laffel LM, Krolewski M, *et al.* Glycosylated hemoglobin and the risk of microalbuminuria in patients with insulin-dependent diabetes mellitus. *N Engl J Med* 1995;**332**:1251–5.

16. UK Prospective Diabetes Study (UKPDS) Group. Intensive blood-glucose control with sulphonylureas or insulin compared with conventional treatment and risk of

complications in patients with type 2 diabetes (UKPDS 33). *Lancet* 1998;**352**:837–53.

17. Patel A, MacMahon S, Chalmers J, *et al.* Intensive blood glucose control and vascular outcomes in patients with type 2 diabetes. *N Engl J Med* 2008;**358**: 2560–72.

18. Patel A, MacMahon S, Chalmers J, Neal B, Woodward M, Billot L, *et al.* Effects of a fixed combination of perindopril and indapamide on macrovascular and microvascular outcomes in patients with type 2 diabetes mellitus (the ADVANCE trial): a randomised controlled trial. *Lancet* 2007;**370**:829–40.

19. UK Prospective Diabetes Study Group. Tight blood pressure control and risk of macrovascular and microvascular complications in type 2 diabetes: UKPDS 38. *BMJ* 1998;**317**:703–13.

20. Remuzzi G, Benigni A, Remuzzi A. Mechanisms of progression and regression of renal lesions of chronic nephropathies and diabetes. *J Clin Invest* 2006;**116**:288–96.

21. Steinke JM, Sinaiko AR, Kramer MS, Suissa S, Chavers BM, Mauer M. The early natural history of nephropathy in Type 1 Diabetes: III. Predictors of 5-year urinary albumin excretion rate patterns in initially normoalbuminuric patients. *Diabetes* 2005;**54**:2164–71.

22. Perkins BA, Ficociello LH, Roshan B, *et al.* In patients with type 1 diabetes and new-onset microalbuminuria the development of advanced chronic kidney disease may not require progression to proteinuria. *Kidney Int* 2010;**77**:57–64.

23. Pezzolesi MG, Poznik GD, Mychaleckyj JC, Paterson AD, Barati MT, Klein JB, *et al.* Genome-wide association scan for diabetic nephropathy susceptibility genes

in type 1 diabetes. *Diabetes* 2009;**58**:1403–10.

24. Böger CA, Haak T, Götz AK, *et al.* Effect of ACE and AT-2 inhibitors on mortality and progression to microalbuminuria in a nested case-control study of diabetic nephropathy in diabetes mellitus type 2: results from the GENDIAN study. *Int J Clin Pharmacol Ther* 2006;**44**: 364–74.

25. Böger CA, Stubanus M, Haak T, *et al.* Effect of MTHFR C677T genotype on survival in type 2 diabetes patients with end-stage diabetic nephropathy. *Nephrol Dial Transplant* 2007;**22**: 154–62.

26. Shimazaki A, Kawamura Y, Kanazawa A, *et al.* Genetic variations in the gene encoding ELMO1 are associated with susceptibility to diabetic nephropathy. *Diabetes* 2005;**54**:1171–8.

27. Tervaert TW, Mooyaart AL, Amann K, *et al.* Pathologic classification of diabetic nephropathy. *J Am Soc Nephrol* 2011;**21**:556–63.

28. Tesch GH. MCP-1/CCL2: a new diagnostic marker and therapeutic target for progressive renal injury in diabetic nephropathy. *Am J Physiol Renal Physiol* 2008;**294**:F697–701.

29. Kimmelstiel P, Wilson C. Intercapillary lesions in the glomeruli of the kidney. *Am J Pathol* 1936;**12**:83–98 7.

30. Haider DG, Peric S, Friedl A, *et al.* Kidney biopsy in patients with diabetes mellitus. *Clin Nephrol* 2011;**76**:180–5.

31. Molitch ME, Steffes M, Sun W, *et al.* Development and progression of renal insufficiency with and without albuminuria in adults with type 1 diabetes in the diabetes control and complications trial and the epidemiology of diabetes interventions and complications study. *Diabetes Care* 2010; **33**:1536–43.

32. Costacou T, Ellis D, Fried L, Orchard TJ. Sequence of progression of albuminuria and decreased GFR in persons with type 1 diabetes: a cohort study. *Am J Kidney Dis* 2007;**50**:721–32.

33. Köttgen A, Pattaro C, Böger CA, *et al.* New loci associated with kidney function and chronic kidney disease. *Nat Genet* 2010;**42**:376–84.

34. Böger CA, Chen MH, Tin A, *et al.* CUBN is a gene locus for albuminuria. *J Am Soc Nephrol* 2011;**22**:555–70.

35. Ellis JW, Chen MH, Foster MC, *et al* Validated SNPs for eGFR and their Associations with Albuminuria. *Hum Mol Genet.* 2012;**21**:3293–8.

36. Berger M, Stassen HH, Kohler K, *et al.* Hidden population substructures in an apparently homogeneous population bias association studies. *Eur J Hum Genet* 2006;**14**:236–44.

37. Zenker M, Mertens PR. Arrest of the true culprit and acquittal of the innocent? Genetic revelations charge APOL1 variants with kidney disease susceptibility. *Int Urol Nephrol* 2010;**42**:1131–4.

38. Genovese G, Friedman DJ, Ross MD, *et al.* Association of trypanolytic ApoL1 variants with kidney disease in African Americans. *Science* 2010;**329**: 841–5.

39. Bacanu SA, Devlin B, Roeder K. The power of genomic control. *Am J Hum Genet* 2000;**66**:1933–44.

40. Hildebrandt F. Genetic kidney diseases. *Lancet* 2010;**375**:1287–95.

41. McCarthy MI, Abecasis GR, Cardon LR, *et al.* Genome-wide association studies for complex traits: consensus, uncertainty and challenges. *Nat Rev Genet* 2008;**9**:356–69.

42. Maeda S. Genetics of diabetic nephropathy. *Ther Adv Cardiovasc Dis* 2008;**2**:363–71.

43. McKnight AJ, Currie D, Maxwell AP. Unravelling the genetic basis of renal diseases; from single gene to multifactorial disorders. *J Pathol* 2010;**220**:198–216.

44. Böger CA, Gorski M, Li M, *et al.* Association of eGFR-Related Loci Identified by GWAS with Incident CKD and ESRD. *PLoS Genet* 2011;**7**:e1002292.

45. Gudbjartsson DF, Holm H, Indridason OS, *et al.* Association of variants at UMOD with chronic kidney disease and kidney stones-role of age and comorbid diseases. *PLoS Genet* 2010;**6**: e1001039.

46. International HapMap Consortium. A haplotype map of the human genome. *Nature* 2005;**437**:1299–320.

47. The 1000 Genomes Project. (http://www1000genomesorg).

48. Marchini J, Howie B, Myers S, *et al.* A new multipoint method for genome-wide association studies by imputation of genotypes. *Nat Genet* 2007;**39**:906–13.

49. Durbin RM, Abecasis GR, Altshuler DL, *et al.* A map of human genome variation from population-scale sequencing. *Nature* 2010;**467**:1061–73.

50. Freedman BI, Bostrom M, Daeihagh P, Bowden DW. Genetic factors in diabetic nephropathy. *Clin J Am Soc Nephrol* 2007;**2**:1306–16.

51. Vardarli I, Baier LJ, Hanson RL, *et al.* Gene for susceptibility to diabetic nephropathy in type 2 diabetes maps to 18q22.3–23. *Kidney Int* 2002;**62**: 2176–83.

52. Janssen B, Hohenadel D, Brinkkoetter P, *et al.* Carnosine as a protective factor in diabetic nephropathy: association with a leucine repeat of the carnosinase gene CNDP1. *Diabetes* 2005;**54**: 2320–7.

53. McDonough CW, Bostrom MA, Lu L, *et al.* Genetic analysis of diabetic

nephropathy on chromosome 18 in African Americans: linkage analysis and dense SNP mapping. *Hum Genet* 2009;**126**:805–17.

54. Tanaka N, Babazono T, Saito S, *et al.* Association of solute carrier family 12 (sodium/chloride) member 3 with diabetic nephropathy, identified by genome-wide analyses of single nucleotide polymorphisms. *Diabetes* 2003;**52**:2848–53.

55. Gumienny TL, Brugnera E, Tosello-Trampont AC, *et al.* CED-12/ELMO, a novel member of the CrkII/Dock180/Rac pathway, is required for phagocytosis and cell migration. *Cell* 2001;**107**:27–41.

56. Craig DW, Millis MP, DiStefano JK. Genome-wide SNP genotyping study using pooled DNA to identify candidate markers mediating susceptibility to end-stage renal disease attributed to Type 1 diabetes. *Diabet Med* 2009;**26**: 1090–8.

57. Leak TS, Perlegas PS, Smith SG, *et al.* Variants in intron 13 of the ELMO1 gene are associated with diabetic nephropathy in African Americans. *Ann Hum Genet* 2009;**73**:152–9.

58. Hanson RL, Craig DW, Millis MP, *et al.* Identification of PVT1 as a candidate gene for end-stage renal disease in type 2 diabetes using a pooling-based genome-wide single nucleotide polymorphism association study. *Diabetes* 2007;**56**:975–83.

59. Millis MP, Bowen D, Kingsley C. Variants in the plasmacytoma variant translocation gene (PVT1) are associated with end-stage renal disease attributed to type 1 diabetes. *Diabetes* 2007;**56**:3027–32.

60. Knowler WC, Coresh J, Elston RC, *et al.* The Family Investigation of Nephropathy and Diabetes (FIND): design and methods. *J Diabetes Complications* 2005;**19**:1–9.

61. Chambers JC, Zhang W, Lord GM, *et al.* Genetic loci influencing kidney function and chronic kidney disease. *Nat Genet* 2010;**42**:373–5.

62. Köttgen A, Glazer NL, Dehghan A, *et al.* Multiple loci associated with indices of renal function and chronic kidney disease. *Nat Genet* 2009;**41**:712–7.

63. Pattaro C, Köttgen A, Teumer A, *et al.* Genome-wide association and functional follow-up reveals new loci for kidney function. *PLoS Genet.* 2012;**8**:e1002584.

64. Kao WH, Klag MJ, Meoni LA, *et al.* MYH9 is associated with nondiabetic end-stage renal disease in African Americans. *Nat Genet* 2008;**40**:1185–92.

65. Kopp JB, Smith MW, Nelson GW, *et al.* MYH9 is a major-effect risk gene for focal segmental glomerulosclerosis. *Nat Genet* 2008;**40**:1175–84.

66. McDonough CW, Palmer ND, Hicks PJ, *et al.* A genome-wide association study for diabetic nephropathy genes in African Americans. *Kidney Int* 2011;**79**: 563–72.

67. Freedman BI, Hicks PJ, Bostrom MA, *et al.* Non-muscle myosin heavy chain 9 gene MYH9 associations in African Americans with clinically diagnosed type 2 diabetes mellitus-associated ESRD. *Nephrol Dial Transplant* 2009;**24**:3366–71.

68. Köttgen A, Hwang SJ, Rampersaud E, *et al.* TCF7L2 variants associate with CKD progression and renal function in population-based cohorts. *J Am Soc Nephrol* 2008;**19**:1989–99.

69. Liu M, Shi S, Senthilnathan S, *et al.* Genetic variation of DKK3 may modify renal disease severity in ADPKD. *J Am Soc Nephrol* 2010;**21**:1510–20.

70. Wheeler HE, Metter EJ, Tanaka T, *et al.* Sequential use of transcriptional profiling,

expression quantitative trait mapping, and gene association implicates MMP20 in human kidney aging. *PLoS Genet* 2009;**5**:e1000685.

71. Gronwald W, Klein MS, Zeltner R, *et al.* Detection of autosomal dominant polycystic kidney disease by NMR spectroscopic fingerprinting of urine. *Kidney Int* 2011;**79**:1244–53.

72. Suhre K, Shin SY, Petersen AK, *et al.* Human metabolic individuality in biomedical and pharmaceutical research. *Nature* 2011;**477**:54–60.

73. Tsaih SW, Pezzolesi MG, Yuan R, *et al.* Genetic analysis of albuminuria in aging mice and concordance with loci for human diabetic nephropathy found in a genome-wide association scan. *Kidney Int* 2010;**77**:201–10.

74. Kretzler M, Cohen CD. Integrative biology of renal disease: toward a holistic understanding of the kidney's function and failure. *Semin Nephrol* 2010; **30**:439–42.

75. Igo RP, Jr., Iyengar SK, Nicholas SB, *et al.* Genomewide linkage scan for diabetic renal failure and albuminuria: the FIND study. *Am J Nephrol* 2011;**33**:381–9.

76. Bowden DW, Colicigno CJ, Langefeld CD, *et al.* A genome scan for diabetic nephropathy in African Americans. *Kidney Int* 2004;**66**:1517–26.

77. Osterholm AM, He B, Pitkaniemi J, *et al.* Genome-wide scan for type 1 diabetic nephropathy in the Finnish population reveals suggestive linkage to a single locus on chromosome 3q. *Kidney Int* 2007;**71**:140–5.

78. Moczulski DK, Rogus JJ, Antonellis A, *et al.* Major susceptibility locus for nephropathy in type 1 diabetes on chromosome 3q: results of novel discordant sib-pair analysis. *Diabetes* 1998;**47**:1164–9.

79. Pezzolesi MG, Katavetin P, Kure M, *et al.* Confirmation of genetic associations at ELMO1 in the GoKinD collection supports its role as a susceptibility gene in diabetic nephropathy. *Diabetes* 2009;**58**:2698–702.

80. Hanson RL, Millis MP, Young NJ, *et al.* ELMO1 variants and susceptibility to diabetic nephropathy in American Indians. *Mol Genet Metab* 2010;**101**:383–90.

81. Iyengar SK, Abboud HE, Goddard KA, *et al.* Genome-wide scans for diabetic nephropathy and albuminuria in multiethnic populations: the family investigation of nephropathy and diabetes (FIND). *Diabetes* 2007;**56**:1577–85.

82. Krolewski AS, Poznik GD, Placha G, *et al.* A genome-wide linkage scan for genes controlling variation in urinary albumin excretion in type II diabetes. *Kidney Int* 2006;**69**:129–36.

83. Placha G, Poznik GD, Dunn J, *et al.* A genome-wide linkage scan for genes controlling variation in renal function estimated by serum cystatin C levels in extended families with type 2 diabetes. *Diabetes* 2006;**55**: 3358–65.

84. Maeda S, Kobayashi MA, Araki S, *et al.* A single nucleotide polymorphism within the acetyl-coenzyme A carboxylase beta gene is associated with proteinuria in patients with type 2 diabetes. *PLoS Genet.* 2010;**6**:e1000842.

85. Maeda S, Araki S, Babazono T, *et al.* Replication study for the association between four Loci identified by a genome-wide association study on European American subjects with type 1 diabetes and susceptibility to diabetic nephropathy in Japanese subjects with type 2 diabetes. *Diabetes* 2010;**59**:2075–9.

86. McDonough CW, Hicks PJ, Lu L, *et al.* The influence of carnosinase gene polymorphisms on diabetic nephropathy risk in African-Americans. *Hum Genet* 2009;**126**: 265–75.

87. Freedman BI, Hicks PJ, Sale MM, *et al.* A leucine repeat in the carnosinase gene CNDP1 is associated with diabetic end-stage renal disease in European Americans. *Nephrol Dial Transplant* 2007;**22**:1131–5.

Pathophysiology of diabetic nephropathy

Ivonne Loeffler

Jena University Hospital, Jena, Germany

Key points

- There are several structural hallmarks of diabetic nephropathy that are specific and related to duration of diabetes, degree of glycemic control, and genetic factors.
- Both the glomerular cells (mesangial cells, glomerular endothelial cells, and podocytes) and the renal interstitial cell types (tubular epithelial cells, peritubular endothelial cells, resident and activated fibroblasts, and mast cells) contribute to the pathogenesis of diabetic nephropathy.
- The most important mediators in diabetic nephropathy are advanced glycation end product, transforming growth factor-β1, connective tissue growth factor, angiotensin II, platelet-derived growth factor, hepatocyte growth factor, bone morphogenic protein-

7, insulin-like growth factor-I, vascular endothelial growth factor, and nitric oxide.
- The excessive accumulation of extracellular matrix, which leads to tubulointerstitial fibrosis in diabetic nephropathy, is mainly mediated by myofibroblasts. These activated fibroblasts can originate from tubular epithelial and/or endothelial cells via epithelial-to-mesenchymal transition and endothelial-to-mesenchymal transition respectively.
- Hypoxia, oxidative stress, and inflammation are important mechanisms in the pathophysiology of diabetic nephropathy.
- Several animal models exist to study the diabetic nephropathy looking at specific aspects.

The changes in kidney structure caused by diabetes are specific, creating a pattern not seen in other renal disease, and the severity of diabetic nephropathy (DN) lesions is related to diabetes duration, degree of glycemic control, and genetic factors [1]. The renal risk of developing nephropathy is with approximately 25–40% similar in patients with type 1 and 2 diabetes mellitus and there are no substantial

---

Diabetes and Kidney Disease, First Edition. Edited by Gunter Wolf.

differences between patients with type 2 and those with type 1 diabetes with respect to the basic pathophysiological mechanisms leading to nephropathy [2–4]. Renal structural abnormalities found in DN such as mesangial expansion, basement membrane thickening, glomerulo- and arteriosclerosis, changes in endothelial and tubular cells, podocyte abnormalities, and interstitial inflammation and fibrosis occur in all renal compartments [5]. However, the excessive deposition of extracellular matrix (ECM) proteins in the mesangium and basement membrane of the glomerulus and in the renal tubulointerstitium are the earliest morphological changes and typical hallmarks of DN [5, 6]. The expansion of the mesangial area, caused by an increase in ECM deposition and mesangial cell (MC) hyperthrophy, appears to be the main cause of reducing glomerular filtration in DN [6, 7]. The extent of these changes, which lead to a reduction in the surface available for filtration and narrowing of the lumen, correlates inversely and highly significantly with the glomerular filtration rate in both types of diabetes [6, 8–10]. Matrix components, typically increased in DN, are collagen types I, III, IV, V, VI, and VIII, tenascin, fibronectin, and laminin [6, 11]. To visualize the thickening of glomerular and tubular basement membranes and the increased amount of mesangial matrix kidney, sections can be stained with periodic acid Schiff (PAS), and immunostaining with specific antibodies unveils the enhanced protein expression of different matrix components, e.g. collagen types I, III, and IV.

Hemodynamic changes and the role of different renal cell types in DN

The earliest clinical evidence that nephropathy exists is the appearance of low, yet abnormal, levels of albumin in the urine, called microalbuminuria [12]. The pathophysiology of albuminuria is complex and likely to be heterogeneous even within a single disease entity such as diabetes, with different cell types in the glomerulus and possibly in the tubule contributing in different degrees and at different stages of disease to the leakage of albumin (Figure 4.1) [13]. However, glomerular hemodynamic changes including hyperperfusion and hyperfiltration facilitate the development of albumin leakage from the glomerular capillary compartment into Bowman's space [14]. The elevation in glomerular capillary pressure and the increase in glomerular plasma flow result from a decrease in both afferent and efferent arteriolar resistances wherein the afferent arteriole is more dilated than the efferent [5, 14, 15].

Many diverse factors, including prostanoids, nitric oxide (NO), growth hormone, insulin, insulin-like growth factors (IGFs), angiotensin II (Ang II), vascular endothelial growth factor (VEGF), and cytokines, have been implicated as agents causing hyperfiltration and hyperperfusion. The enhanced intraglomerular pressure leads subsequently to the development of MC matrix overexpression and podocyte injury, because the glomerular capillary basement membrane is in continuum with both podocytes and MCs (Figure 4.1) [5, 14]. Thus changes in capillary pressure cause abnormal shear stress or stretching of glomerular cells, which in turn stimulate the production of cytokines and growth factors in an autocrine and/or paracrine manner. For instance, exposure of glomerular cells (e.g. MCs, podocytes, and glomerular endothelial cells) *in vitro* to stretching or shear stress can activate certain signal transduction systems, growth response, cytokine synthesis, and increased production of ECM proteins [5, 14–16]. MCs, which are located in the intercapillary space, share many characteristics with vascular smooth muscle cells; they possess an abundant number of actin filaments and they contract and proliferate in response to numerous vasoactive sub-

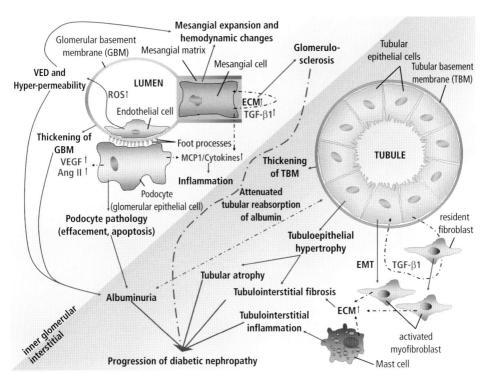

Involvement of different renal cell types in pathogenesis of diabetic nephropathy (DN). Multiple factors contribute to the pathogenesis of DN. Via "crosstalking" the glomerular cell types (mesangial cells, glomerular endothelial cells, and podocytes) are involved in thickening of the glomerular basement membrane and mesangial expansion as well as via upregulation of various mediators, such as transforming growth factor (TGF)-β1, vascular endothelial growth factor, angiotensin II, reactive oxygen species (ROS), and MCP-1, in glomerular inflammation, glomerulosclerosis, and vascular endothelial dysfunction (VED). In addition to some of these glomerular changes and the pathology of podocytes, tubules also contribute to the development of albuminuria, a hallmark of DN. Increased extracellular matrix (ECM) production by the renal interstitial cell types (tubular cells, resident fibroblasts, activated myofibroblasts, and mast cells) leads to tubulointerstitial fibrosis, another characteristic feature of DN. See text for details. Reproduced from D'Agati V, *et al*. RAGE, glomerulosclerosis and proteinuria: roles in podocytes and endothelial cells. *Trends Endocrinol Metab* 2010;**21**:50–6. (See also Plate 4.1.)

stances and growth factors/cytokines [17, 18]. After initial injury, the activated MCs may change phenotype, expressing fibroblast-like myosin [18]. Loss and disassembly of actin fibers in the mesangial area are found in diabetic glomeruli with an impaired contractility in response to vasoconstrictive agents [16]. MCs play an important role in the regulation of glomerular hemodynamics and are the principal glomerular cells involved in ECM deposi-

tion in the mesangium (Figure 4.1) [16, 17]. Although both stretching and high glucose induce gene expression and protein secretion of ECM components in MCs *in vitro*, stretching also stimulates collagen synthesis at all glucose concentrations, whereas it is only at high glucose levels that net collagen accumulation in the medium can be demonstrated [16]. Furthermore, in response to hyperglycemia and stretch, MCs undergo a short period of proliferation followed by cell hypertrophy, and after prolonged exposure to high glucose MCs arrest in the G_1 phase of the cell cycle, which is mediated by p27[Kip1], an inhibitor of cyclin-dependent kinases [5, 16].

Ang II plays a pivotal role in this growth process. Although mesangial cell pathophysiology has long been considered at the heart of development of DN, podocytes have been identified more recently as a central target for the effects of the metabolic milieu in the development and progression of albuminuria in both type 1 and type 2 diabetes mellitus [14, 19]. Podocytes are highly differentiated cells with a complex cellular morphology which directly cover the glomerular basement membrane (GBM) (Figure 4.1) [5, 16]. The podocyte cell body bulges into the urinary space and gives rise to long primary processes that extend toward the capillaries to which they affix by numerous foot processes [16]. The foot processes of neighboring podocytes interconnected by several slit diaphragm molecules, such as nephrin, form the final barrier for filtration. Proteins that anchor foot processes to the GBM (e.g. α3β1-integrin, integrin-linked kinase (ILK), and α-actinin-4 (ACTN4)) and those associated with the slit diaphragm (e.g. nephrin, podocin, ACTN4, and CD2-associated protein) are crucial for normal function of the filtration barrier [20]. Podocytes are the principal glomerular cell type involved in the formation of the GBM, as they produce and assemble most of the components of the GBM, such as the α3 chain of collagen type IV, fibronectin, laminin, agrin, and heparin sulfate proteoglycan. Whereas collagen type IV, fibronectin and laminin in diabetic glomeruli are increased, the expression of agrin and heparin sulfate proteoglycan is reduced [16]. The decrease in the GBM content of these negatively charged molecules contributes to the loss of charge selectivity in the glomerular filtration barrier and to the development and progression of proteinuria [21]. Furthermore, structural abnormalities of podocyte foot processes, such as foot process widening, effacement, and narrower filtration slits, have been described in DN, in which the foot process width directly correlates with the urinary albumin excretion rate (Figure 4.1) [16, 21]. In addition to foot process widening, the number and density of podocytes have been reported to be markedly reduced (podocytopenia) in diabetic patients with type 1 or 2 diabetes [21]. In the adult kidney, podocytes are unable to undergo regenerative proliferation to compensate for a loss of podocytes or an increase in GBM surface area. Therefore, it is not clear whether in DN there is an absolute reduction in podocyte number or a relative reduction due to the increased surface area of GBM [16]. Broadening of foot processes would be a compensatory response of the remaining podocytes in an attempt to cover areas of bare GBM [16]. In fact, podocytopenia worsens with the progression from normoalbuminuria to microalbuminuria to overt proteinuria, in which the loss of cell anchorage to the GBM may result from downregulation of α3β1-integrin, the principal adhesion complex that attaches the podocyte to the GBM, which has been shown in several studies [21]. Furthermore, in DN nephrin protein production is downregulated, and the decrease in nephrin, which is exclusively expressed by podocytes and predominantly localized to the slit diaphragm, leads to broadening of the foot process widths and subsequently increased proteinuria [16, 21]. Many of these processes are mediated by Ang II.

An alternative explanation for proteinuria in DN is disturbed handling of proteins by proximal tubular cells [19, 22]. The albumin and other ultrafiltered proteins are normally reabsorbed in the tubular system by endocytosis via megalin and cubulin, and only traces of protein are found in the urine under physiological conditions. Albuminuria in pathophysiological states such as DN might be due to attenuated tubular reabsorption of albumin (Figure 4.1)

[19]. Furthermore, it has been clearly demonstrated that an increase in tubular basement membrane (TBM) width is an integral component of early nephropathy, and a direct effect of hyperglycemia on the turnover of the TBM matrix components has been shown. For example, exposure of human renal proximal tubular cells to high glucose increases the amount of collagen IV and fibronectin in the culture supernatant and decreases the pathways which are responsible for their degradation [23]. Diabetic tubules show a higher intracellular glucose concentration and one consequence resulting from this intracellular glucose accumulation is activation of the polyol pathway. The metabolism of hexose or pentose sugars by this pathway is of great importance in glucose-mediated alterations in proximal tubular cell matrix generation, but it has also been shown that there is a significant amount of variability in the ability of cultured proximal tubular cells from different individuals to activate the polyol pathway; this may be one factor, which explains the heterogeneous nature of DN [23]. A further early renal structural feature of diabetes is tubular hypertrophy. In contrast to alterations in matrix generation, cell hypertrophy is not mediated by the polyol pathway, but some effects are linked to increasing proximal tubular sodium absorption [23]. Tubuloepithelial hypertrophy, characterized by cell cycle arrest in the G_1 phase, is one of the precursors of the later irreversible changes in the tubulointerstitial architecture leading to tubular atrophy and interstitial fibrosis (Figure 4.1). Part of this association between growth and fibrogenesis may be because similar networks of cytokines and growth factors that induce cellular hypertrophy can also stimulate ECM synthesis and deposition [24]. The biological functions of endothelium, an interior covering of blood vessels, are numerous and in DN vascular endothelial dysfunction (VED) has been shown (Figure 4.1) [25]. VED results in reduced production of NO, reduced activation of nitric oxide synthase (NOS), and increased production of reactive oxygen species (ROS). The deranged endothelial function upregulates the expression of prothrombotic and proinflammatory mediators, which are implicated in the pathogenesis of DN [25]. Hyperglycemia induces endothelial apoptotic cell death and scavenges NO and induces VED, which, in turn, increases the deposition of the ECM leading to glomerulosclerosis and progressive decline in the glomerular filtration rate to produce nephropathy. More precisely, high concentration of glucose alters endothelial glycocalyx permeability, and the expression and activity of NOS is downregulated through glucose-mediated production of ROS, which play a major role in the changes of intraglomerular hemodynamics in DN [25]. Furthermore, interaction of glomerular endothelial cells with other glomerular cells, such as MCs and podocytes, determine the overall balance of cell growth and matrix accumulation, and in disease states where sclerosis results there is a shift toward abnormal cell growth and matrix synthesis (Figure 4.1) [18]. In addition, endothelial cells, together with tubular cells, are involved in two other mechanisms, called endothelial-to-mesenchymal transition (EndMT) and epithelial-to-mesenchymal transition (EMT). In both mechanisms the cells undergo biochemical changes which lead to a transdifferentation to activated myofibroblasts. The myofibroblasts, in turn, contribute to the development of diabetic renal interstitial fibrosis via synthesis and secretion of ECM (see below). Mast cells, which play a key role in inflammatory processes, are also associated with human DN (Figure 4.1) [26]. The number of these infiltrating cells in the interstitium is significantly increased in DN compared with normal kidney tissue. Mast cells are often found in periglomerular and peritubular locations, but never within glomeruli, and they contribute directly to ECM accumulation and also influence fibroblast activity in DN [26]

Several growth factors, cytokines, chemokines, and vasoactive agents have been implicated in the pathogenesis of DN [24]. These factors are stimulated by high glucose and its metabolites, non-enzymatic glycation products, and hemodynamic changes, and are released from resident renal cells. They may, in turn, through autocrine and paracrine mechanisms, stimulate either proliferation or hypertrophy of cells, and increase their production of ECM proteins [24].

Advanced glycation end products

Non-enzymatic and irreversible reactions between sugars and the free amino groups on proteins, lipids, and nucleic acids by the Maillard reaction result in dysfunction through the formation of AGEs [27, 28]. These chemically heterogeneous compounds induce many of the pathogenic changes that occur in DN. For instance, AGEs directly stimulate ECM production, reduce the expression and activity of degradative matrix metalloproteinases, and significantly interact with the renin–angiotensin system (RAS) [27]. AGEs result in the expression and activation of a number of transcription factors implicated in the development of DN, including nuclear factor κB (NF-κB) and protein kinase C (PKC). This effect can be both direct (through AGE receptors) and indirect, via generation of ROS [27]. However, AGEs contribute to the release of proinflammatory cytokines and expression of growth factors, such as TGF-β1 and CTGF, by interacting via specific receptors with, for example, monocytes/macrophages and endothelial cells [28]. Although present at low levels in homeostasis, the multiligand receptor for AGEs (RAGE) expression is increased in diabetic kidney, especially in podocytes [29, 30]. AGEs and signaling via RAGE is strongly implicated

in podocyte effacement, in the upregulation of podocyte expression of monocyte chemoattractant protein-1 (MCP-1), and podocyte apoptosis [29]. Podocyte RAGE activation also increases the expression/activation of VEGF, which, in turn, leads to both hyperpermeability and proteinuria (Figure 4.1) [30]. An activation of RAGE in endothelial cells is involved in the generation of ROS, which then promote endothelial dysfunction [31]. In MCs, RAGE activation inhibits cell proliferation and promotes MC hypertrophy as well as increasing the mesangial synthesis of ECM, such as fibronectin and collagen types I and IV, and the mesangial secretion of MCP-1, which participates in the inflammatory process (Figure 4.1) [31]. In addition to podocytes, mesangial, and endothelial cells, RAGE has also been identified on the surface of tubular cells in kidneys, where activation leads to increased expression of TGF-β1, which is responsible for development of activated myofibroblasts via EMT (Figure 4.2) [31].

Transforming growth factor-β1

TGF-β1, a potent profibrotic cytokine, and its type II receptor are increased in type 1 and 2 diabetes [5, 6, 32]. In DN in tubular cells and MCs, TGF-β1 is induced by mechanisms involving high glucose, AGEs and ROS, and Ang II (Figure 4.2) [5, 19]. Although in MCs TGF-β1 is induced by high glucose, TGF-β1 blockade prevents glucose-induced MC hypertrophy and ECM production, indicating that these effects are mediated by TGF-β1 via an autocrine mechanism [5, 16]. It is obvious that TGF-β1 is the key cytokine inducing the production of different ECM proteins in renal cells and inhibiting ECM degradation (Figure 4.2) [6, 14, 21, 33]. The TGF-β system in the podocyte also stimulates ECM production by the podocyte (contributing to GBM thickening) and promotes apoptosis and decreases integrin expression, which can lead to podo-

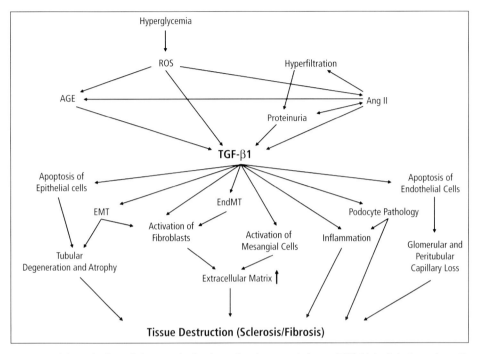

Schematic view of the central role of transforming growth factor (TGF)-β1 in diabetic nephropathy (DN). Various mechanisms relevant to hyperglycemia-induced activation of TGF-β1 lead to tissue destruction in DN. The multifunctional cytokine TGF-β1, induced by advanced glycation end products, angiotensin II, proteinuria, and reactive oxygen species, acts as the key mediator of tubulointerstitial and glomerular pathobiology in DN. See text for details. Modified after Wolf G. New insights into the pathophysiology of diabetic nephropathy: from haemodynamics to molecular pathology. *Eur J Clin Invest* 2004;**34**:785–96. and Böttinger EP, *et al*. TGF-beta signaling in renal disease. *J Am Soc Nephrol* 2002;**13**:2600–10.

cyte detachment and podocytopenia [14, 21]. In diabetic kidneys, TGF-β1 expression is associated with increased tubular cell apoptosis, which leads to tubular degeneration and atrophy [34]. Epithelial cells of the proximal tubule have the potential to contribute to the pathogenesis of renal fibrosis by the production of TGF-β1, because the proximal tubular cell-derived TGF-β1 on the one hand regulates the terminal differentiation of interstitial fibroblasts associated with induction of interstitial collagen gene expression and its protein incorporation into the ECM, and on the other hand stimulates marked alterations in cell morphology, such that the epithelial cells acquire an elongated, spindle shape, fibroblastic appearance associated with rearrangement of their actin cytoskeleton [23]. Loss of glomerular and peritubular capillaries is associated with increased apoptosis of endothelial cells, which is directly induced by TGF-β1 (Figure 4.2) [34]. Furthermore, TGF-β1 may also indirectly promote endothelial cell apoptosis by depleting cell types that produce VEGF. This angiogenic survival factor is expressed in podocytes and tubular cells in normal kidneys, and TGF-β1-induced apoptosis of podocytes and tubular cells may be causing the described loss of expression of VEGF in progressive renal disease [34].

Connective tissue growth factor

CTGF is another prosclerotic cytokine and has also been shown to be involved in both the early and the later stages of DN [6]. In support of the hypothesis of the relevance of CTGF in DN, it has been shown that CTGF is scarcely expressed in the normal kidney, but it is strongly induced in both human and experimental DN [16]. CTGF, originally identified as a growth factor secreted by vascular endothelial cells in culture, is exclusively induced by TGF-β1 in fibroblasts and therefore a crucial downstream mediator of TGF-β1-stimulated matrix protein expression and the profibrotic effects of TGF-β1 [35–38]. Downstream of a cascade of events induced by hyperglycemia, CTGF and TGF-β1 work in a coordinated manner to promote increased expression of ECM proteins. CTGF mediates the TGF-β1-induced increases in ECM proteins (collagen types I, III, IV, and fibronectin) [6]. Furthermore, CTGF indirectly plays a role in the pathogenesis of DN by modulating the bioactivity of other cytokines implicated in the pathogenesis of the glomerular damage, because CTGF appears to enhance IGF-I prosclerotic effects and to increase the binding of TGF-β1 to its receptors [16].

Angiotensin II

Ang II plays a pivotal role as a mediator of proteinuria in DN through the induction of various cytokines and chemokines via autocrine and paracrine pathways [5, 19]. Circulating Ang II is formed in the blood by RAS, which is activated in DN [16, 24]. Ang II, in the diabetic kidney stimulated by hyperglycemia and metabolic and hemodynamic processes, mediates glomerular hyperfiltration and, via enhancing the uptake of glucose by cells, enhanced oxidative stress, which is important for the formation of AGEs (Figure 4.2) [19]. Specifically, a local increase in Ang II in the podocyte

microenvironment by hyperglycemia leads to suppression of nephrin expression in podocytes, and thereby increases the ultrafiltration of proteins, which further contribute to podocyte damage [5]. In addition, Ang II, also induced in tubular cells by hyperglycemia, increases tubular reabsorption of ultrafiltered proteins as well, contributing thereby to tubular inflammation and fibrosis [5, 6]

Platelet-derived growth factor

In addition to TGF-β, another growth factor implicated in progressive renal injury is platelet-derived growth factor (PDGF) [39] The PDGF system, which is upregulated in glomeruli from diabetic rats and MCs in culture exposed to high glucose medium, stimulates TGF-β synthesis in renal cells and the subsequent hypertrophy and increased collagen production. For example, PDGF mediates both high glucose- and AGE-dependent induction of collagen III in cultured MCs through augmenting the production of TGF-β1, suggesting that PDGF acts as an intermediate factor [24].

Hepatocyte growth factor and bone morphogenic protein-7

Hepatocyte growth factor (HGF), a multifunctional polypeptide, and its specific tyrosine kinase receptor play an important role in renal development [40]. In the kidney, HGF expression is limited to mesenchyme-derived cells, including glomerular MCs, endothelial cells, interstitial fibroblasts, and macrophages [40]. Although HGF and its receptor are stimulated in kidneys of diabetic rats and the expression of HGF is induced by high glucose in cultured proximal tubular and inner medullary collecting duct cells, [24] there is emerging evidence that administration of HGF protein, or its gene, in various animal models of chronic renal disease suppresses the profibrogenic cytokine

TGF-β1 and its receptor, inhibits the activation of myofibroblasts, and attenuates ECM deposition and interstitial fibrosis [40]. In recent years, another protein, called bone morphogenic protein-7 (BMP-7), is gaining increasing scientific attention in diabetic kidneys. BMP-7, a homodimeric member of the TGF-β superfamily, is primarily expressed in kidney tubules and glomeruli [41]. In human and experimental DN, the renal cortical expression of BMP-7 is progressively decreased in both tubules and glomeruli [42, 43]. Furthermore, in cultured tubular cells, BMP-7 expression is reduced by TGF-β1 and moreover BMP-7 reverses TGF-β1-induced EMT in association with reversal of chronic renal injury [42, 44]. In addition, the upregulation of CTGF by TGF-β1 inhibits BMP-7 signaling *in vitro* and *in vivo* and reduces important features of DN, such as GBM thickening and albuminuria [45, 46].

Insulin-like growth factor-I

IGF-I is a potent mitogenic polypeptide and although circulating IGF-I levels are normal or reduced in patients with diabetes, the local renal IGF-I system is upregulated in key diabetic kidney tissues and glomerular ultrafiltrate as well as in renal fibroblasts under hyperglycemic conditions, suggesting a role for IGF-I in the pathogenesis of both glomerular hypertrophy and hyperfiltration in diabetes [6, 16, 24, 47, 48]. The enhanced renal IGF-I levels are correlated with pathological alterations, such as increased proliferation of mesangial and tubular cells and increased migration of podocytes and MCs [48] Further effects of IGF-I in the kidney at the cellular level are the promotion of ECM accumulation in MCs, tubular cells, and also fibroblasts, and the increase in DNA synthesis and protein synthesis in tubular cells [48] In addition, IGF-I together with CTGF, both produced by human renal fibroblasts, have been shown to cooperate the induction of collagen type I and type III production

by high glucose, whereas CTGF alone has no effect on collagen secretion [47].

Vascular endothelial growth factor

VEGF, a homodimeric glycoprotein, is an endothelial-specific growth factor that promotes glomerular and peritubular endothelial cell proliferation, differentiation, and survival, and furthermore is a potent inducer of vascular permeability and dilation [5, 16, 49]. In the kidney, VEGF is predominantly expressed by podocytes and tubular cells, but also in MCs and the collecting duct [5, 16, 49]. VEGF and its receptors are upregulated in patients with type 1 and type 2 diabetes and also in experimental animals [49]. Whereas hypoxia is the main stimulus of VEGF, several other factors, such as hyperglycemia, TGF-β1, PDGF, IGF-I, Ang II, AGEs, and ROS, also have the potential to upregulate VEGF expression [49]. A functional role of VEGF in the pathophysiology of DN is most likely, because inhibition of VEGF has beneficial effects on diabetes-induced functional and structural alterations, such as hyperfiltration, albuminuria, and glomerular hypertrophy [5, 16, 49].

Nitric oxide

NO, produced by the NOS, is an important modulator of renal function and morphology [50]. Several factors and mechanisms, such as VEGF, TGF-β1, leptin, and shear stress, stimulate the expression and activity of NOS in the diabetic kidney [50]. Indeed, both expression and activity of endothelial NOS are increased in DN, and endothelial NOS inhibitors prevent glomerular hyperfiltration in diabetic animals, [16] but it has also been shown that VED, which leads to albuminuria in DN, results in reduced activation of endothelial NOS and reduced generation and bioavailability of NO [25]. These confusing and contradictory findings can be explained by different diabetic metabolic milieus, occurring either during early phases of nephropathy or during moderate glycemic control with some degree of treatment with exogenous insulin, representing more the clinically applicable state of DN [50]

Tubulointerstitial fibrosis, EMT, and EndMT in diabetic nephropathy

The pathophysiology of tubulointerstitial fibrosis is divided into four arbitrary phases: (1) cellular activation and injury phase, (2) the fibrogenic signaling phase, (3) the fibrogenic phase, and (4) the destructive phase [51]. In the first phase, tubular, perivascular, and mononuclear cells are activated; they begin to populate in the interstitium and release proinflammatory and injurious molecules. The second phase is characterized by the production of fibrosis-promoting factors, such as TGF-β1, CTGF, Ang II, and PDGF. In the third phase, ECM production increases and matrix degradation decreases, which results in the fourth phase, in that the number of intact nephrons progressively declines resulting in a continuous reduction in glomerular filtration [51]. Proximal tubular cells are the predominant cell type in the normal renal interstitium, in which there are relatively few resident interstitial fibroblasts. These resident interstitial fibroblasts lie in close apposition to the proximal TBM and their numbers increase in progressive DN [23]. Furthermore, the cells take on the phenotypic appearance of activated myofibroblasts, which are positive for α-smooth muscle actin (α-SMA) and fibroblast-specific protein 1 (FSP-1), and are the major source of the expanded ECM, the direct cause of fibrosis [23]. Although in renal fibrosis, the role of matrix-producing myofibroblasts, which contribute to progression of fibrosis in DN by facilitating deposition of interstitial ECM, is widely accepted, their origin is yet controversial discussed [52–54]. First Strutz et al [55]

hypothesized and then Iwano et al [56] confirmed that up to 36% of all interstitial fibroblasts are derived from tubular cells by EMT (Figure 4.3). EMT is a highly regulated process, which is defined by four key events: (1) loss of epithelial cell adhesion (e.g. E-cadherin adhesion complex), (2) de novo α-SMA expression and actin reorganization, (3) disruption of TBM, and (4) enhanced cell migration and invasion of the interstitium (Figure 4.3) [57, 58]. Several factors are known to play an important role in the induction of EMT and subsequently of tubulointerstitial fibrosis. For example, chronic hypoxia in the tubulointerstitium, AGEs, CTGF, and metalloproteinases have been shown to stimulate EMT in models of renal disease, but, above all, the enhanced multifunctional cytokine TGF-β1 has been identified as a central mediator of the fibrotic response in diabetic kidneys and as a regulator for EMT [59–62]. Another novel mechanism for generation of myofibroblasts in early diabetic renal fibrosis is EndMT (Figure 4.3). Here, in contrast to the EMT mechanism, the activated myofibroblasts are of endothelial origin. Different research groups showed that in models for DN a significant number of α-SMA- and FSP-1-positive cells (myofibroblasts) coexpressed the endothelial marker CD31, suggesting that these fibroblasts are likely of endothelial origin [63, 64]. Similar to EMT, EndMT can be induced by TGF-β1 and be inhibited by BMP-7 [44, 65, 66].

Hypoxia

Chronic hypoxia in the interstitium, an important hallmark of DN, is multifactorial and occurs via several mechanisms acting in concert, such as anemia in the early stage and loss of peritubular capillaries in the tubulointerstitium in the late stage [67, 68]. Hypoxia

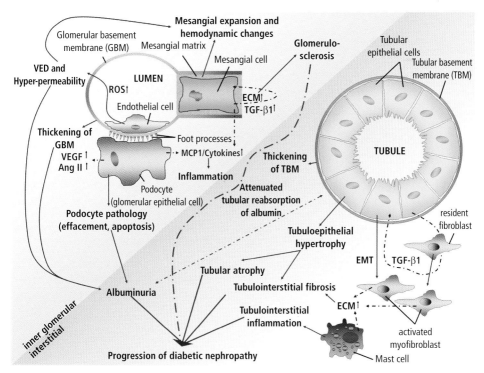

Plate 4.1 Involvement of different renal cell types in pathogenesis of diabetic nephropathy (DN). Multiple factors contribute to the pathogenesis of DN. Via "crosstalking" the glomerular cell types (mesangial cells, glomerular endothelial cells, and podocytes) are involved in thickening of the glomerular basement membrane and mesangial expansion as well as via upregulation of various mediators, such as transforming growth factor (TGF)-β1, vascular endothelial growth factor, angiotensin II, reactive oxygen species (ROS), and MCP-1, in glomerular inflammation, glomerulosclerosis, and vascular endothelial dysfunction (VED). In addition to some of these glomerular changes and the pathology of podocytes, tubules also contribute to the development of albuminuria, a hallmark of DN. Increased extracellular matrix (ECM) production by the renal interstitial cell types (tubular cells, resident fibroblasts, activated myofibroblasts, and mast cells) leads to tubulointerstitial fibrosis, another characteristic feature of DN. See text for details. Reproduced from D'Agati V, et al. RAGE, glomerulosclerosis and proteinuria: roles in podocytes and endothelial cells. *Trends Endocrinol Metab* 2010;**21**:50–6.

Diabetes and Kidney Disease, First Edition. Edited by Gunter Wolf.
© 2013 John Wiley & Sons, Ltd. Published 2013 by John Wiley & Sons, Ltd.

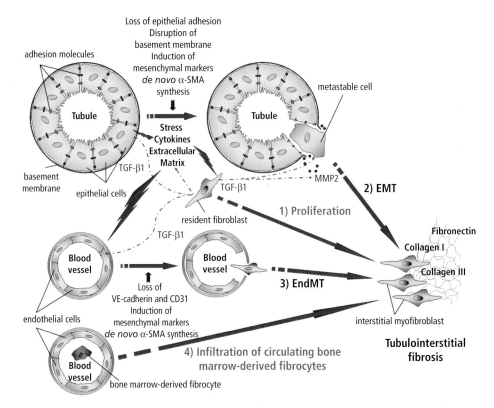

Plate 4.2 Hypothesis of progression of tubulointerstitial fibrosis by EMT and EndMT. Interstitial myofibroblasts responsible for synthesis of ECM and contribution to fibrosis have been proposed to be derived from more sources: (1) proliferation/activation of resident fibroblasts, (2) epithelial-to-mesenchymal transition (EMT), (3) endothelial-to-mesenchymal transition (EndMT), and/or (4) infiltration of circulating bone marrow-derived fibrocytes. Initiated by external stimuli (e.g., hyperglycemia, cytokines, extracellular matrix) tubular or endothelial cells lose their cell-cell contacts and start to express mesenchymal markers (e.g. α-smooth muscle actin, vimentin) and undergo EMT and EndMT, respectively. The initially metastable cells, which coexpress tubular/endothelial and mesenchymal markers, disengage themselves from cell connective and transdifferentiate to interstitial myofibroblasts. These mesenchymal cells derived from epithelium or endothelium in the tubulointerstitium contribute to progression of DN. Modified and supplemented according to Kizu A, *et al.* Endothelial-mesenchymal transition as a novel mechanism for generating myofibroblasts during diabetic nephropathy. *Am J Pathol* 2009;**175**:1371–3, and Barnes JL, *et al.* Myofibroblast differentiation during fibrosis: role of NAD(P)H oxidases. *Kidney Int* 2011;**79**:944–56.

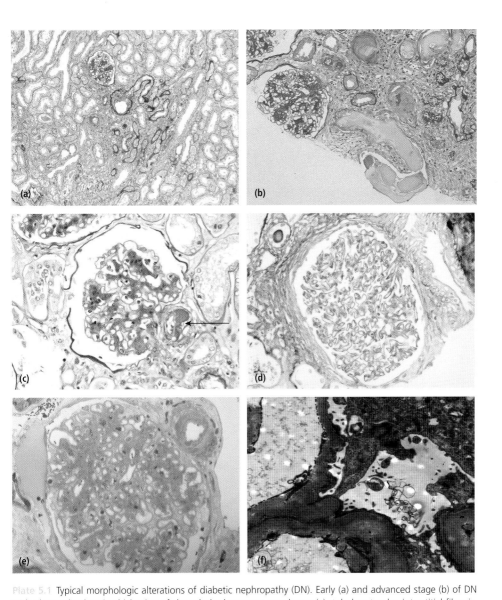

Plate 5.1 Typical morphologic alterations of diabetic nephropathy (DN). Early (a) and advanced stage (b) of DN with glomerulosclerosis, thickening of the tubular basement membrane (a), tubular atrophy, interstitial fibrosis, signs of acute tubular damage with cast-like intratubular material and mild interstitial inflammation (b). Periodic acid Schiff (PAS) stain ×100. (c) Characteristic glomerular and vascular changes in DN with mild to moderate diffuse to nodular glomerulosclerosis and arteriolar hyalinosis (arrow). PAS stain, ×400. (d) Pseudolinear positivity for IgG in DN (×400). (e) Semithin section with moderate mesangial matrix expansion and marked thickening of the glomerular basement membrane (GBM) as well as hyalinosis of the Vas afferens (×400). (f) Electron microscopy (×7750) confirming marked thickening of GBM together with foot process effacement of podocytes.

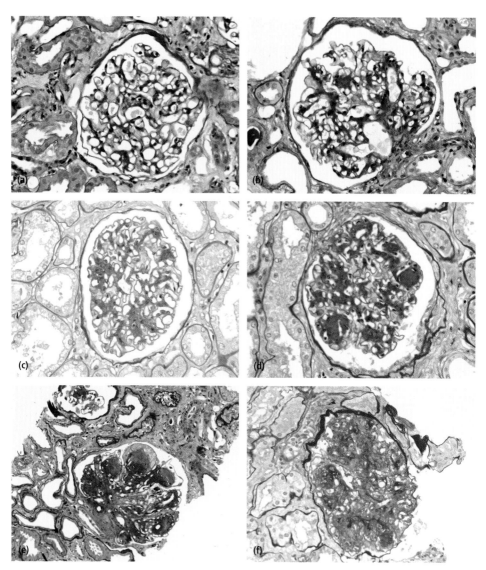

Plate 5.2 Classes of diabetic nephropathy (DN) according to Tervaert et al. (2010) [periodic acid Schiff (PAS), ×400]. (a) Class I, i.e. mild or non-specific light microscopic changes. (b, c) Class II with mild mesangial expansion >25% and patent capillary lumen (class IIa, b) or severe mesangial expansion with mesangium > capillary lumen (class IIb, c). (d, e) Class III, i.e., nodular type glomerulosclerosis (Kimmelstiel–Wilson lesion). (f) Class IV, i.e. advanced diabetic nephropathy with lesions from class I–III in >50% of glomeruli with lesions from class I–III. Classes of diabetic nephropathy (DN) according to Tervaert TW, Mooyaart AL, Amann K, Cohen AH, Cook HT, Drachenberg CB, Ferrario F, Fogo AB, Haas M, de Heer E, Joh K, Noel LH, Radhakrishnan J, Seshan SV, Bajema IM, Bruijn JA: Pathologic classification of diabetic nephropathy. J Am Soc Nephrol 2010;**21**:556–63.

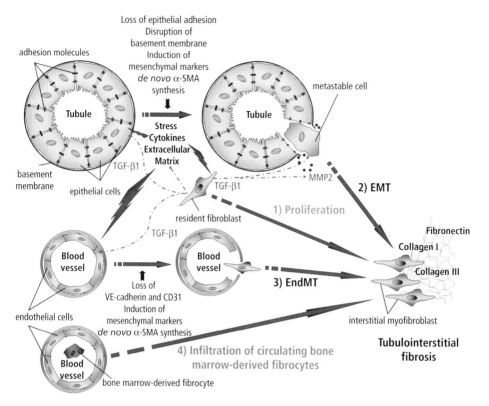

Hypothesis of progression of tubulointerstitial fibrosis by EMT and EndMT. Interstitial myofibroblasts responsible for synthesis of ECM and contribution to fibrosis have been proposed to be derived from more sources: (1) proliferation/activation of resident fibroblasts, (2) epithelial-to-mesenchymal transition (EMT), (3) endothelial-to-mesenchymal transition (EndMT), and/or (4) infiltration of circulating bone marrow-derived fibrocytes. Initiated by external stimuli (e.g., hyperglycemia, cytokines, extracellular matrix) tubular or endothelial cells lose their cell-cell contacts and start to express mesenchymal markers (e.g. α-smooth muscle actin, vimentin) and undergo EMT and EndMT, respectively. The initially metastable cells, which coexpress tubular/endothelial and mesenchymal markers, disengage themselves from cell connective and transdifferentiate to interstitial myofibroblasts. These mesenchymal cells derived from epithelium or endothelium in the tubulointerstitium contribute to progression of DN. Modified and supplemented according to Kizu A, *et al.* Endothelial-mesenchymal transition as a novel mechanism for generating myofibroblasts during diabetic nephropathy. *Am J Pathol* 2009;**175**:1371–3, and Barnes JL, *et al.* Myofibroblast differentiation during fibrosis: role of NAD(P)H oxidases. *Kidney Int* 2011;**79**:944–56. (See also Plate 4.2.)

is a potent regulator of gene expression for a broad spectrum of molecules and in DN an important factor aggravating interstitial fibrosis, partly by the induction of factors such as TGF-β1 and VEGF, which lead to apoptosis of tubular cells or EMT [5, 67, 68]. This induction of growth factors and cytokines is mediated by hypoxia-inducible factor-1 (HIF-1), and Ang II can further increase this important transcription factor [5]. Administration of erythropoietin (EPO) to correct anemia and blockade of RAS to preserve peritubular capillary flow and reduce oxidative stress are key to the improvement of kidney oxygenation [68].

Oxidative stress

Hyperglycemia leads to an increase in mitochondrial ROS formation, which mediate many negative biological effects, including oxidation of proteins and damage to DNA. Oxidative stress in the form of increased production of ROS represents a pathophysiological link between hyperglycemia and other major pathways responsible for diabetic complications [28]. ROS are capable of activating PKC in vascular endothelial cells, which increases the production of cytokines and ECM [28]. Oxidative stress is a leading initiator of cellular dysfunction in diabetes complications, and increased ROS generation can induce podocyte dysfunction [21]. Furthermore, antioxidants blocks glucose-induced increase in fibronectin and collagen type IV gene expression in MCs and attenuates hyperglycemia-induced apoptosis in human tubular cells [1].

Inflammation

Inflammatory pathways have a central role in the development of diabetic complications, such as DN [69]. Inflammation in the diabetic kidney is characterized by increased synthesis of proinflammatory cytokines [e.g. interleukin (IL)-1, IL-6, and IL-18, tumor necrosis factor (TNF)], upregulation of adhesion molecules, and enhanced expression of chemoattractant cytokines (e.g. MCP-1 and RANTES), with subsequent transmigration of monocytes, neutrophils, and lymphocytes into renal tissue [69]. MCP-1 is an important chemokine for macrophages/monocytes and its expression in MCs is stimulated by high glucose, but also a increased tubular expression of MCP-1 has been found in experimental models and in renal biopsies from patients with DN [5]. The expression of proinflammatory cytokines could be further stimulated in podocytes and tubular cells by proteinuria acting in concert with hyperglycemia and AGEs (Figure 4.1) [5].

One of the major elements implicated in this inflammatory reaction is NF-κB, a ubiquitous transcription factor that is activated by many stimuli relevant to DN [69]. The accumulation of macrophages and neutrophils are features of the development of DN and these cells and their products (e.g. ROS, cytokines and proteases) exacerbate inflammation in the kidneys of patients with diabetes mellitus [69]. The diabetes-associated induction of proinflammatory and profibrotic cytokines, including TGF-β1, is partly dependent on Ang II and contributes to the destruction of nephrons in DN (Figure 4.2) [5].

Rodent models of DN

The Animal Models of Diabetic Complications Consortium (AMDCC), created in 2001 by the National Institutes of Health, was initiated to develop and characterize models of DN and other complications [70]. Although no current strain of type 1 or type 2 diabetes reliably develops all the features of human DN, AMDCC investigators and other investigators in the field have found a number of exciting new models, in addition to standard models, that replicate various features of DN [70]. Some leading murine models of this disorder will be briefly illustrated, noting that considerably more models are available.

Streptozotocin model

Streptozotocin (STZ)-induced diabetes is an overall recognized model for type 1 diabetes mellitus. By injection of the islet toxin STZ, the animals develop type 1 diabetes and exhibit a broad spectrum of renal diabetic pathophysiology including kidney enlargement, diffuse mesangial expansion, glomerular hypertrophy, basement membrane thickening, ECM accumulation, glomerulosclerosis, and upregulation of TGF-β1 mRNA and protein expression [39]. Although much knowledge about DN has been found using the STZ model, it is not perfect, because one important feature of this model is that the renal functional and morphological changes will not lead to progressive renal insufficiency even when followed for up to 18 months [39].

db/db mouse model

The *db/db* mouse model of leptin deficiency is currently the most widely used mouse for modeling DN in settings of type 2 diabetes [71]. The *db/db* mice have a mutation deletion of the leptin receptor, and leptin deficiency confers susceptibility to obesity and insulin resistance [71]. The underlying genetic background is susceptible to diabetic complications such as nephropathy, and DN in these mice is manifest by albuminuria, podocyte loss, and mesangial matrix expansion [71]. Although these mice do not develop progressive renal insufficiency and therefore fail to recapitulate later and morphologically advanced features of DN, the *db/db* mice are a good model of early changes of human DN [71].

Endothelial nitric oxide synthase-deficient mice

The endothelial cell-derived vasodilator NO is an important mediator in DN, and combination of endothelial nitric oxide synthase (eNOS) deficiency with either the STZ-induced type 1 diabetes or the *db/db* model for diabetes type 2 induces nephropatic changes that mimic many aspects of human DN [70, 71]. In particular, the introduction of eNOS deficiency into the *db/db* mice background has shown as a major advance in DN model development, because these mice develop obesity, hypertension, albuminuria, marked mesangial expansion, and mesangiolysis, which offers great potential for studying mechanisms underlying progression [71].

BTBR *ob/ob* mice

The characteristics of the BTBR (*b*lack and *t*an *b*rachyuric, i.e., short tailed) *ob/ob* mice are insulin resistant with elevated serum insulin levels and pancreatic islet hypertrophy and subsequent sustained hyperglycemia [71]. The kidney phenotype of these mice includes early loss of podocytes, chronologically coinciding with onset of proteinuria. Furthermore, this mouse model develops on later stage progressive, advanced DN with features of more extensive mesangial expansion, mesangiolysis, persistent podocyte loss, basement membrane thickening, and interstitial fibrosis [71].

Further helpful mouse models to study the pathophysiology of DN are (1) bradykinin B2 receptor-deficient mice, (2) decorin deficient mice, (3) mice that overexpress renin, (4) mice that overexpress calmodulin in pancreatic β cells (OVE26 mouse), (5) mice with a single nucleotide substitution in the gene encoding for insulin (Akita mouse), and (6) podocyte-specific insulin receptor knockout mice [70, 71].

1. Caramori ML, Mauer M. Diabetes and nephropathy. *Curr Opin Nephrol Hypertens* 2003;**12**:273–82.
2. Hasslacher C, Ritz E, Wahl P, Michael C. Similar risks of nephropathy in patients with type I or type II diabetes mellitus. *Nephrol Dial Transplant* 1989;**4**:859–63.
3. Berger M, Mönks D, Wanner C, Lindner TH. Diabetic nephropathy: an inherited disease or just a diabetic complication? *Kidney Blood Press Res* 2003;**26**:143–54.
4. Parving HH. Diabetic nephropathy: prevention and treatment. *Kidney Int* 2001;**60**:2041–55.
5. Wolf G. New insights into the pathophysiology of diabetic nephropathy: from haemodynamics to molecular

pathology. *Eur J Clin Invest* 2004;**34**: 785–96.

6. Mason RM, Wahab NA. Extracellular matrix metabolism in diabetic nephropathy. *J Am Soc Nephrol* 2003;**14**:1358–73.

7. Steffes MW, Osterby R, Chavers B, Mauer SM. Mesangial expansion as a central mechanism for loss of kidney function in diabetic patients. *Diabetes* 1989;**38**:1077–81.

8. Mauer SM, Steffes MW, Ellis EN, *et al.* Structural-functional relationships in diabetic nephropathy. *J Clin Invest* 1984; **74**:1143–55.

9. Osterby R, Tapia J, Nyberg G, *et al.* Renal structures in type 2 diabetic patients with elevated albumin excretion rate. *APMIS* 2001;**109**:751–61.

10. Osterby R, Hartmann A, Nyengaard JR, Bangstad HJ. Development of renal structural lesions in type-1 diabetic patients with microalbuminuria. Observations by light microscopy in 8-year follow-up biopsies. *Virchows Arch* 2002;**440**:94–101.

11. Gerth J, Cohen CD, Hopfer U, *et al.* Collagen type VIII expression in human diabetic nephropathy. *Eur J Clin Invest* 2007;**37**:767–73.

12. Shumway JT, Gambert SR. Diabetic nephropathy-pathophysiology and management. *Int Urol Nephrol* 2002; **34**:257–64.

13. Karalliedde J, Viberti G. Proteinuria in diabetes: bystander or pathway to cardiorenal disease? *J Am Soc Nephrol* 2010;**21**:2020–7.

14. Wolf G, Ziyadeh FN. Cellular and molecular mechanisms of proteinuria in diabetic nephropathy. *Nephron Physiol* 2007;**106**:26–31.

15. Hostetter TH. Hyperfiltration and glomerulosclerosis. *Semin Nephrol* 2003; **23**:194–9.

16. Gruden G, Perin PC, Camussi G. Insight on the pathogenesis of diabetic nephropathy from the study of podocyte and mesangial cell biology. *Curr Diabetes Rev* 2005;**1**:27–40.

17. Shigeta Y, Kikkawa R. A role of mesangial dysfunction in the development of diabetic nephropathy. *Jpn J Med* 1991;**30**: 622–4.

18. Fogo AB. Mesangial matrix modulation and glomerulosclerosis. *Exp Nephrol* 1999;**7**:147–59.

19. Ziyadeh FN, Wolf G. Pathogenesis of the podocytopathy and proteinuria in diabetic glomerulopathy. *Curr Diabetes Rev* 2008;**4**:39–45.

20. Diez-Sampedro A, Lenz O, Fornoni A. Podocytopathy in diabetes: a metabolic and endocrine disorder. *Am J Kidney Dis* 2011;**58**:637–46.

21. Wolf G, Chen S, Ziyadeh FN. From the periphery of the glomerular capillary wall toward the center of disease: podocyte injury comes of age in diabetic nephropathy. *Diabetes* 2005;**54**: 1626–34.

22. Russo LM, Sandoval RM, McKee M, *et al.* The normal kidney filters nephrotic levels of albumin retrieved by proximal tubule cells: retrieval is disrupted in nephrotic states. *Kidney Int* 2007;**71**:504–13.

23. Phillips AO, Steadman R. Diabetic nephropathy: the central role of renal proximal tubular cells in tubulointerstitial injury. *Histol Histopathol* 2002;**17**:247–52.

24. Wolf G, Ziyadeh FN. Molecular mechanisms of diabetic renal hypertrophy. *Kidney Int* 1999;**56**:393–405.

25. Balakumar P, Chakkarwar VA, Krishan P, Singh M. Vascular endothelial dysfunction: a tug of war in diabetic nephropathy? *Biomed Pharmacother* 2009; **63**:171–9.

26. Rüger BM, Hasan Q, Greenhill NS, *et al.* Mast cells and type VIII collagen in

human diabetic nephropathy. *Diabetologia* 1996;**39**:1215–22.

27. Forbes JM, Cooper ME, Oldfield MD, Thomas MC. Role of advanced glycation end products in diabetic nephropathy. *J Am Soc Nephrol* 2003;**14**:S254–8.

28. Locatelli F, Canaud B, Eckardt KU, *et al.* The importance of diabetic nephropathy in current nephrological practice. *Nephrol Dial Transplant* 2003 ;**18**:1716–25.

29. D'Agati V, Yan SF, Ramasamy R, Schmidt AM. RAGE, glomerulosclerosis and proteinuria: roles in podocytes and endothelial cells. *Trends Endocrinol Metab* 2010;**21**:50–6.

30. Wendt TM, Tanji N, Guo J, *et al.* RAGE drives the development of glomerulosclerosis and implicates podocyte activation in the pathogenesis of diabetic nephropathy. *Am J Pathol* 2003;**162**:1123–37.

31. Daroux M, Prévost G, Maillard-Lefebvre H, *et al.* Advanced glycation end-products: implications for diabetic and non-diabetic nephropathies. *Diabetes Metab* 2010;**36**:1–10.

32. Yamamoto T, *et al.* Expression of transforming growth factor beta is elevated in human and experimental diabetic nephropathy. *Proc Natl Acad Sci U S A* 1993;**90**:1814–8.

33. Ziyadeh FN, Nakamura T, Noble NA, *et al.* Involvement of transforming growth factor-beta and its receptors in the pathogenesis of diabetic nephrology. *Kidney Int Suppl* 1997;**60**:S7–11.

34. Böttinger EP, Bitzer M. TGF-beta signaling in renal disease. *J Am Soc Nephrol* 2002;**13**:2600–10.

35. Bradham DM, Igarashi A, Potter RL, Grotendorst GR. Connective tissue growth factor: a cysteine-rich mitogen secreted by human vascular endothelial cells is related to the SRC-induced

immediate early gene product CEF-10. *J Cell Biol* 1991;**114**:1285–94.

36. Igarashi A, Okochi H, Bradham DM, Grotendorst GR. Regulation of connective tissue growth factor gene expression in human skin fibroblasts and during wound repair. *Mol Biol Cell* 1993;**4**:637–45.

37. Okada H, Kikuta T, Kobayashi T, *et al.* Connective tissue growth factor expressed in tubular epithelium plays a pivotal role in renal fibrogenesis. *J Am Soc Nephrol* 2005;**16**:133–43.

38. Duncan MR, Frazier KS, Abramson S, *et al.* Connective tissue growth factor mediates transforming growth factor beta-induced collagen synthesis: down-regulation by cAMP. *FASEB J* 1999;**13**: 1774–86.

39. Phillips A, Janssen U, Floege J. Progression of diabetic nephropathy. Insights from cell culture studies and animal models. *Kidney Blood Press Res* 1999;**22**:81–97.

40. Liu Y. Hepatocyte growth factor and the kidney. *Curr Opin Nephrol Hypertens* 2002;**11**:23–30.

41. Zhang Y, Zhang Q. Bone morphogenetic protein-7 and Gremlin: New emerging therapeutic targets for diabetic nephropathy. *Biochem Biophys Res Commun* 383;2009:1–3.

42. Wang SN, Lapage J, Hirschberg R. Loss of tubular bone morphogenetic protein 7 in diabetic nephropathy. *J Am Soc Nephrol* 2001;**12**:2392–99.

43. De Petris L, Hruska KA, Chiechio S, Liapis H. Bone morphogenetic protein-7 delays podocyte injury due to high glucose. *Nephrol Dial Transplant* 2007;**22**:3442–50.

44. Zeisberg M, Hanai J, Sugimoto H, *et al.* BMP-7 counteracts TGF-beta1-induced epithelial-to-mesenchymal transition and reverses chronic renal injury. *Nat Med* 2003;**9**:964–8.

45. Xu Y, Wan J, Jiang D, Wu X. BMP-7 counteracts TGF-beta1-induced epithelial-to-mesenchymal transition in human renal proximal tubular epithelial cells. *J Nephrol* 2009;**22**:403–10.

46. Nguyen TQ, Roestenberg P, van Nieuwenhoven FA, *et al.* CTGF inhibits BMP-7 signaling in diabetic nephropathy. *J Am Soc Nephrol* 2008;**19**:2098–2107.

47. Lam S, van der Geest RN, Verhagen NA, *et al.* Connective tissue growth factor and IGF-I are produced by human renal fibroblasts and cooperate in the induction of collagen production by high glucose. *Diabetes* 2003;**52**:2975–83.

48. Vasylyeva TL, Ferry RJ Jr.Novel roles of the IGF-IGFBP axis in etiopathophysiology of diabetic nephropathy. *Diabetes Res Clin Pract* 2007;**76**:177–86.

49. Schrijvers BF, Flyvbjerg A, De Vriese AS. The role of vascular endothelial growth factor (VEGF) in renal pathophysiology. *Kidney Int* 2004;**65**:2003–17.

50. Komers R, Anderson S. Paradoxes of nitric oxide in the diabetic kidney. *Am J Physiol Renal Physiol* 2003;**284**:F1121–37.

51. Eddy AA. Molecular basis of renal fibrosis. *Pediatr Nephrol* 2000;**15**:290–301.

52. Essawy M, Soylemezoglu O, Muchaneta-Kubara EC, *et al.* Myofibroblasts and the progression of diabetic nephropathy. *Nephrol Dial Transplant* 1997;**12**:43–50.

53. Zeisberg M, Kalluri R. The role of epithelial-to-mesenchymal transition in renal fibrosis. *J Mol Med* 2004;**82**:175–82.

54. Meran S, Steadman R. Fibroblasts and myofibroblasts in renal fibrosis. *Int J Exp Path* 2011;**92**:158–67.

55. Strutz F, da H, Lo CW, *et al.* Identification and characterization of a fibroblast marker: FSP1. *J Cell Biol* 1995;**130**:393–405.

56. Iwano M, Plieth D, Danoff TM, *et al.* Evidence that fibroblasts derive from epithelium during tissue fibrosis. *J Clin Invest* 2002;**110**:341–50.

57. Yang J, Liu, Y. Dissection of key events in tubular epithelial to myofibroblast transition and its implications in renal interstitial fibrosis. *Am J Pathol* 2001; **159**:1465–75.

58. Liu Y. Epithelial to mesenchymal transition in renal fibrogenesis: pathologic significance, molecular mechanism, and therapeutic intervention. *J Am Soc Nephrol* 2004; **15**:1–12.

59. Hills CE, Squires PE. TGF-β1-induced epithelial-to-mesenchymal transition and therapeutic intervention in diabetic nephropathy. *Am J Nephrol* 2010;**31**: 68–74.

60. Sharma K, Ziyadeh FN. The emerging role of transforming growth factor-beta in kidney diseases. *Am J Physiol* 1994; **266**:F829–42.

61. Iwano M, Neilson EG. Mechanisms of tubulointerstitial fibrosis. *Curr Opin Nephrol Hypertens* 2004;**13**:279–84.

62. Burns WC, Twigg SM, Forbes JM, *et al.* Connective tissue growth factor plays an important role in advanced glycation end product-induced tubular epithelial-to-mesenchymal transition: implications for diabetic renal disease. *J Am Soc Nephrol* 2006;**17**:2484–94.

63. Zeisberg EM, Potenta SE, Sugimoto H, *et al.* Fibroblasts in kidney fibrosis emerge via endothelial-to-mesenchymal transition. *J Am Soc Nephrol* 2008;**19**: 2282–7.

64. Li J, Qu X, Bertram JF. Endothelial-myofibroblast transition contributes to the early development of diabetic renal interstitial fibrosis in streptozotocin-induced diabetic mice. *Am J Pathol* 2009; **175**:1380–8.

65. Kizu A, Medici D, Kalluri R. Endothelial-mesenchymal transition as a novel

mechanism for generating myofibroblasts during diabetic nephropathy. *Am J Pathol* 2009;**175**:1371–3.

66. Barnes JL, Gorin Y. Myofibroblast differentiation during fibrosis: role of NAD(P)H oxidases. *Kidney Int* 2011; **79**:944–56.

67. Singh DK, Winocour P, Farrington K. Mechanisms of disease: the hypoxic tubular hypothesis of diabetic nephropathy. *Nat Clin Pract Nephrol* 2008;**4**:216–26.

68. Nangaku M. Chronic hypoxia and tubulointerstitial injury: a final common pathway to end-stage renal failure. *J Am Soc Nephrol* 2006;**17**:17–25.

69. Navarro-González JF, Mora-Fernández C, Muros de Fuentes M, García-Pérez J. Inflammatory molecules and pathways in the pathogenesis of diabetic nephropathy. *Nat Rev Nephrol* 2011;**7**:327–40.

70. Brosius FC 3rd, Alpers CE, Bottinger EP, *et al*. Mouse models of diabetic nephropathy. *J Am Soc Nephrol* 2009; **20**:2503–12.

71. Alpers CE, Hudkins KL. Mouse models of diabetic nephropathy. *Curr Opin Nephrol Hypertens* 2011;**20**:278–84.

Chapter 5

Histology of human diabetic nephropathy

Kerstin Amann and Christoph Daniel

Universität Erlangen-Nürnberg, Erlangen, Germany

Key points

- Diabetic nephropathy is the leading cause of end-stage renal failure in adults.
- Diabetic nephropathy shows a typical clinical course of proteinuria and a spectrum of characteristic morphologic alterations of the glomeruli, the tubulointerstitium and the renal vasculature.
- Ultrastructurally, even in the very early stages of diabetic nephropathy a marked thickening of the glomerular basement membrane can be observed.
- Advanced diabetic nephropathy is histologically characterized by nodular glomerulsclerosis, so-called Kimmelstiel–Wilson glomerulosclerosis, progressive tubular atrophy, interstitial fibrosis, and arteriolar hyalinosis.
- The increased knowledge about the morphology of diabetic nephropathy is reflected by the recent

proposal for a new classification of diabetic nephropathy.
- The most important differential diagnoses of diabetic nephropathy are diseases that are also associated with marked proteinuria, i.e., amyloidosis, light-chain deposition disease and membranoproliferative glomerulonephritis.
- Rarely, in addition to pre-existing diabetic nephropathy, other glomerular diseases may be present, i.e., immunecomplex glomerulonephritis or renal involvement in systemic disease like vasculitis.
- Whenever the clinical course of diabetic nephropathy is atypical or changes rapidly, a kidney biopsy is strongly recommended to rule out other concurrent disease that would require different therapeutic options.

Involvement of the kidney, i.e., diabetic nephropathy, is a major complication of diabetes mellitus and certainly one of the most devastating [1]. Renal dysfunction develops in about one-third of patients with diabetes, yielding an estimated number of about 150 million patients worldwide, with the number increasing to 300 million in the year 2025 [2]. Renal involvement in the two major types of diabetes

---

Diabetes and Kidney Disease, First Edition. Edited by Gunter Wolf.
© 2013 John Wiley & Sons, Ltd. Published 2013 by John Wiley & Sons, Ltd.

mellitus, i.e., type 1 or insulin-dependent diabetes mellitus (IDDM), and type 2, or non-insulin dependent diabetes mellitus (NIDDM), is morphologically similar, but occurs with different incidence and follows a different time course. About 15–20% of type 1 diabetic patients and 30–40% of type 2 diabetic patients will eventually develop end-stage renal failure. The natural history of diabetic nephropathy is characterized by five stages. Stages 1 and 2, i.e., the prediabetic stages, are characterized by renal hypertrophy and hyperfiltration. Stage 3, i.e., incipient diabetic nephropathy, is functionally characterized by microalbuminuria, defined as >30 mg but <300 mg of albumin in the urine per day, and hypertension. On the morphologic level, glomerular basement thickening, mesangial matrix expansion, and arteriolar hyalinosis can be observed (Plate 5.1). In stage 4, i.e., overt diabetic nephropathy, proteinuria and/or nephrotic syndrome are paralleled by a decrease in glomerular filtration rate (GFR), which further declines when end-stage renal disease (stage 5) is reached. Histologically, advanced diabetic nephropathy is characterized by nodular glomerulosclerosis, so-called Kimmelstiel–Wilson glomerulosclerosis, and progressive tubular atrophy and interstitial fibrosis (Box 5.1, Plate 5.1a–c) [3, 4].

Long-known risk factors for diabetic nephropathy are hypertension, hyperglycemia, dyslipidemia, obesity, and genetic factors [5]. Clinical trials have shown that strict control of hyperglycemia and hypertension can slow the progression of diabetic nephropathy and that insulin resistance correlates with the onset and severity of albuminuria. Moreover, there is recent evidence that altered insulin signaling in glomerular cells and particularly podocytes may contribute to the development of diabetic nephropathy [6]. Microalbuminuria, which is the initial clinical indicator of diabetic nephropathy, reflects a functional and potentially reversible abnormality initiated by glomerular hyperfiltration. Microalbuminuria induces a specific genetic program in tubular epithelial cells, which orchestrate tubular atrophy, interstitial inflammation, and fibrosis.

Renal morphologic changes in diabetes mellitus are summarized under diabetic nephropathy(DN), which represents a combination of characteristic glomerular, tubulointerstitial, and vascular changes. In parallel to the varying clinical course of renal involvement in diabetes mellitus with microalbuminuria, proteinuria, and renal failure the histologic alterations are also very variable. DN usually starts with subtle thickening of the glomerular basement membrane, which can only be seen on electron microscopy, and progresses to so-called nodular diabetic glomerulosclerosis (Kimmelstil–Wilson type) that ends up with

---

Characteristic light microscopy and electron microscopy alterations in the course of diabetic nephropathy

Light microscopy

Diffuse or nodular expansion of mesangial matrix with formation of diffuse or nodular type glomerulosclerosis (Kimmelstiel–Wilson)

Intima thickening and hyalinosis if arteries and arterioles

Tubular atrophy and interstitial fibrosis

Changes have similar prognostic significance

Electron microscopy

Thickening of GBM and TBM

Glomerular enlargement (hypertrophy of glomeruli)

Podocyte damage leading to loss of podocytes

complete glomerular obliteration and further sclerosis of the kidney. Often there is not a good correlation between the clinical and the morphologic appearance of the disease.

Full-blown DN can usually be expected after 10–15 years of diabetes mellitus. Diabetic patients who present with such a history and typical clinical symptoms usually do not undergo a kidney biopsy. However, indications for a kidney biopsy in the setting of suspected DN are (1) onset of proteinuria <5 years of diabetes mellitus, (2) acute onset/progressive course of DN, (3) nephritic urine sediment with erythrocytes and cylinders, and (4) renal symptoms in the absence of diabetic retinopathy in type I diabetes mellitus. Of note, DN can recur in the transplanted kidney or can occur *de novo*, usually presenting with a much more progressive course of the disease [7].

Morphology and pathogenesis of characteristic histologic alterations of the kidney in diabetic nephropathy

Macroscopically, the earliest visible alteration is a bilateral increase in kidney size that can be seen on ultrasound and that is due to a combination of hyperfiltration and structural adaptation (Box 5.1). The kidney structure on ultrasound, however, is not yet altered at that point in time. Ultrastructurally, even in very early stages a marked thickening of the glomerular basement membrane (GBM) can be observed [3, 4].

On *light microscopy* the following characteristic changes can be seen occurring as early, on average, as 2 years after the onset of diabetes mellitus and comprise glomerular, tubulointerstitial, and vascular alterations (Plate 5.1a–c).

1. *Glomeruli*: Glomeruli show various structural alterations that can present in variable combinations: glomerular enlargement (so-called glomerular hypertrophy) and thickening of GBM, both typical of nodular glomeruloscle-

rosis (Kimmelstiel–Wilson sclerosis), and a more diffuse increase in the mesangial matrix with variable degrees of sclerosis (Plate 5.1b,c,e). Other characteristic findings are so-called hyalin lesions or fibrin caps and the so-called capsular drops. These findings represent different underlying pathomechanisms, i.e., thickening of the GBM is due to basement membrane modifications by glycation or deposition of advanced glycation end products (AGEs) whereas the increase in mesangial matrix production is due to stimulation of mesangial cells by hyperglycemia [8]. The characteristic Kimmelstiel–Wilson noduli that often show a lammellated structure and contain fragments of erythrocytes may derive from microaneurysms of glomerular capillaries or from mesangiolysis, i.e., dissolution of the mesangium due to hydrostatic or metabolic damage [9–11].

For a long time pathophysiologic changes in mesangial cells have been considered as the heart of diabetic kidney disease, but recent evidence implicates the podocyte as an important player in the development and progression of DN. Podocytes are terminally differentiated epithelial cells and are critically important for the integrity of the GBM. During DN, different histopathologic changes on podocytes can be observed, ranging from ultrastructural changes to the loss of podocytes.

Podocyte loss occurs by apoptosis [12–14] or detachment [15] and was found to be the strongest predictor for disease progression [16]. In particular, the significant loss of podocytes in early DN may explain the onset of microalbuminuria [17]. Detached podocytes could be detected in the urine of 53% Japanese type 2 diabetic patients with microalbuminuria and in 80% with macroalbuminuria [18]. Apoptosis of podocytes is induced by a variety of mechanisms, including formation of AGEs and the production of reactive oxygen species (ROS). Glucose can also effect podocyte survival by inducing the renin–angiotensin system (RAS) leading to increased angiotensin II (Ang II) levels and induction of proapoptotic transforming growth factor (TGF)-β. In addition, Ang II increases ROS production by activation of NADPH oxidase and stimulates receptor advanced glycation end products (RAGE) expression via its AT2 receptors [19]. The interaction of AGEs with its receptor, RAGE, mediates podocyte apoptosis by alteration of forkhead box O (Foxo4) acetylation, as shown in a recent study [12]. Consequently, podocyte loss could be prevented in experimental DN by treatment with angiotensin-converting enzyme (ACE) inhibitors [20]. Podocyte damage is not only due to high glucose levels but also due to reduced insulin concentrations, insulin resistance, or changes in insulin sensitizing agents like adiponectin and leptin [21]. However, not all detached podocytes must necessarily undergo apoptosis. Alterations of the podocyte cytoskeleton and anchoring within the GBM are suggested mechanisms leading to podocyte loss during DN. Diabetic conditions, for example, modulate expression of integrins and decrease binding of podocytes to the GBM [19]. Nephrin, the key component of the slit diaphragm, is crucial for maintaining the integrity of the glomerular filtration barrier but also regulates the actin cytoskeleton of the podocyte. In a study by Doublier *et al.* [22] nephrin immunostaining was extensively reduced in renal biopsies from patients with DN. In addition, protein kinase C-α, which is upregulated in podocytes in DN, also mediates endocytosis of nephrin from the slit membrane [23].

2. *Tubulointerstitium*: The tubuli and the renal interstitium in DN can also show variable lesions, which for a long time were attributed to glomerular injury although they do not correlate well with the degree of glomerular alterations. Recent studies provided evidence for early tubular apoptosis and atrophy as separate pathomechanisms in DN [24, 25]. In addition, marked uniformly thickening of non-atrophic tubules can be regarded as a typical, but not

100% specific, sign of DN (Plate 5.1a). In advanced DN there is usually a combination of advanced tubular atrophy, interstitial fibrosis and a variable degree of concomitant interstitial inflammation. The latter may comprise lymphocytes, plasma cells, and neutrophilic and eosinophilic granulocytes, making the distinction from interstitial nephritis sometimes difficult. Rarely, marked vacuolization of tubular epithelial cells, i.e., Armanni–Ebstein cells, can be seen. A study in patients with DN who had undergone pancreas transplantation documented that advanced tubulointerstitial damage, like tubular atrophy and interstitial fibrosis, is partly reversible over a long period of time (5–10 years) if the underlying stimulus, i.e., hyperglycemia, had been stopped [26]. This has not been shown, however, for the accompanying vascular changes.

3. *Renal vasculature*: In the kidney diabetic macro- and microangiopathy can also be seen: Most characteristic for DN is a combination of arteriolar hyalinosis of the vasa afferentia and efferentia with the above-mentioned glomerular changes, i.e., nodular glomerulosclerosis (Plate 5.1c, arrow). It is important to know that in some patients vascular changes can precede glomerular alterations.

The increased knowledge about the morphology of DN is reflected by the recent proposal for classification of diabetic nephropathy (Box 5.2, Plate 5.2) that takes into account most of the above-mentioned changes, bringing them into an easy to handle scoring system and algorithm for daily routine [27]. Here, the morphologic picture is used for categorization of the lesions into I (Plate 5.2a), IIa and IIb (Plate 5.2b,c), III (Plate 5.2d,e), and IV (Plate 5.2f). Also, the interstitial and vascular changes can be scored semiquantitatively (0–2). This new classification proposal is currently being analyzed for interobserver variation and its prognostic value.

Additional investigations using *immunhistology* on paraffin sections or *immunofluorescence*

Box 5.2 **Classes of diabetic nephropathy**

I   Mild or non-specific light microscopic changes and thickening of the GBM on electron microscopy (females: >395 nm; males: >430 nm, older than 9 years of age)
IIa Mild mesangial expansion
IIb Severe mesangial expansion
III Nodular sclerosis (Kimmelstiel–Wilson lesion)
IV   Advanced diabetic glomerulosclerosis

According to Tervaert TW, Mooyaart AL, Amann K, Cohen AH, Cook HT, Drachenberg CB, Ferrario F, Fogo AB, Haas M, de Heer E, Joh K, Noel LH, Radhakrishnan J, Seshan SV, Bajema IM, Bruijn JA: Pathologic classification of diabetic nephropathy. *J Am Soc Nephrol* 2010;**21**:556–63.

---

on frozen sections are important to rule out concurrent renal and in particular glomerular disease (see below). Moreover, in DN one can see the more or less typical pseudolinear staining for immunoglobulin (Ig)G (rarely also for IgM and C3c) of the thickened GBM that has to be distinguished from the very similar linear staining pattern in anti-GBM glomerulonephritis (GN) and the more granular pseudolinear staining pattern in membranous GN (Plate 5.1D). Here, it can be of some help that in DN similar staining can also be seen in thickened tubular basement membranes. In advanced glomerulosclerosis, unspecific trapping of IgG, IgM, and C3c can be seen in the mesangium.

Electron microscopy (EM) is routinely performed on most native kidney biopsies. In DN, the presence and degree of thickening of the GBM and of podocyte damage with increased size, marked vacuolization of the cytoplasm, and effacement or loss of foot processes can be visualized by EM (Plate 5.1f). Here, an up to 10-fold increase in normal GBM thickness can occur together with splicing and crinkling of the GBM. At the onset of DN, when microalbuminuria can be detected in patients, the first structural changes were found in podocytes. These early changes include widening of podocyte foot processes and increased width of filtration slits in podocytes from patients with DN [28]. Such structural changes could be reported in histomorphometric studies investi-

gating both NIDDM [29] and IDDM [28] patients. The width of the foot processes in DN patients is increased about 20–40% compared with healthy controls [28, 29]. Interestingly, the width of filtration slits also changes during development of DN. The width is still increased in DN patients before onset of microalbuminuria and persists in DN patients with microalbuminuria compared with non-diabetic control subjects. In contrast, in diabetic patients with proteinuria, the width of filtration slits were similar to normal control subjects. Of note, the width of the filtration slits positively correlate with the GFR [28].

Years ago, EM investigations had already made major contributions to understanding the pathophysiology and sequence of alterations in DN [3, 4]. Quantitative ultrastructural methods were also instrumental for a study where regression of existing glomerulosclerosis and interstitial fibrosis was documented for 10 years and the diabetic milieu was corrected by pancreas transplantation [30].

The three most important morphologic differential diagnoses of DN are those diseases that can occur histologically with a diffuse or nodular glomerulosclerosis that looks similar to that in DN:

- amyloidosis (Congo +)
- light-chain deposition disease (LCDD; with deposition of kappa/lambda light chains)
- membranoproliferative GN (MPGN; immuno-histology, immunofluorescence).

Here, additional stains like the Congo red stain are most helpful to either confirm or rule out amyloidosis.

Clinically, differential diagnoses that morphologically can usually be easily distinguished from DN are

- minimal change glomerulonephritis (MCGN)
- focal segmental glomerulosclerosis (FSGS)
- membranous GN/MPGN
- hypertensive GN
- ischemic nephropathy.

In addition to the above-mentioned alterations in DN, patients with diabetes mellitus may present additional renal diseases such as minimal change GN, IgA-GN or if there is an acute onset of disease also crescentic GN as in vasculitis. Moreover, the kidney in patients with DN can also be involved in systemic diseases such as, for example, cast nephropathy in multiple myeloma. Of note, in up to 20% of diabetic patients, glomerular diseases such as membranous GN or postinfectious GN or interstitial diseases such as interstitial nephritis can occur even in the absence of any sign of DN. It depends on the symptoms and clinical judgment whether patients with diabetes mellitus undergo kidney biopsy to confirm DN or another concurrent renal disease.

The typical morphologic spectrum of diabetic nephropathy, i.e., glomerular, vascular, and tubulointerstitial alterations, usually develops after 10–15 years of clinically apparent diabetes mellitus. In exceptional cases, renal disease may start earlier, i.e., after 3–5 years of diabetic disease. Patients with existing diabetic nephropathy are not safe from other renal diseases, in particular immunecomplex glomerulonephritides, and renal involvement in systemic diseases like vasculitis may occur. If this is clinically suspected or the course of diabetic nephropathy rapidly changes, a kidney biopsy is necessary to make a final diagnosis which in most cases requires additional therapeutic options than pure diabetic nephropathy.

1. Groop PH, Thomas MC, Moran JL, *et al*. The presence and severity of chronic kidney disease predicts all-cause mortality in type 1 diabetes. *Diabetes* 2009;**58**: 1651–8.

2. Tang SC. Diabetic nephropathy: A global and growing threat. *Hong Kong Med J* 2010;**16**:244–245.

3. Osterby R, Hartmann A, Nyengaard JR, Bangstad HJ. Development of renal structural lesions in type-1 diabetic patients with microalbuminuria. Observations by light microscopy in 8-year follow-up biopsies. *Virchows Arch* 2002;**440**:94–101.

4. Osterby R, Tapia J, Nyberg G, *et al*. Renal structures in type 2 diabetic patients with elevated albumin excretion rate. *APMIS* 2001;**109**:751–1.

5. Dronavalli S, Duka I, Bakris GL. The pathogenesis of diabetic nephropathy. *Nat Clin Pract Endocrinol Metab* 2008; **4**:444–52.

6. Jauregui A, Mintz DH, Mundel P, Fornoni A. Role of altered insulin signaling pathways in the pathogenesis of podocyte malfunction and microalbuminuria. *Curr Opin Nephrol Hypertens* 2009;**18**:539–45.

7. Bhalla V, Nast CC, Stollenwerk N, *et al*. Recurrent and de novo diabetic

nephropathy in renal allografts. *Transplantation* 2003;**75**:66–71.

8. Lin S, Sahai A, Chugh SS, *et al.* High glucose stimulates synthesis of fibronectin via a novel protein kinase c, rap1b, and b-raf signaling pathway. *J Biol Chem* 2002;**277**:41725–41735.

9. Najafian B, Alpers CE, Fogo AB. Pathology of human diabetic nephropathy. *Contrib Nephrol* 2011;**170**:36–47.

10. Saito Y, Kida H, Takeda S, *et al.* Mesangiolysis in diabetic glomeruli: Its role in the formation of nodular lesions. *Kidney Int* 1988;**34**:389–96.

11. Stout LC, Kumar S, Whorton EB. Focal mesangiolysis and the pathogenesis of the Kimmelstiel-Wilson nodule. *Hum Pathol* 1993;**24**:77–89.

12. Chuang PY, Dai Y, Liu R, *et al.* Alteration of forkhead box o (foxo4) acetylation mediates apoptosis of podocytes in diabetes mellitus. *PLoS One* 2011;**6**: e23566.

13. Isermann B, Vinnikov IA, Madhusudhan T, *et al.* Activated protein c protects against diabetic nephropathy by inhibiting endothelial and podocyte apoptosis. *Nat Med* 2007;**13**:1349–58.

14. Susztak K, Raff AC, Schiffer M, Bottinger EP. Glucose-induced reactive oxygen species cause apoptosis of podocytes and podocyte depletion at the onset of diabetic nephropathy. *Diabetes* 2006;**55**:225–33.

15. Wolf G, Chen S, Ziyadeh FN. From the periphery of the glomerular capillary wall toward the center of disease: Podocyte injury comes of age in diabetic nephropathy. *Diabetes* 2005;**54**:1626–34.

16. Meyer TW, Bennett PH, Nelson RG. Podocyte number predicts long-term urinary albumin excretion in Pima Indians with type ii diabetes and microalbuminuria. *Diabetologia* 1999;**42**:1341–4.

17. Pagtalunan ME, Miller PL, Jumping-Eagle S, *et al.* Podocyte loss and progressive glomerular injury in type ii diabetes. *J Clin Invest* 1997;**99**:342–8.

18. Nakamura T, Ushiyama C, Suzuki S, *et al.* The urinary podocyte as a marker for the differential diagnosis of idiopathic focal glomerulosclerosis and minimal-change nephrotic syndrome. *Am J Nephrol* 2000; **20**:175–9.

19. Lewko B, Stepinski J. Hyperglycemia and mechanical stress: targeting the renal podocyte. *J Cell Physiol* 2009;**221**:288–95.

20. Gross ML, El-Shakmak A, Szabo A, *et al.* Ace-inhibitors but not endothelin receptor blockers prevent podocyte loss in early diabetic nephropathy. *Diabetologia* 2003;**46**:856–68.

21. Welsh GI, Coward RJ. Podocytes, glucose and insulin. *Curr Opin Nephrol Hypertens* 2010;**19**:379–84.

22. Doublier S, Salvidio G, Lupia E, *et al.* Nephrin expression is reduced in human diabetic nephropathy: Evidence for a distinct role for glycated albumin and angiotensin ii. *Diabetes* 2003;**52**: 1023–30.

23. Tossidou I, Teng B, Menne J, *et al.* Podocytic pkc-alpha is regulated in murine and human diabetes and mediates nephrin endocytosis. *PLoS One* 2010;**5**:e10185.

24. Brezniceanu ML, Liu F, Wei CC, *et al.* Catalase overexpression attenuates angiotensinogen expression and apoptosis in diabetic mice. *Kidney Int* 2007;**71**:912–23.

25. Bagby SP. Diabetic nephropathy and proximal tubule ROS: Challenging our glomerulocentricity. *Kidney Int* 2007;**71**: 1199–202.

26. Fioretto P, Sutherland DE, Najafian B, Mauer M. Remodeling of renal interstitial and tubular lesions in pancreas transplant recipients. *Kidney Int* 2006;**69**:907–12.

27. Tervaert TW, Mooyaart AL, Amann K, *et al*. Pathologic classification of diabetic nephropathy. *J Am Soc Nephrol* 2010;**21**: 556–63.

28. Bjorn SF, Bangstad HJ, Hanssen KF, *et al*. Glomerular epithelial foot processes and filtration slits in IDDM patients. *Diabetologia* 1995;**38**: 1197–204.

29. White KE, Bilous RW. Structural alterations to the podocyte are related to proteinuria in type 2 diabetic patients. *Nephrol Dial Transplant* 2004;**19**:1437–40.

30. Fioretto P, Steffes MW, Sutherland DE, *et al*. Reversal of lesions of diabetic nephropathy after pancreas transplantation. *N Engl J Med* 1998;**339**: 69–75.

Chapter 6

Natural history and diagnosis of diabetic kidney disease

Bethany Karl and Kumar Sharma

University of California San Diego, La Jolla, CA, USA

Key points

- Diabetic kidney disease encompasses diabetic nephropathy, incipient nephropathy, and diabetic glomerulopathy.
- Type 1 diabetic patients who develop persistent microalbuminuria are at high risk of progression to overt nephropathy and renal failure.
- Type 2 diabetic patients with nephropathy progress to renal failure at a similar rate to type 1 diabetic patients

- Early screening for diabetic kidney disease includes measuring the albumin–creatinine ratio and assessing renal function either with serum creatinine or the glomerular filtration rate.
- Diabetic kidney disease is a complex interplay between genetic, metabolic, and hemodynamic factors.

Patients with diabetes continue to lead the population of those requiring renal replacement therapy and renal transplantation. Diabetic kidney disease, formerly referred to as diabetic nephropathy, has shown to be a complex interplay between genetic, metabolic and hemodynamic factors [1]. Much of the prior work has focused on the hemodynamic and genetic components leading to renal dysfunction, with little attention paid to the metabolic effects of diabetes on the kidney. This chapter will present the currently accepted natural history and diagnosis of diabetic kidney disease, including investigations based on metabolic understandings that could provide future insight into discoveries.

The diagnosis of diabetic nephropathy has historically been clinical, based on the

---

Diabetes and Kidney Disease, First Edition. Edited by Gunter Wolf.

presence of overt proteinuria; however, studies reveal a more heterogeneous state of diabetic kidney disease leading to a change in terminology [2]. It was once thought that if a patient with longstanding diabetes had associated kidney disease without overt proteinuria, the cause was not diabetes. It has since been shown that this clinical scenario could very well be a variant form of diabetic kidney disease. Biopsy-proven diabetic glomerulopathy exists in diabetic patients with incipient nephropathy, a term that represents those with evidence of microalbuminuria; and in some without any trace of proteinuria [2, 3]. Brocco *et al.* [4] performed kidney biopsies on type 2 diabetics with microalbuminuria and concluded that only one-third of patients had "typical" diabetic glomerulopathy. The other two-thirds showed a spectrum from near-normal structure to severe tubulointerstitial lesions and arterial hyalinosis. Studies have also challenged the current definition of a diabetic patient, as diabetic kidney disease has been seen in prediabetics. Mac-Moune *et al.* [5] showed glomerular basement membrane thickening in patients with metabolic syndrome and proteinuria up to 2 years prior to their formal diagnosis of diabetes. In this same patient population, Sucurro *et al.* [6] found decreased glomerular filtration rates prior to overt diabetes.

Therefore, it has been shown that the broad definition of diabetic kidney disease has come to represent a characteristic set of structural and functional kidney abnormalities in patients with impaired glucose handling and overt diabetes [7]. Diabetic kidney disease can encompass the compilation of pathologic changes seen in many parts of the kidney, including the glomerulus, the tubules, the interstitial compartment, and vasculature [4]. It is imperative for clinicians to be familiar with the natural course of diabetic kidney disease and diagnostic tools, as currently understood, complete with their limitations. Through this understanding, clinicians will be better prepared to evaluate, diagnosis and treat their patients accordingly.

The natural history of a disease is defined as the course of disease if it is not treated or manipulated in any way. Clinical observation of the natural history of diabetic kidney disease in humans, both in type 1 and type 2 diabetics, is often confounded as patients are started on forms of therapy to control glucose, hypertension, and proteinuria. Thus, historical studies are referred to for large cohorts that develop diabetic complications with diabetes. However, the historical experience is limited as most patients are treated in one form or another for diabetes, hypertension, and abnormal lipid profiles or even with low-dose aspirin or vitamins. Therefore, it is worth evaluating what is the natural history of diabetic kidney disease with common therapies. Surprisingly, at least in many cohorts of well-characterized patients, there does not appear to be a substantial abatement of progressive kidney disease in patients with type 1 diabetes.

The pediatric literature has long reported on the natural history diabetic kidney disease seen in type 1 diabetic patients. Of note, the data are primarily from before the use of renin–angiotensin system blockade, which is likely to affect the course of disease. At onset of diagnosis patients may present with hyperfiltration. As their baseline glomerular filtration rate (GFR) is now higher, any decline in kidney function may be viewed as a normalization of kidney function with control of diabetes versus a progressive decline in kidney function leading to complications. Typically, onset of diabetic nephropathy is considered when microalbuminuria is persistent within 7–10 years of diagnosis [8, 9]. Patients with persistent micro-albuminuria have associated increased risk of progression to overt proteinuria and renal failure [10]. Approximately 80% of those with persistent microalbuminuria show a 10–20% increase per year of urinary albumin excretion to overt proteinuria in 10–15 years. Andersen *et al.* [11] followed type 1 diabetics and found two peak incidences for developing evidence of proteinuria, after 16 and 32 years of diabetes. After overt proteinuria, the GFR gradually falls at a highly variable rate estimated between 2 and 20 mL/min/year, with renal failure in greater than 75% after 20 years [12]. The importance of observing GFR along with proteinuria in these patients was highlighted by Caramori *et al.* [13], who biopsied type 1 diabetics with normoalbuminuria and revealed that those who had associated decreased GFR already had evidence of advanced diabetic glomerulopathy.

Although the natural history of type 1 diabetic kidney disease has a strong correlation with renal failure, only a minority, 30–40%, of type 1 diabetics will fall victim to this complication [11, 14]. This low prevalence continues to drive research into exploring different receptors and proteins that might be involved with predisposition.

Type 2 diabetes and kidney disease

In contrast to type 1 diabetic kidney disease, albuminuria may be less specific for type 2 associated diabetic kidney disease. Approximately 20–40% of patients with type 2 diabetes and microalbuminuria will progress to overt nephropathy. Of this small number, only an estimated 20% will progress to renal failure, with the GFR falling at a parallel rate compared with type 1 patients [12], again with the caveat that these statistics predate renin–angiotensin system blockade. Non-progressors have increased risk of expiring secondary to cardiovascular disease prior to needing renal replacement therapy [15].

Remission/reversal of proteinuria

Although proteinuria predicts a high risk of progression, studies have shown evidence of remission, in both type 1 and type 2 patients, with varying degrees of proteinuria to normoalbuminuria after medical interventions. Although not always sustained, it proves intervention can alter the natural history of disease. One of the best interventions we have for albuminuric diabetic kidney disease is the use of the renin–angiotensin–aldosterone system (RAAS) blockade. Many studies support the use of angiotensin-converting enzyme (ACE) inhibitors or angiotensin-receptor blockers (ARB) in decreasing albuminuria, which have both been shown to reduce progression of diabetic kidney disease. Lewis *et al.* [16] proved that reduced progression was independent of blood pressure control in type 2 diabetics given irbesartan. Barnett *et al.* [17] addressed the question of whether ACE inhibitor or ARB is better, and found telmisartan not to be inferior to enalipril in achieving renal protection in type 2 diabetics with early diabetic kidney disease.

Other than RAAS blockade alone, others have looked at glycemic and blood pressure control in achieving proteinuric control. Hovind *et al.* [18, 19] showed 39% of type 1 diabetics reverting to albuminuria with aggressive blood pressure control. Rossing *et al.* [20] showed this was similarly possible in 25% of nephrotic-range albuminuric type 2 diabetics. Hsieh *et al.* [21] showed 35% of type 2 diabetic patients reverting to normoalbuminuria after controlling blood pressure and glycemia to American Diabetes Association goals. For glycemic control, it was recently shown that pancreas transplantation can lead to reversal of diabetic nephropathy. This was shown by Fioretto *et al.* [22], who performed native kidney biopsies at 10 years after pancreas transplantation, revealing reversal of not only the glomerular but also the tubulointerstitial lesions of diabetic kidney disease. They hypothesized that these ends were possible with achieving long-term euglycemia.

Understanding the course of diabetic kidney disease and the associated pathology lends to research in therapeutics. Research over 30 years ago has shown that hyperglycemia alone is not the cause of diabetic kidney disease, and initial alterations of renal hemodynamics likely have a role to play [23]. This led to investigation of the role of RAAS in the GFR and the current top medical therapeutic recommendation in those at risk for diabetic kidney disease, RAAS inhibition. Despite this intervention, many still progress to end-stage disease, leaving the way open for a more novel therapeutic approach. As in most diseases, prevention of disease is most effective. This mantra has led to the discovery of the "salt paradox" and insight into early disease, when hyperfiltration in the proximal tubule and renal hypertrophy are seen as initial pathologic changes [24, 25]. Early proximal tubular changes can set the stage for oxidative stress, inflammation, hypoxia, and tubulointerstitial fibrosis, and thereby progression of diabetic kidney disease [23].

Hannedouche and colleagues [26] studied the GFR, renal hemodynamics, and segmental tubular handling of sodium in type 1 diabetics without kidney disease compared with control subjects. They found proximal sodium reabsorption was higher and significantly correlated with GFR in type 1 patients. Because of this, there was a decrease in distal sodium delivery and proposed that deactivation of tubuloglomerular feedback led to vasodilation and higher GFR. The "salt paradox" in early diabetic kidney disease was initially discovered during an investigation into RAAS control in the diabetic kidney. Based on the premise that reabsorption of salt leads to hyperfiltration Vallon *et al.* [27–29] questioned if decreasing dietary salt would cause a decrease in hyperfiltration and the GFR. They found the opposite to be true, that decreasing dietary salt led to an increase in hyperfiltration and the GFR. The clinical relevance of this has not been determined; however, it offers strong support for tubuloglomerular feedback at work in early diabetic kidney disease [30]. This question of how clinically relevant early hyperfiltration is connected to progression of kidney disease in type 1 diabetics in the setting of RAAS inhibitors has been raised in several studies [31, 32].

The nidus for initial change in renal hemodynamics is thought secondary to the presence of increased glucose in the proximal tubule and by action of the sodium–glucose cotransporters [33]. Specifically, SGLT2 is known to reabsorb nearly all filtered glucose load at its location in the early proximal tubule, independent of insulin [23, 34]. Inhibition of this cotransporter results in increased urinary glucose excretion and may prove to be an important addition to glucose management in diabetic patients [34–36].

Risk factors

When approaching any diagnosis it is important to consider common risk factors for the disease and its progression. For diabetic kidney disease, these include longer duration, poor glycemic control, hypertension, and the presence of proteinuria [37]. Other factors include race, genetic susceptibility (family history), advanced age, and male sex [7]. In addition, there is now evidence that elevated uric acid in diabetic kidney disease patients may predict faster progression [37, 38].

Guidelines for diagnosis

The following recommendations are based on the clinical practice guidelines for diabetic kidney disease outlined by the Kidney Disease Outcomes Quality Initiative (KDOQI), last updated 2007 [39]. They acknowledge that these are generalizations for identifying most cases. They also had difficulty recommending criteria for non-albuminuric cases. Although the gold standard for diagnosis of diabetic kidney disease is renal biopsy, most of the time it is still made on clinical grounds. Based on the knowledge of its natural history, it is recommended to start screening for albuminuria at 5 years in type 1 diabetics and at time of diagnosis in type 2 diabetics.

The early screening test should be an albumin-to-creatinine ratio (ACR) with a first morning void spot collection. The reason for the ratio is that the urinary concentration of albumin alone is highly variable and may lead concerns about accuracy. Studies have been carried out to confirm the sensitivity and specificity of ACR to be greater than 85% compared with timed collections. Despite confidence in ACR, studies have shown differences among age, race, and sex groups [40, 41]. One must also question accuracy when dealing with low muscle mass or obese patients [42, 43]. Interestingly, Wada *et al.* [44] showed that the ACR of urine shows a seasonal variation with higher values in the winter, paralleling the group's earlier finding of seasonal variation of elevated blood pressure.

If a positive result is obtained, the test should be confirmed for persistence with two of three positive repeat measurements within 6 months. Diabetic kidney disease should be considered in (1) type 1 diabetics with microalbuminuria (ACR 30–300 mg/g) and duration of diabetes >10 years; and (2) type 1 or type 2 diabetics with macroalbuminuria (ACR >300 mg/g).

Albuminuria should raise concern for diabetic kidney disease; however, this test should not stand alone. The KDOQI committee encourages the interpretation of albuminuria in relation to the estimation of renal function to risk-stratify patients. Renal function should be assessed through measured serum creatinine or estimated GFR, with knowledge of their limitations. On the basis of natural history, it is important to remember that patients with early nephropathy may have evidence of hyperfiltration and may have a normal to elevated GFR (Table 6.1).

Other clues that support diabetic nephropathy aside from evidence of albuminuria and impaired renal function include large kidneys on ultrasound and the existence of diabetic retinopathy or neuropathy; however absence in type 2 diabetics does not rule out nephropathy (Table 6.2).

As diabetes affects the microvascular circulation, the presence of retinopathy, which can

Likelihood of diabetic kidney disease based on knowing estimated glomerular (eGFR) and albuminuria

eGFR (mL/min/1.73 m^2)	Normoalbuminuria (ACR <30 mg/g)	Microalbuminuria (ACR 30–300 mg/g)	Macroalbuminuria (ACR >300 mg/g)
>60	Possible	Possible	Likely
30–60	Unlikely	Possible	Likely
<30	Unlikely	Unlikely	Likely

ACR, albumin-to-creatinine ratio.

Adapted from KDOQI Clinical Practice Guidelines and Clinical Practice Recommendations for Diabetes and Chronic Kidney Disease. *American journal of kidney diseases*: the official journal of the National Kidney Foundation. 2007;**49**(2 Suppl 2):S12–154. Epub 2007/02/06.

Assessing criteria for diabetic kidney disease

Inclusion	Exclusion
Pre-existing diabetes, impaired glucose	Other systemic disease process
Persistent albuminuria, proteinuria	Rapid increase in proteinuria, nephrotic syndrome
Elevated Cre, decreased GFR	Rapid decrease in GFR
Normal to large kidneys on ultrasound	Presence of active urinary sediment
Diabetic retinopathy or neuropathy	Refractory hypertension
	Greater than expected drop in GFR with ACE inhibitor/ARB

ACE inhibitor, angiotensin-converting enzyme inhibitor; ARB, angiotensin-receptor blockers; GFR, glomerular filtration rate.

be evaluated with a routine ophthalmologic examination, was thought to predict nephropathy. Studies have shown that retinopathy correlates well with overt nephropathy; however it is less supportive in early diabetic kidney disease. A Danish study noted proliferative retinopathy predicted nephropathy in type 1 diabetics [45]. Pedro et al. [46] performed an epidemiologic study in Spain from an ophthalmologic standpoint on the prevalence of microangiopathy, and found microalbuminuria associated with risk of diabetic retinopathy in type 1 diabetics but not in type 2 diabetics. An American study estimated that 30% of type 2 diabetics with renal insufficiency had no evidence of retinopathy or albuminuria [47].

Exclusion criteria for diabetic kidney disease include rapidly decreasing renal function, rapidly increasing proteinuria, active urinary sediment, refractory hypertension, or large reduction in GFR after the start of an ACE inhibitor or ARB. If a patient has any one of the exclusion criteria, further investigation for another cause of kidney disease should be investigated because of the high prevalence of diabetes in the world population. One recent investigation by Chong et al. [48] performed a retrospective analysis of kidney biopsies in type 2 diabetics, showing 62.7% had diabetic kidney disease, 18.2% had non-diabetic kidney disease, and 19.1% had mixed lesions. There have also been investigations into the prevalence of

hematuria associated with diabetic kidney disease, as is it often thought hematuria would suggest an alternative diagnosis. Mazzucco et al. [49] found 62% of patients with biopsy-proven diabetic kidney disease had hematuria on urinalysis; however, only 4% of them had evidence of dysmorphic erythrocytes, which are more often seen in glomerulonephritis. If a patient meets any of the noted exclusion criteria above, it may be worth a discussion with the patient about the risk and benefits of kidney biopsy.

Non-albuminuric diabetic kidney disease is harder to stratify. One group from Italy tried to look at the clinical significance of non-albuminuric disease in type 2 diabetics with a GFR less than $60 \, mL/min/1.73^2$. They found no association between the presence of disease and glycemic control and low correlation with hypertension and retinopathy. The best correlation was with cardiovascular disease, hypothesizing that the renal pathology of non-albuminuric diabetic kidney disease may represent macroangiopathy [50].

The nature of diabetic kidney disease calls into question whether or not we should classify patients in relation to the five clinical stages of chronic kidney disease, which is an estimated GFR scale, or if diabetic kidney disease should have its own classification system. As already mentioned, diabetic patients are not often biopsied to confirm their diabetic

Table 6.3 Diabetic kidney disease pathologic classes

Diabetic kidney disease class	Pathologic criteria on light microscopy
1	Isolated glomerular basement membrane thickening
2 (a) (b)	Mesangial expansion (mild) (severe) Without nodular sclerosis Global glomerulosclerosis <50% of glomeruli
3	+nodular sclerosis >1 glomerulus with nodular increase in mesangial matrix
4	Advanced diabetic glomerulosclerosis Global glomerulosclerosis >50% of glomeruli

kidney disease; however, Tervaert and colleagues [51] have challenged the current pathologic evaluation of diabetic kidney disease. They have published pathologic criteria after grading diabetic kidney disease glomerular lesions to identify four classes of diabetic glomerulopathy with separate evaluations of interstitial and vascular involvement. The criteria are independent of type of diabetes, albuminuria and measured GFR (Table 6.3).

Future insights

As one can appreciate, there is no exacting formula for diagnosis of diabetic kidney disease. The varied clinical presentations of diabetic kidney disease make its diagnosis difficult and may delay therapeutics despite the consensus that early treatment is necessary to prevent progression [52–54]. Current research is attempting to better align a set of biomarkers or tests for diagnosis, in addition to ACR and GFR, and to better evaluate progression. Some of the current investigations include high

urinary mindin levels in type 2 diabetic kidney disease patients which correlate with eGFR [55, 56]; high sensitivity C-reactive protein (CRP) levels in offspring of type 2 diabetic kidney disease patients that were directly associated with ACR [57]; adding cystatin C as a third measured marker increased predictive accuracy of mortality and renal failure [58]; low levels of adiponectin that predicted high ACR in type 2 diabetic patients [59]; inflammatory markers including CRP, interleukin-6, serum amyloid A protein, fibrinogen correlated with higher glomerular basement membrane thickening in type 2 diabetics [60]; higher urinary IgM levels predicting renal and cardiovascular death in type 2 diabetics [61].

One promising platform is knowledge of the kidney as a metabolic organ and diabetes as an abnormal metabolic process. The kidney's role in gluconeogenesis was elucidated by Mutel et al. [62], who disregarded the contribution of liver glycogenolysis and proved there was a compensatory increase in kidney gluconeogenesis during fasting in mice to maintain euglycemia. The role of the kidney as a gluconeogenic organ may be linked to pathways associated with chronic diabetic kidney disease. Insulin action and resistance of the kidney may play a dominant role in pathogenesis. Welsh and colleagues [63] have looked at the role of insulin signaling in the kidney and found that podocyte-specific deficiency in insulin receptors leads to glomerular pathologic changes in the kidney that resemble diabetic kidney disease lesions in the absence of sustained hyperglycemia. Their experiments challenge the cause of albuminuria intrinsically to the podocyte. Perhaps therapy targeting expression of insulin receptors in podocytes can lend to novel therapeutics for prevention of albuminuria [64, 65].

Diabetics are known to possess decreased mitochondrial oxidative phosphorylation capacity [66]. Studies evaluating the renal mitochondria of diabetics show this dysfunction despite their increased number [67, 68]. Achilli *et al.* [69] investigated mitochondrial DNA in diabetics and identified specific haplotypes that may predispose to one diabetic complication over another, including separate haplotypes for diabetic nephropathy and renal failure. Covington *et al.* [70] identified that mitochondrial calpain 10, a resident protease responsible for mitochondrial homeostasis, was reduced after exposure to high glucose resulting in observed renal cell apoptosis and renal dysfunction.

Owing to the kidney's participation in gluconeogenesis, insulin signaling and overall high metabolic activity, the field of metabolomics shows promise in assisting early novel identification of diabetic kidney disease through biomarkers and related therapeutic interventions. Investigation into the urine metabolome of diabetic kidney disease has begun to explore patterns of metabolism that might lend to precise signatures of disease [71, 72]. Metabolomics may provide important clues to better understanding the pathogenesis of diabetic kidney disease in addition to novel means to monitor progression of established disease.

1. Decleves AE, Sharma K. New pharmacological treatments for improving renal outcomes in diabetes. *Nat Rev Nephrol* 2010;**6**: 371–80.
2. Fioretto P, Mauer M, Brocco E, *et al.* Patterns of renal injury in NIDDM patients with microalbuminuria. *Diabetologia* 1996;**39**:1569–76.
3. Dalla Vestra M, Saller A, Bortoloso E, *et al.* Structural involvement in type 1 and type 2 diabetic nephropathy. *Diabetes Metab* 2000;**26**(Suppl 4):8–14.
4. Brocco E, Fioretto P, Mauer M, *et al.* Renal structure and function in non-insulin dependent diabetic patients with microalbuminuria. *Kidney Int Suppl* 1997; **63**:S40–4.
5. Mac-Moune Lai F, Szeto CC, Choi PC, *et al.* Isolate diffuse thickening of glomerular capillary basement membrane: a renal lesion in prediabetes? *Mod Pathol* 2004;**17**:1506–12.
6. Succurro E, Arturi F, Lugara M, *et al.* One-hour postload plasma glucose levels are associated with kidney dysfunction. *Clin J Am Soc Nephrol* 2010;**5**:1922–7.
7. Ayodele OE, Alebiosu CO, Salako BL. Diabetic nephropathy—a review of the natural history, burden, risk factors and treatment. *J Natl Med Assoc* 2004;**96**: 1445–54.
8. Chiarelli F, Verrotti A, Morgese G. Glomerular hyperfiltration increases the risk of developing microalbuminuria in diabetic children. *Pediatr Nephrol* 1995;**9**: 154–8.
9. Mogensen CE, Schmitz O. The diabetic kidney: from hyperfiltration and microalbuminuria to end-stage renal failure. *Med Clin N Am* 1988;**72**:1465–92.
10. Caramori ML, Kim Y, Huang C, *et al.* Cellular basis of diabetic nephropathy: 1. Study design and renal structural-functional relationships in patients with long-standing type 1 diabetes. *Diabetes* 2002;**51**:506–13.
11. Andersen AR, Christiansen JS, Andersen JK, *et al.* Diabetic nephropathy in Type 1 (insulin-dependent) diabetes: an epidemiological study. *Diabetologia* 1983; **25**:496–501.
12. Molitch ME, DeFronzo RA, Franz MJ, *et al.* Nephropathy in diabetes. *Diabetes care.* 2004;**27**(Suppl 1):S79–83.
13. Caramori ML, Fioretto P, Mauer M. Low glomerular filtration rate in normoalbuminuric type 1 diabetic patients: an indicator of more advanced glomerular lesions. *Diabetes* 2003;**52**: 1036–40.

14. Lehmann R, Spinas GA. [Diabetic nephropathy: significance of microalbuminuria and proteinuria in Type I and Type II diabetes mellitus]. *Praxis* 1995;**84**:1265–71. (In German)

15. Rossing K, Christensen PK, Hovind P, *et al.* Progression of nephropathy in type 2 diabetic patients. *Kidney Int* 2004;**66**: 1596–605.

16. Lewis EJ, Hunsicker LG, Clarke WR, *et al.* Renoprotective effect of the angiotensin-receptor antagonist irbesartan in patients with nephropathy due to type 2 diabetes. *N Engl J Med* 2001;**345**:851–60.

17. Barnett AH, Bain SC, Bouter P, *et al.* Angiotensin-receptor blockade versus converting-enzyme inhibition in type 2 diabetes and nephropathy. *N Engl J Med* 2004;**351**:1952–61.

18. Hovind P, Rossing P, Tarnow L, *et al.* Remission of nephrotic-range albuminuria in type 1 diabetic patients. *Diabetes Care* 2001;**24**:1972–7.

19. Hovind P, Rossing P, Tarnow L, *et al.* Remission and regression in the nephropathy of type 1 diabetes when blood pressure is controlled aggressively. *Kidney Int* 2001;**60**:277–83.

20. Rossing K, Christensen PK, Hovind P, Parving HH. Remission of nephrotic-range albuminuria reduces risk of end-stage renal disease and improves survival in type 2 diabetic patients. *Diabetologia* 2005;**48**:2241–7.

21. Hsieh MC, Hsieh YT, Cho TJ, *et al.* Remission of diabetic nephropathy in type 2 diabetic Asian population: role of tight glucose and blood pressure control. *Eur J Clin Invest* 2011;**41**:870–8.

22. Fioretto P, Mauer M. Effects of pancreas transplantation on the prevention and reversal of diabetic nephropathy. *Contrib Nephrol* 2011;**170**:237–46.

23. Vallon V. The proximal tubule in the pathophysiology of the diabetic kidney. *Am J Physiol Regul Integr Comp Physiol* 2011;**300**:R1009–22.

24. Vallon V, Blantz RC, Thomson S. Glomerular hyperfiltration and the salt paradox in early [corrected] type 1 diabetes mellitus: a tubulo-centric view. *J Am Soc Nephrol* 2003;**14**:530–7.

25. Seyer-Hansen K, Hansen J, Gundersen HJ. Renal hypertrophy in experimental diabetes. A morphometric study. *Diabetologia* 1980;**18**:501–5.

26. Hannedouche TP, Delgado AG, Gnionsahe DA, *et al.* Renal hemodynamics and segmental tubular reabsorption in early type 1 diabetes. *Kidney Int* 1990;**37**:1126–33.

27. Vallon V, Wead LM, Blantz RC. Renal hemodynamics and plasma and kidney angiotensin II in established diabetes mellitus in rats: effect of sodium and salt restriction. *J Am Soc Nephrol* 1995; **5**:1761–7.

28. Vallon V, Kirschenmann D, Wead LM, *et al.* Effect of chronic salt loading on kidney function in early and established diabetes mellitus in rats. *J Lab Clin Med* 1997;**130**:76–82.

29. Vallon V, Schroth J, Satriano J, *et al.* Adenosine A (1) receptors determine glomerular hyperfiltration and the salt paradox in early streptozotocin diabetes mellitus. *Nephron Physiol* 2009;**111**: 30–8.

30. Vallon V, Blantz R, Thomson S. The salt paradox and its possible implications in managing hypertensive diabetic patients. *Curr Hypertens Rep* 2005;**7**:141–7.

31. Thomas MC, Moran JL, Harjutsalo V, *et al.* Hyperfiltration in type 1 diabetes: does it exist and does it matter for nephropathy? *Diabetologia* 2012;**55**: 1505–13.

32. Rosolowsky ET, Niewczas MA, Ficociello LH, *et al*. Between hyperfiltration and impairment: demystifying early renal functional changes in diabetic nephropathy. *Diabetes Res Clin Pract* 2008; **82**(Suppl 1):S46–53.

33. Vallon V, Richter K, Blantz RC, *et al*. Glomerular hyperfiltration in experimental diabetes mellitus: potential role of tubular reabsorption. *J Am Soc Nephrol* 1999;**10**:2569–76.

34. Nomura S. Renal sodium-dependent glucose cotransporter 2 (SGLT2) inhibitors for new anti-diabetic agent. *Curr Top Med Chem* 2010;**10**:411–8.

35. Duijzer E, Zwakenberg M, Heerspink HJ. [The kidney: target for blood glucose-lowering therapy]. *Nederlands Tijdschrift voor Geneeskunde* 2011;**155**:A3667. (In Dutch)

36. Bailey CJ. Renal glucose reabsorption inhibitors to treat diabetes. *Trends Pharmacol Sci* 2011;**32**:63–71. E

37. Altemtam N, Russell J, El Nahas M. A study of the natural history of diabetic kidney disease (DKD). *Nephrol Dial Transplant* 2012;**27**:1847–54.

38. Hovind P, Rossing P, Johnson RJ, Parving HH. Serum uric acid as a new player in the development of diabetic nephropathy. *J Ren Nutr* 2011;**21**:124–7.

39. KDOQI Clinical Practice Guidelines and Clinical Practice Recommendations for Diabetes and Chronic Kidney Disease. *Am J Kidney Dis* 2007;**49**(Suppl 2):S12–154.

40. Xu R, Zhang L, Zhang P, *et al*. Gender-specific reference value of urine albumin-creatinine ratio in healthy Chinese adults: results of the Beijing CKD survey. *Clin Chim Acta* 2008;**398**:125–9.

41. Methven S, MacGregor MS, Traynor JP, *et al*. Assessing proteinuria in chronic kidney disease: protein-creatinine ratio versus albumin-creatinine ratio. *Nephrol Dial Transplant* 2010;**25**:2991–6.

42. Ellam TJ. Albumin:creatinine ratio—a flawed measure? The merits of estimated albuminuria reporting. *Nephron Clin Pract* 2011;**118**:c324–30.

43. Guidone C, Gniuli D, Castagneto-Gissey L, *et al*. Underestimation of urinary albumin to creatinine ratio in morbidly obese subjects due to high urinary creatinine excretion. *Clin Nutr* 2012;**31**:212–6.

44. Wada Y, Hamamoto Y, Ikeda H, *et al*. Seasonal variations of urinary albumin creatinine ratio in Japanese subjects with Type 2 diabetes and early nephropathy. *Diabet Med* 2012;**29**:506–8.

45. Karlberg C, Falk C, Green A, Sjolie AK, Grauslund J. Proliferative retinopathy predicts nephropathy: a 25-year follow-up study of type 1 diabetic patients. *Acta Diabetol* 2012;**49**:263–8.

46. Pedro RA, Ramon SA, Marc BB, *et al*. Prevalence and relationship between diabetic retinopathy and nephropathy, and its risk factors in the North-East of Spain, a population-based study. *Ophthalmic Epidemiol* 2010;**17**:251–65.

47. Kramer HJ, Nguyen QD, Curhan G, Hsu CY. Renal insufficiency in the absence of albuminuria and retinopathy among adults with type 2 diabetes mellitus. *JAMA* 2003;**289**:3273–7.

48. Chong YB, Keng TC, Tan LP, *et al*. Clinical predictors of non-diabetic renal disease and role of renal biopsy in diabetic patients with renal involvement: a single centre review. *Ren Fail* 2012;**34**:323–8.

49. Mazzucco G, Bertani T, Fortunato M, *et al*. Different patterns of renal damage in type 2 diabetes mellitus: a multicentric study on 393 biopsies. *Am J Kidney Dis* 2002;**39**:713–20.

50. Penno G, Solini A, Bonora E, *et al.* Clinical significance of nonalbuminuric renal impairment in type 2 diabetes. *J Hypertens* 2011;**29**:1802–9.

51. Tervaert TW, Mooyaart AL, Amann K, *et al.* Pathologic classification of diabetic nephropathy. *J Am Soc Nephrol* 2010;**21**:556–63.

52. McGowan T, McCue P, Sharma K. Diabetic nephropathy. *Clin Lab Med* 2001;**21**:111–46.

53. Caramori ML, Mauer M. Diabetes and nephropathy. *Curr Opin Nephrol Hypertens* 2003;**12**:273–82.

54. Kovesdy CP, Sharma K, Kalantar-Zadeh K. Glycemic control in diabetic CKD patients: where do we stand? *Am J Kidney Dis* 2008;**52**:766–77.

55. Murakoshi M, Gohda T, Tanimoto M, *et al.* Role of mindin in diabetic nephropathy. *Exp Diabetes Res* 2011; **2011**:486305.

56. Murakoshi M, Tanimoto M, Gohda T, Hagiwara S, Takagi M, Horikoshi S, *et al.* Mindin: a novel marker for podocyte injury in diabetic nephropathy. *Nephrol Dial Transplant* 2011;**26**: 2153–60.

57. Zambrano-Galvan G, Rodriguez-Moran M, Simental-Mendia LE, *et al.* C-reactive Protein Is Directly Associated with Urinary Albumin-to-Creatinine Ratio. *Arch Med Res* 2011;**42**:451–6.

58. Peralta CA, Shlipak MG, Judd S, *et al.* Detection of chronic kidney disease with creatinine, cystatin C, and urine albumin-to-creatinine ratio and association with progression to end-stage renal disease and mortality. *JAMA* 2011;**305**: 1545–52.

59. Kacso I, Lenghel A, Bondor CI, *et al.* Low plasma adiponectin levels predict increased urinary albumin/creatinine ratio in type 2 diabetes patients. *Int Urol Nephrol* 2011.

60. Dalla Vestra M, Mussap M, Gallina P, *et al.* Acute-phase markers of inflammation and glomerular structure in patients with type 2 diabetes. *J Am Soc Nephrol* 2005;**16**(Suppl 1):S78–82.

61. Tofik R, Torffvit O, Rippe B, Bakoush O. Urine IgM-excretion as a prognostic marker for progression of type 2 diabetic nephropathy. *Diabetes Res Clin Pract* 2012;**95**:139–44.

62. Mutel E, Gautier-Stein A, Abdul-Wahed A, *et al.* Control of blood glucose in the absence of hepatic glucose production during prolonged fasting in mice: induction of renal and intestinal gluconeogenesis by glucagon. *Diabetes* 2011;**60**:3121–31.

63. Welsh GI, Hale LJ, Eremina V, *et al.* Insulin signaling to the glomerular podocyte is critical for normal kidney function. *Cell Metab* 2010;**12**:329–40.

64. Fornoni A. Proteinuria, the podocyte, and insulin resistance. *N Engl J Med* 2010;**363**:2068–9.

65. Rask-Madsen C, King GL. Diabetes: podocytes lose their footing. *Nature* 2010;**468**:42–4.

66. Szendroedi J, Phielix E, Roden M. The role of mitochondria in insulin resistance and type 2 diabetes mellitus. *Nat Rev Endocrinol* 2012;**8**:92–103.

67. Ma ZA, Zhao Z, Turk J. Mitochondrial dysfunction and beta-cell failure in type 2 diabetes mellitus. *Experimental diabetes research.* 2012;**2012**:703538.

68. Malik AN, Czajka A. 10 Mitochondrial dysfunction in diabetic nephropathy. *Heart* 2011;**97**:e8.

69. Achilli A, Olivieri A, Pala M, *et al.* Mitochondrial DNA backgrounds might modulate diabetes complications rather than T2DM as a whole. *PloS one* 2011;**6**:e21029.

70. Covington MD, Schnellmann RG. Chronic high glucose downregulates

mitochondrial calpain 10 and contributes to renal cell death and diabetes-induced renal injury. *Kidney Int* 2011.

71. van der Kloet FM, Tempels FW, Ismail N, *et al*. Discovery of early-stage biomarkers for diabetic kidney disease using MS-based metabolomics (FinnDiane study). *Metabolomics* 2012;**8**:109–19.

72. Ng DP, Salim A, Liu Y, *et al*. A metabolomic study of low estimated GFR in non-proteinuric type 2 diabetes mellitus. *Diabetologia* 2012;**55**:499–508.

Part II

Special Situations, Risk Factors and Complications

Cardiovascular disease in diabetic nephropathy: pathophysiology and treatment

Martin Busch

Jena University Hospital, Jena, Germany

Key points

- Cardiovascular disease (CVD) is the leading cause of mortality in diabetes.
- Chronic kidney disease (CKD) is an independent cardiovascular risk factor.
- The multiple presence of conventional risk factors, together with diabetes and CKD explains the excessive risk for CVD in patients with diabetic nephropathy.
- Therapeutic strategies should focus on lowering and treatment of classical risk factors (i.e., obesity, dyslipidemia, arterial hypertension), treatment of diabetes mellitus, and best-possible management of CKD, especially in advanced CKD.
- Specific therapeutic efforts should consider the pathophysiologic features of vascular disease in diabetic nephropathy, i.e., during the management of coronary artery disease.

Cardiovascular disease (CVD) has a large impact on the prognosis of patients with diabetes mellitus, especially when chronic kidney disease (CKD) occurs. Atherosclerotic risk in diabetic nephropathy is characterized by different risk scenarios (Figure 7.1). First, diabetic patients are susceptible to classical atherosclerotic risk factors. Many of these risk factors (i.e., obesity, hypertension, dyslipidemia, higher age) are to be found in diabetic patients, often several together. Around 50% of the additive cardiovascular (CV) risk in diabetes can be explained by the presence of such risk factors. But, second, diabetic patients undergo risk potentiation due to diabetes mellitus itself. CVD is the leading cause of mortality in diabetic patients, 75% die from CV complications. Their risk for a primary myocardial infarction is similar to non-diabetic

Diabetes and Kidney Disease, First Edition. Edited by Gunter Wolf.
© 2013 John Wiley & Sons, Ltd. Published 2013 by John Wiley & Sons, Ltd.

Diabetes mellitus	**Common CV risk**	**Chronic kidney disease**
	• Arterial hypertension/ Left ventricular hypertrophy	
	• Dyslipidemia	
• Enhanced dyslipidemia	• Smoking	• Progressive hypertension
• Insulin resistance	• Obesity	• RAAS activation
• Abnormal platelet function	• Higher age	• Sodium retention
• Hyperglycemia	• Male gender	• Increased sympathetic activity
• Advanced glycation end products/carbonyl stress	• Genetic factors/family history of CV events	• Endothelial dysfunction
• Endothelial dysfunction	• Absence of exercise	• Proteinuria
• Diabetic microangiopathy	• Menopause	• Advanced glycation end products/oxidative stress
• Diabetic neuropathy		• Asymmetric dimethylarginine
• Diabetic foot syndrome/inflammation		• Homocysteine
• Albuminuria		• Volume overload
• Hypoglycemia		• Mineral disorders/ potassium
• Autonomic neuropathy		• Renal anemia
• Silent ischemia		• Left ventricular hypertrophy
• Small vessel disease		• Hyperphosphatemia
		• Vitamin D deficiency
		• Hyperparathyreoidism
		• Vascular calcification
		• Enhanced vascular stiffness
		• Chronic inflammation
		• Upregulation of proinflammatory cytokines and growth factors
		• Malnutrition
		• Multiple biomarkers

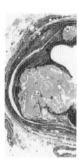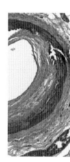

Diabetic nephropathy and the burden of CV risk from different origin. Cardiovascular disease in the general population and in diabetes mellitus leads to classical atherosclerotic plaque formation (left), whereas chronic kidney disease is additionally associated with vascular calcification processes, mainly located in the media (right). Adapted from Pasterkamp G, *et al*. [7] (left) and courtesy of Dr. Kerstin Amann, University of Erlangen (right), with permission.

patients who have already experienced such an event [1]. Typical macrovascular manifestations of diabetic vascular disease are coronary artery disease (CAD), cerebrovascular disease, and peripheral arterial disease (PAD). According to meta-analysis in 2010, diabetes confers about a twofold excess risk for CAD, major stroke subtypes, and other vascular deaths [2]. Compared with 1999–2000, the estimated 10-year risk for developing CAD among people with diabetes in the USA was 22% lower by 2007–2008 indicating that efforts in improving CV risk factors should further benefit the health status of people with diabetes [3]. In patients with diabetic nephropathy, vascular disease will be complicated further by albuminuria and chronic kidney disease (CKD). CKD of all kind results in CV risk potentiation dependent on its stage (Table 7.1). Around one-quarter of patients with type 2 diabetes

Cardiovascular risk according to stages of chronic kidney disease

Stage	CV risk (odds ratio, univariate)
1	Depending on degree of proteinuria
2	1.5
3	2–4
4	4–10
5	10–50
ESRD	20–1000

The increase in risk compared with people free of chronic kidney disease depends on the age of the population studied: The younger the person, the higher the relative risk. Microalbuminuria increases the cardiovascular risk two- to fourfold.
Reproduced with permission from Schiffrin EL, Lipman ML, Mann JF. Chronic kidney disease: effects on the cardiovascular system. *Circulation* 2007;**116**:85–97.

develop microalbuminuria within 10 years of the diagnosis of diabetes. With the diagnosis of microalbuminuria, the risk of death rises up to 3% annually, increasing further if macroalbuminuria occurs (4.6% annually). If plasma creatinine is elevated [including end-stage renal disease (ESRD)], the risk of death is estimated to be nearly 20% per year [4].

Based on the definition by the World Health Organization (WHO), arteriosclerosis is a combination of vascular changes of the intima and media. The term atherosclerosis emphasizes the intimal accumulation of lipids. The endothelium plays a central role in pathogenesis. The classical "reaction to injury" hypothesis describes endothelial dysfunction that is caused by atherosclerotic risk factors [5].

Endothelial dysfunction supports the intimal deposition of lipoproteins, especially low-density lipoprotein (LDL). Lipoproteins are modified by reactive oxygen species. Endothelial defects lead to the expression of adhesion molecules, which attract monocytes, macrophages, T-cells, and mast cells. These cells migrate to the intima, forming early plaque. Immunocompetent cells in the plaque define atherosclerosis as an inflammatory disease [5, 6]. Macrophages incorporate LDL-bound cholesterol esters and oxidized LDL via their scavenger receptors. In lysosomes, LDLs are cleaved into cholesterol and free fatty acids. Cholesterol is re-esterified or bound to apolipoprotein E and high-density lipoprotein (HDL) in the blood. HDL will be transported to the liver. Esters are deposited in the cytoplasm leading to foam cells, which are the subendothelial lipid deposits of the early atherosclerotic lesion [5]. Macrophages secrete interleukin (IL)-1β and tumor necrosis factor (TNF)-α, which attract leukocytes and activate vascular smooth muscle cells (VSMCs) and fibroblasts. Thrombocytes are a further source of proinflammatory mediators and growth factors (platelet-derived growth factor). VSMCs and the collagen matrix define the fibrous plaque [5]. In the plaque, there is necrosis of foam cells, extracellular deposition of lipids and cholesterol crystals, detritus of cells, and secondary calcification (see also Figure 7.1) [7]. Such plaque with vascular stenosis is denoted as a complex lesion [5]. Proinflammatory and proteolytic processes reduce the stability of the plaque [6]. During plaque rupture, prothrombotic materials such as phospholipids, platelet adhesion factor, and tissue factor (TF) are secreted. Local thrombosis with occlusion of the vessel results in clinically remarkable acute events [6]. Thus, activation and aggregation of platelets play a major role. Thromboxane A_2 derived from platelets stimulates proagglutination and vasoconstriction. Low doses of acetylsalicylic acid (aspirin) reduce the cyclooxygenase-dependent production of thromboxane A_2 in humans by 97–99% [8]. Thienopyridines like clopidogrel are blockers of the platelet type 2 purinergic receptor.

They inhibit the binding of adenosine diphosphate (ADP) to this receptor, which prevents the activation of the glycoprotein (Gp) IIb–IIIa receptor and the subsequent binding of fibrinogen. Thus, the formation of stable platelet aggregates is blocked. The direct inhibition of the fibrinogen binding site by GpIIb–IIIa blockers like integrilin is also a therapeutic tool, especially in acute coronary syndrome [8].

Pathophysiological conditions of vascular disease in diabetic nephropathy

Diabetic vascular disease refers mostly to the classical theory of atherosclerosis. Endothelial dysfunction in diabetes is enhanced by insulin resistance, dyslipidemia/free fatty acid liberation, hyper-/hypoglycemia, disturbed platelet function, decreased fibrinolysis/increased procoagulation, or abnormalities in blood flow [9]. The involvement of small vessels and multiple lesions and a multivessel disease are common, even in younger patients.

Endothelial dysfunction

Endothelium-dependent nitric oxide (NO)-mediated vascular relaxation is impaired in diabetes. Hyperglycemia decreases the availability of endothelium-derived NO. The loss of NO increases the activity of the proinflammatory transcription factor nuclear factor kappa B (NF-κB) promoting inflammation, cell migration into the intima, and foam cell formation [9]. NO balance is defined by its production from endothelial NO synthase (eNOS) and its degradation or inactivation, particularly by oxygen-derived free radicals. Hyperglycemia may induce such oxidative stress. In CKD, endothelial dysfunction exists too. Whether albuminuria is an expression of generalized endothelial and vascular dysfunction rather than a genuine source of further vascular complications remains controversial. Nevertheless, albuminuria is correlated with endothelial dysfunction [10]. It increases the relative risk for total and CV mortality as well as for renal end points [11].

Insulin resistance

Insulin resistance is a typical sign of type 2 diabetes. Primarily, the accumulation of visceral fat is accompanied by insulin resistance and disturbed lipid metabolism. Insulin resistance is associated with elevations in free fatty acid levels [9]. The production of vasoconstrictors such as prostanoids and endothelin is increased. Endothelin promotes inflammation and causes VSMC growth. Endothelin-1 concentration in plasma increases after administration of insulin. Drugs that increase insulin sensitivity improve vasodilation. Diabetes enhances the migration of VSMC into atherosclerotic lesions. Apoptosis of VSMC in the plaque is increased, influencing the propensity for plaque rupture. Elevated protein kinase C (PKC) activity, NF-κB production, and generation of free radicals have also been described for VSMC in diabetes [9].

Hyperglycemia/hypoglycemia

Before the diagnosis of diabetes mellitus, abnormal glucose tolerance is a strong predictor of CV complications and death [12]. Hyperglycemia and glucose fluctuations are closely associated with oxidative stress generation and inflammation [13]. Inflammation leads to enhanced insulin resistance and β-cell dysfunction. Acute hyperglycemia rapidly attenuated endothelium-derived vasodilation and reduced myocardial perfusion. Hyperglycemia is a risk factor for micro- and macrovascular complication and all-cause mortality [12]. Hypoglycemia is also associated with adverse clinical outcomes, including vascular events and death in patients with type 2 diabetes. However, the presence of severe hypoglycemia may represent the patient's status (i.e., for multimorbidity) and should raise clinical suspicion of the patient's susceptibility to adverse outcomes [14]. A higher risk for hypoglycemia in patients with albuminuria/CKD or neuropathy should be considered [15].

Dyslipidemia

Levels of circulating free fatty acids are elevated in diabetes because of excess liberation from adipose tissue and decreased uptake in muscles. Free fatty acids and glucose activate PKC, which contributes to superoxide generation. Elevated free fatty acids lead to an increase in very low-density lipoprotein (VLDL) production and cholesteryl ester synthesis in the liver. These triglyceride-rich proteins and the diminished clearance by lipoprotein-lipase result in elevated triglycerides as observed in diabetes. Elevated triglycerides contribute to lower HDL levels. Moreover, LDL morphology is changed: increasing the amount of small, dense LDL contributes to atherogenesis [9]. Dyslipidemia in CKD is evident as well. Increased VLDL, prolonged persistence of postprandial chylomicron remnants, accumulation of small dense LDL, modification of apolipoproteins by glycation or oxidation, elevated lipoprotein (a), or accumulation of non-cardioprotective acute-phase HDL have been described [16].

Platelet function

Platelet function in diabetes mellitus is abnormal. Platelets are involved in thrombus formation [8]. Prostacyclin and NO derived from the endothelium inhibit platelet activation and relax VSMC. However, patients with diabetes have reduced release of prostacyclin and NO from the endothelium and the platelets as well. Moreover, the release of thromboxane A_2 from platelets is increased, and adhesion molecules are highly expressed. Thus, platelet turnover and platelet aggregation are acceler-

ated in diabetes. Enhanced fibrinogen-binding is caused by increased expression of GpIIb–IIIa [17]. Based on the predominating role of platelet activation in diabetic CVD, prevention strategies with aspirin or thienopyridines are recommended.

Another factor influencing diabetic CVD is impaired fibrinolytic balance, which is caused by an increase in plasma coagulation factors and lesion-based coagulants and a decrease in endogenous anticoagulants [9]. In type 2 diabetes, levels of plasminogen activator inhibitor (PAI) are increased and associated with impairment of fibrinolytic activity.

Advanced glycation end products

Since the discovery of glycosylated hemoglobin (HbA1c) in the blood of diabetic patients, advanced glycation end products (AGEs) have become a topic of growing interest. Formed during complex pathways, AGEs are chemical modifications of proteins, lipids, peptides, amino acids, and nucleic acids by carbohydrates/reducing sugars, including reactive carbonyl compounds (RCOs) as metabolic intermediates. AGEs are present as residues in plasma proteins such as albumin, free in plasma, and in peptide fragments of proteins enriched with AGEs [18]. AGEs are formed during aging as a physiological process. They accumulate in chronic diseases such as diabetes mellitus, atherosclerosis, Alzheimer's disease, and CKD. AGEs like N^ε-carboxymethyllysine (CML) and pentosidine are formed by combined non-enzymatic glycation and oxidation. Although the role of oxidative stress in diabetes mellitus remains controversial, CKD increases oxidative stress, especially in ESRD. Moreover, RCO clearance is impaired. AGEs are related to a decrease in the glomerular filtration rate (GFR). AGEs in plasma are significantly increased in CKD compared to healthy controls. Detoxification of AGEs during dialysis treatment is limited [18, 19].

AGEs elicit receptor-mediated effects. The most well-known is the receptor for AGEs (RAGE). Physiological expression of RAGE has been detected in endothelial cells, VSMC, mononuclear cells, and macrophages. RAGE–ligand interaction results in the release of interleukins and TNF-α leading to the activation of NF-κB and generation of reactive oxygen species. Endothelial RAGE is considered to serve as a link between AGE accumulation and endothelial dysfunction. AGEs are found in atherosclerotic plaques [18].

Although the AGE concept is meaningful, clinical data showing an association of increased AGEs with CV end points are scarce. AGE protein residues in plasma such as CML and pentosidine were not an independent CV or renal risk factor [18, 19]. However, AGEs in plasma are affected by fluctuations, i.e., from nutritional sources, whereas tissue accumulation serves as a long-term memory of AGE formation [18]. The formation of AGEs can be prevented or AGEs may be broken down by certain drugs. Nevertheless, these principles have not culminated in market-ready drugs until now. Experimental AGE-inhibiting properties of angiotensin-converting enzyme (ACE) inhibitors or angiotensin II type 1 receptor blockers (ARBs) could not be confirmed in patients with type 2 diabetic nephropathy [18].

Asymmetric dimethylarginine

Asymmetric dimethylarginine (ADMA) is a competitive inhibitor of eNOS and therefore may be involved in disturbed NO generation and endothelial dysfunction [9, 20]. Moreover, ADMA may block the entry of L-arginine into the cells, with a resulting decrease in synthesis of NO [20]. ADMA is derived from proteins which contain arginine residues. These residues are methylated by the enzyme protein arginine methyltransferase (PRMT) type I and released as the proteins are hydrolyzed. PRMT type II forms symmetric dimethylarginine (SDMA), which is a stereoisomer of ADMA and not an inhibitor of NOS. ADMA is metabolized mainly by dimethylarginine dimethylaminohydrolase (DDAH), only a small amount is cleared by the kidney [20]. SDMA is completely eliminated renally. Oxidative stress may increase the concentration of ADMA by interacting as it degrades. The concentration of both dimethylarginines is increased in CKD, with that of SDMA being more pronounced. DDAH is also expressed in the kidney. Thus, it is unclear whether an increase in ADMA is caused by a reduction in GFR or a lower metabolization rate. Systemic administration of ADMA leads to a rapid lowering in cardiac output and an increase in systemic vascular resistance. Data from patients with CKD suggest that ADMA is an independent marker for vascular complications, death, and renal outcome [20].

C-reactive protein

Atherosclerosis is an inflammatory disease [5, 6]. During acute coronary syndrome (ACS), concentration of cytokines is increased. Because of this, acute-phase proteins like C-reactive protein (CRP) are increasingly produced in the liver. CRP is said to reflect the vulnerability of atherosclerotic lesions or the probability of plaque rupture [5]. Moreover, CRP contributes to the progression of atherosclerosis via several mechanisms, i.e., foam cell formation. High sensitivity CRP was investigated as a CV risk factor in the general population as well as in diabetes and CKD. CKD is a chronic inflammatory state due to increased oxidative stress, chronic infections, and comorbidities. In ESRD, the extracorporal blood flow as well as the biocompatibility of the dialyzers and the purity of the dialysate have an additional impact [10]. CRP is a predictor of total and CV mortality in CKD patients. In CKD, the determination of standard CRP seems to be adequate for risk stratification and has been recommended [19].

Lowering of CRP by aspirin was disappointing. In the general population, treatment with statins lowered CRP and prevented vascular events independently of lipid lowering [21], whereas treatment with rosuvastatin 10 mg daily versus placebo in dialysis patients (28% with diabetes, 40% with CVD) did not result in CV risk reduction [22]. Thus, statin therapy for CRP-lowering in CKD cannot be recommended as yet.

Homocysteine

Elevated total homocysteine (Hcy) is another but moderate cofactor linked with CVD. Hcy acts pro-oxidatively by the generation of hydrogen peroxide and free radicals. A deficiency in vitamins B6, B12, and folic acid causes hyperhomocysteinemia in healthy people, and mutations of enzymes which are involved in Hcy metabolism, i.e. methylenetetrahydrofolate reductase (MTHFR) [23]. Serum concentration of total Hcy (tHcy) is increased in CKD, especially in ESRD [19]. The lowering of tHcy by vitamin supplementation did not reduce CV end points in the general population or in CV risk populations [23]. Nevertheless, loss of water-soluble vitamins is evident in chronic hemodialysis patients. Thus, multivitamin supplementation (i.e., B12, B6, folic acid), at least after each hemodialysis session, is recommended and has Hcy-lowering properties. A further increase in the intake of folic acid, vitamin B12, and vitamin B6 did not reduce total mortality and CV events [24]. Owing to meta-analysis, folic acid therapy can reduce CV risk in patients with ESRD or advanced CKD by 15% [25].

Renin–angiotensin system/hypertension

The impact of hypertension for vascular disease in diabetes and CKD is enhanced by the role of the renin–angiotensin–aldosterone system (RAAS). Progression of CKD leads to the stimulation of RAAS. Increased blood pressure harms the endothelium. Angiotensin II (Ang II) stimulates NAD(P)H contributing to oxidative stress. Moreover, Ang II is associated with upregulation of several cytokines, inflammatory mediators, chemokines, or adhesion molecules promoting endothelial dysfunction and vascular remodeling [10]. Sodium retention and sympathetic nervous system activation contribute to the elevation of blood pressure as well. Plasma catecholamine concentrations are elevated in CKD. Hypertension and hormonal mechanisms play a pivotal role in the induction of left ventricular hypertrophy (LVH), which is a strong predictor of mortality in the early stages of CKD [26].

Vascular calcification

In CKD, besides atherosclerotic vascular damage, vascular calcification occurs. In diabetes, calcification is noted too. Vascular calcification is closely related to CKD-associated bone and mineral disorders (CKD-MBD). It is denoted by sclerosis and calcification of the media in elastic arteries and arterioles [27]. Plaque formation is not so typical for CKD-related vascular disease as for conventional atherosclerosis (see Figure 7.1). Calcification of intimal lesions is also augmented [27]. Calcification of the media leads to increased vascular stiffness along with increased systolic and decreased diastolic blood pressure values (increased pulse pressure), further progression of left ventricular hypertrophy, and reduced coronary perfusion. Bone matrix proteins were found in calcified vessels. Osteogenetic differentiation of VSMC into osteoblast-like cells is a key mechanism of calcification. These cells generate a collagen extracellular matrix in which minerals, e.g., calcium and phosphate, are deposited. This process is enhanced by hyperphosphatemia [28]. Calcification is inhibited *in vivo*. However, there is a deficiency of calcification inhibitors during CKD. Functional vitamin K deficiency is said to be causative. Several inhibitors of calcification are activated vitamin K dependent [28]. Therefore, it has been recommended to circumvent treatment with vitamin K antagonists as oral anticoagulants in ESRD [29]. In this regard, antithrombotic agents like oral thrombin- or factor Xa inhibitors might offer new therapeutic horizons. Fetuin-A (α2-Schmid Heremans glycoprotein), a transporter of γ-carboxylated matrix Gla protein (MGP), is an inhibitor of calcification. Low serum fetuin-A and MGP levels are associated with vascular calcification [10]. Calcification is inversely correlated with bone mineral density [28]. Besides secondary hyperparathyreoidism, vitamin D deficiency and hyperphosphatemia, several other factors (i.e., osteoprotegerin, bone morphogenetic protein and its receptor, pyrophosphate, and leptin) are closely related to vascular calcification in CKD [10]. Poor vitamin D status indicates an increased CV risk, since vitamin D has antihypertrophic, antiatherosclerotic, antihypertensive, renoprotective, antiinflammatory, antioxidative, and antidiabetic effects [30].

Clinical evidence, prevention, and treatment strategies

By the 1960s, using the Framingham risk score, patients who exhibited certain risk factors for CVD could be identified. These factors were higher age, male gender, higher systolic blood pressure, dyslipidemia, diabetes mellitus, smoking and an ECG showing left ventricular hypertrophy. These factors are called "classical risk factors." Nowadays, also genetic predisposition (i.e., any familial history for CV events), heavy alcohol consumption, lifestyle factors, like absence of motion or sedentary living, obesity and associated insulin resistance, or early menopause in women are considered to be risk markers. Diabetes mellitus

and CKD go along with the presence of multiple conventional risk factors. Some of these risk factors can be influenced by a change of lifestyle or treatment issues, others not.

Aspirin use

Pre-existing CVD is a strong predictor for future CV events defining the difference between primary and secondary prevention strategies. In secondary prevention, risk markers should be monitored and treated more stringently. Type 2 diabetes is a CAD risk equivalent. Hence, the presence of diabetes permits a secondary prevention concept. Regarding antiplatelet agents, a 2010 ACC/ADA/AHA Joint Scientific Statement recommends low-dose aspirin (75–162 mg/day) for men over age 50 years and women over 60 years with diabetes who have one or more additional risk factors (such as family history of coronary heart disease, smoking, hypertension, microalbuminuria or higher stages of CKD, dyslipidemia). In the remaining patients, the potential adverse effects from gastrointestinal bleeding offsets potential benefits of treatment [31]. Low-dose aspirin is strongly recommended for all patients who have previously experienced coronary heart disease, stroke, or suffer from chronic forms of large-vessel disease, including peripheral arterial occlusive disease [17]. Low-dose aspirin appears to be associated with an absolute risk of hemorrhagic stroke of one per 10000 people annually [31]. In primary prevention, a 15% additional CV risk reduction over that seen with antihypertensive treatment has been shown. The secondary prevention strategy results in a reduction in the incidence of vascular events of around 20% [17]. In hypertensive patients with CKD (estimated GFR <60 mL/min), the use of low-dose aspirin was also successful for primary prevention [32]. This may further support aspirin therapy, even if nephropathy occurs. The risk for bleeding is moderately increased.

Lipid lowering

Increased LDL or decreased HDL is considered to indicate dyslipidemia. In type 2 diabetes, dyslipidemia is characterized by elevated triglycerides and low HDL [33]. In several trials, the effects of LDL lowering were mostly studied. By meta-analysis of 14 randomized trials with a total of 90056 patients (21% diabetes, 62% with previous vascular disease), it was shown that lowering LDL reduced the 5-year incidence of coronary events, coronary revascularization, or stroke by about one-fifth per mmol/L reduction in LDL cholesterol [34]. Lipid-lowering drugs are recommended for primary and of course for secondary prevention in all patients having diabetes [35]. The use of statins in patients with diabetic nephropathy is discussed in depth in Chapter 8. The impact of fibric acid derivatives, such as peroxisome proliferator-activated receptor-α agonists, which raise HDL and lower triglycerides seems to be low in the light of statin treatment. In type 2 diabetes, there was no significant CV risk reduction in treatment with fenofibrate versus placebo [36]. In the Action to Control Cardiovascular Risk in Diabetes (ACCORD) lipid trial, the combination of simvastatin and fenofibrate was not better than simvastatin alone [37]. Niacin, another drug which increases HDL cholesterol and lowers triglycerides, can be considered at most as a second-line agent because of a variety of adverse effects [33]. Both substances, fibrate and niacin, should be monitored very careful, especially in CKD. In ESRD, lower cholesterol concentrations may be associated with a higher mortality as a result of malnutrition and chronic inflammation [38].

Antihypertensive treatment

Repeat measurement of systolic blood pressure ≥140 mmHg and/or a diastolic blood pressure of ≥90 mmHg confirms the diagnosis of arterial hypertension. In the general population, lowering of blood pressure to 115/75 mmHg is nearly linearly associated with reduced total and CV mortality [39]. The effect is detectable until old age (80–89 years). Patients with diabetes mellitus and patients having proteinuria profit from treatment with ACE inhibitors or ARBs. The ACE inhibitor perindopril (4 mg per day) together with the diuretic indapamide (1.25 mg per day) reduced the risk of major vascular events, including death, in patients with type 2 diabetes mellitus (26% with microalbuminuria) [40]. Renal protection by different antihypertensive strategies leads to a further CV risk reduction (see Chapter 15). After myocardial infarction, treatment with beta-blockers in combination with ACE inhibitors or ARBs is recommended, including patients with diabetes [41]. Beta-blockade in diabetes mellitus is safe. For blood pressure targets, there is a J-shaped curve. In type 2 diabetics at high risk for CV events, a systolic blood pressure target of less than 120 mmHg, compared with less than 140 mmHg, did not reduce the rate of fatal and non-fatal major CV events with the exception of stroke [42]. Thus, patients with type 2 diabetes should be treated for hypertension when their blood pressure is above 140 and/or 90 mmHg, aiming at a systolic BP well below this threshold but not below 120 mmHg [43]. Blood pressure therapy comprises dietary sodium restriction to no more than 2–3 g daily, only moderate alcohol intake, regular exercise, and weight loss in those with a body mass index >25 kg/m^2 (Table 7.2). Blood pressure should be monitored closely and home blood pressure measurements are recommended. Different treatment strategies are discussed in Chapter 15.

Management of diabetes in the face of vascular disease

Hyperglycemia is one marker for CV risk potentiation in diabetes. HbA1c reflects changes in glycemic control status over the previous 1–2

Table 7.2 Management of cardiovascular risk factors in advanced chronic kidney disease (GFR <60 mL/min)

Factor	Suggested activities
Follow-up	Estimation of GFR every 1–6 months, depends on progression, patients should be referred to a nephrologist
Diet	Sodium chloride restriction, at least ≤6 g/day, better ≤3 g/day
Smoking	Smoking cessation whenever possible
Exercise/weight	30–60 min moderate daily exercise, maintain BMI <25 kg/m^2, waist circumference <102 cm (men), <88 cm (women)
Hypertension	Target blood pressure <130/80 mmHg, treat with an ACE inhibitor or ARB, in addition with a loop diuretic, a beta-blocker, or a calcium channel blocker, or some combination
Proteinuria	Try to gain proteinuria <1 g/day, treat with an ACE inhibitor or ARB
Diabetes mellitus	Target HbA1c level <7% and fasting glucose between 5.0–8.9 mmol/L, avoid hypoglycemia
Dyslipidemia	Statin therapy is recommended in all patients, targets for LDL cholesterol should follow guidelines for the general population
Aspirin	Low-dose aspirin (75–100 mg daily) is recommended in patients with age >50 years if CV risk is high and if there is no contraindication to aspirin, add PPI if needed
Anemia	Iron supplementation is recommended, vitamin B12 and folic acid supplementation if needed, if Hb-target is not achieved, add ESA to gain a Hb level of 11–12 g/dL (6.8–7.5 mmol/L)
CKD-MBD	Maintain serum phosphorus in the normal range, supplement vitamin D if 25-hydroxyvitamin D levels fall <30 ng/mL, avoid hypercalcemia, if parathyroid hormone is still increased above twice the upper reference limit, consider treatment with active vitamin D, vitamin D analogues, or calcimimetics following current guidelines [52]

GFR, glomerular filtration rate; BMI, body-mass index; ACE, angiotensin converting enzyme; ARB, angiotensin II type 1-receptor blocker; LDL, low-density lipoprotein; Hb, hemoglobin; ESA, erythropoiesis-stimulating agents; HbA1c, glycosylated hemoglobin; PPI, proton pump inhibitor; CKD-MBD, chronic kidney disease-related mineral bone disorders.
Adapted from Abboud H, Henrich WL. Clinical practice. Stage IV chronic kidney disease. *N Engl J Med* 2010; **362**:56–65.

months. Since hypoglycemia also influences HbA1c levels, the quality of glucose-lowering treatment cannot be monitored by measuring HbA1c alone. Meta-analysis has shown that there is an increment in CV risk of around 18% per increase of 1 unit (%) HbA1c [44]. Intensive glycemic control resulted in a 15% reduction in events of coronary heart disease but had no significant effect on stroke or all-cause mortality [45]. In the ACCORD trial, the intensive glucose-lowering approach (HbA1c 6.4% versus 7.5% in standard therapy) increased mortality and did not reduce major CV events. Moreover, it led to higher rates of hypoglycemia, weight gain, and fluid retention [15]. The risk of severe hypoglycemia is doubled during intensive treatment. Thus, a clinical approach might be to reduce HbA1c concentration steadily and to avoid severe hypoglycemia [45]. The American Diabetes Association recommends an HbA1c goal of <7%. Less stringent HbA1c goals may be appropriate for patients with a history of severe hypoglycemia, limited life expectancy, advanced microvascular or macrovascular complications, or extensive comorbid conditions including longstanding diabetes [46]. Whether several oral or insulin therapies influence CV risk to a greater extent is questionable, since clinical intervention studies have focused mainly on glycemic control. Therapy with insulin, the sulfonylureas, and the thiazolidinediones is associated with weight gain, whereas metformin and the dipeptidyl-peptidase-4 inhibitors are considered weight neutral [47]. See also Chapters 13 and 14.

The challenge of nephropathy

In 2009, diabetes mellitus was the leading cause, by nearly 40%, for ESRD in the USA [48]. CV risk starts to increase early in CKD; patients with microalbuminuria are also affected [26] (Table 7.1). In ESRD, CV mortality is responsible for up to 45% of total mortality [49]. In CKD, conventional risk factors should be treated as described above. However, mortality in CKD often cannot be attributed to classical atherothrombotic events but rather to progressive congestive heart failure, sudden out of hospital death, lung edema, cardiac arrhythmias, or inflammatory complications [48]. In ESRD, sudden cardiac death is responsible for up to 62% of CV and around one-quarter of total mortality [48, 49]. Table 7.2 shows risk factors and consequences arising from CKD which should be considered during the care of patients with advanced CKD [50] (Figure 7.1). In addition, signs of progressive inflammation, malnutrition, or vascular disease should be noted and prompt diagnostic and therapeutic action carried out. The time point when renal replacement therapy needs to be initiated should be set very carefully. The K/DOQI and the upcoming K/DIGO guidelines give distinct recommendations for the management of patients with

CKD. Regarding treatment of renal anemia with erythropoiesis-stimulating agents (ESAs), reaching normal hemoglobin (Hb) levels did not result in better survival. Hence, therapy with ESA should not start until Hb falls below 10 g/dL. The Hb target level is 11–12 g/dL at a maximum; values above 13 g/dL should be avoided [51].

In the case of vitamin D deficiency, native vitamin D should be supplemented with a target 25-OH-vitamin D concentration of >30 ng/mL [52]. Hyperphosphatemia is another CV risk factor supporting calcification and endothelial damage [28]. In CKD, phosphate levels should be kept within the normal range by dietary measures and treatment with phosphate binders [52]. The use of calcium-free phosphate binders may be associated with better outcome, especially in patients with proven calcification [52]. These issues and the treatment of secondary hyperparathyreoidism will be discussed in Chapter 16. Metabolic acidosis in advanced CKD should also prompt therapeutic efforts. A serum bicarbonate concentration of ≥22 mmol/L is recommended. In order to minimize CV risk of patients with ESRD, renal transplantation should be considered whenever possible.

Coronary artery disease

CAD is accelerated in diabetes mellitus and CKD. Patients with known CAD and diabetes had a 75% rate of death over 10 years; up to 50% die 5 years after a myocardial infarction (MI) [33]. CAD in diabetes is often a silent disease without typical symptoms of angina pectoris. Symptoms of heart failure like dyspnea and physical stress insufficiency may occur alone. In cases suspicious for CAD, the diagnosis can be proven by the use of cardiac stress tests (i.e., ergometry, stress echocardiography, or myocardial perfusion scintigraphy).

If the diagnostic tests are positive, coronary angiography should be undertaken to assure the diagnosis and severity of CAD. Even if stress tests are negative, one cannot totally exclude relevant CAD, especially in diabetic patients with ESRD. Thus, diabetic patients eligible for renal transplantation should undergo pretransplant coronary angiography independently of age.

Based on diagnostic findings, the question needs to be answered whether intensive medical therapy is adequate (i.e., in the case of coronary sclerosis without relevant stenosis) or whether coronary revascularization is necessary. For revascularization, percutaneous coronary intervention (PCI) or coronary artery bypass grafting (CABG) are possible. There are two different conditions: treatment of chronic, symptomatic, or asymptomatic CAD without acute coronary syndrome (ACS) *and* treatment of ST segment elevation MI (STEMI), non-STEMI (NSTEMI), or unstable angina (UA) within ACS. In the last group, revascularization should be implemented to reduce morbidity and mortality [53]. Diabetic patients with ACS benefit from primary PCI. In selected cases with UA, or NSTEMI, revascularization can be carried out more deliberately if there is a prompt response to medical therapy, but angiographic assessment should be undertaken within 24 hours [53]. Patients with chronic CAD benefit from revascularization by CABG. However, advances in PCI techniques (i.e., drug-eluting stents) have made PCI a good alternative dependent on the extent of the disease. Mortality after PCI is comparable with that after CABG. However, the need for future revascularization procedures is greater after PCI [53]. Decision-making about the optimal treatment should be made by an interdisciplinary team consisting of cardiologists and cardiac surgeons. The individual perioperative risk, the future risk for major adverse cardiac events and a higher rate of cerebrovascular events in CABG should be taken into account. Patients with ACS should be controlled stringently to prevent hyper- and hypoglycemia [53].

Cerebrovascular disease

Similar to CAD, the risk for a cerebrovascular disease in diabetics is more than double that of non-diabetics. Diabetes and hyperglycemia predicted the future risk of ischemic stroke but not hemorrhagic stroke [54]. Efforts for the modulation of CV risk include the prevention of cerebrovascular disease too. Current guidelines advise lowering of blood glucose after stroke but disagree on the threshold or treatment targets. However, if glucose should be lowered, the prevention of hypoglycemia is important and requires strict monitoring. In patients with CKD at risk for vascular calcification, macrovascular changes like carotid stenosis should be considered as a source of cerebral embolism.

Peripheral arterial disease

Patients with diabetic nephropathy are at high risk for peripheral arterial disease (PAD). Ten years after the diagnosis of diabetes, the cumulative incidence of PAD was 15%, which had increased to 45% 20 years later [55]. Patients with PAD may be asymptomatic or may develop intermittent claudication or critical limb ischemia. Patients with PAD should be screened for CAD, since PAD predicts CAD. Diabetic PAD often affects distal limb vessel, such as the tibial and peroneal arteries. The potential for collateralization is limited [33]. In particular, vascular calcification worsens the options for revascularization. PAD should imply a consequent management of risk factors. In dialysis patients, a previous diagnosis of PAD, elevated serum phosphorus levels, and mean systolic blood pressure were the predictors of amputation within 2 years [56]. If distal ulcers are found, there is often uncertainty about the distinction between micro- or macrovascular disease. When there is doubt, angiographic screening is recommended. Patients with disabling claudication and those with critical limb ischemia (often diagnosed when ulcers or persistent foot infection occur) should undergo revascularization if treatable lesions are found. The decision about endovascular or open surgery depends on the severity and the localization of the lesions. Percutaneous iliac interventions in diabetic patients have been reported as similar to those in non-diabetic patients [57]. Nevertheless, the rate of foot or limb loss is high in diabetic patients, especially in those having diabetic nephropathy. Amputation rates following revascularization are much higher [57]. Mostly, non-healing ulcers, persistent foot infection, or necrosis oblige to the amputation. Additional microvascular changes are often jointly responsible for such an outcome.

Microvascular complications

Besides diabetic nephropathy, diabetic retinopathy and diabetic foot syndrome (DFS) are microvascular complications. In observational study, there was a strong association between the stage of CKD and DFS [58]. Diabetics with DFS undergo a higher rate of amputation. Besides screening for retino- and nephropathy, diabetic patients with CKD should be regularly screened for the presence of DFS aiming at the prevention of amputations [58]. Congestive heart failure in the absence of visible coronary heart disease can also be attributed to cardiac small-vessel disease as a microvascular complication (besides the possibility of hypertensive heart disease). Cognitive decline and its progression to vascular dementia results from microvascular disease and carotid stenosis.

1. Haffner SM, Lehto S, Ronnemaa T, *et al.* Mortality from coronary heart disease in subjects with type 2 diabetes and in nondiabetic subjects with and without prior myocardial infarction. *N Engl J Med* 1998;**339**:229–34.

2. Sarwar N, Gao P, Seshasai SR, *et al.* Diabetes mellitus, fasting blood glucose concentration, and risk of vascular disease: a collaborative meta-analysis of 102 prospective studies. *Lancet* 2010; **375**:2215–22.

3. Ford ES. Trends in the risk for coronary heart disease among adults with diagnosed diabetes in the U.S.: findings from the National Health and Nutrition Examination Survey, 1999–2008. *Diabetes Care* 2011;**34**:1337–43.

4. Adler AI, Stevens RJ, Manley SE, *et al.* Development and progression of nephropathy in type 2 diabetes: the United Kingdom Prospective Diabetes Study (UKPDS 64). *Kidney Int* 2003;**63**: 225–32.

5. Ross R. Atherosclerosis—an inflammatory disease. *N Engl J Med* 1999;**340**:115–26.

6. Hansson GK. Inflammation, atherosclerosis, and coronary artery disease. *N Engl J Med* 2005;**352**: 1685–95.

7. Pasterkamp G, Falk E, Woutman H, *et al.* Techniques characterizing the coronary atherosclerotic plaque: influence on clinical decision making? *J Am Coll Cardiol* 2000;**36**:13–21.

8. Davi G, Patrono C. Platelet activation and atherothrombosis. *N Engl J Med* 2007; **357**:2482–94.

9. Creager MA, Luscher TF, Cosentino F, *et al*. Diabetes and vascular disease: pathophysiology, clinical consequences, and medical therapy: Part I. *Circulation* 2003;**108**:1527–32.

10. Schiffrin EL, Lipman ML, Mann JF. Chronic kidney disease: effects on the cardiovascular system. *Circulation* 2007; **116**:85–97.

11. Levey AS, de Jong PE, Coresh J, *et al.* The definition, classification, and prognosis of chronic kidney disease: a KDIGO Controversies Conference report. *Kidney Int* 2011;**80**:17–28.

12. Pistrosch F, Natali A, Hanefeld M. Is hyperglycemia a cardiovascular risk factor? *Diabetes Care* 2011;**34**(Suppl 2): S128–31.

13. Brownlee M. Biochemistry and molecular cell biology of diabetic complications. *Nature* 2001;**414**:813–20.

14. Zoungas S, Patel A, Chalmers J, *et al.* Severe hypoglycemia and risks of vascular events and death. *N Engl J Med* 2010;**363**:1410–8.

15. Gerstein HC, Miller ME, Byington RP, *et al.* Effects of intensive glucose lowering in type 2 diabetes. *N Engl J Med* 2008; **358**:2545–59.

16. Ritz E, Wanner C. Lipid changes and statins in chronic renal insufficiency. *J Am Soc Nephrol* 2006;**17**:S226–30.

17. Colwell JA, Nesto RW. The platelet in diabetes: focus on prevention of ischemic events. *Diabetes Care* 2003;**26**:2181–8.

18. Busch M, Franke S, Ruster C, *et al.* Advanced glycation end-products and the kidney. *Eur J Clin Invest* 2010;**40**: 742–55.

19. Busch M, Franke S, Muller A, *et al.* Potential cardiovascular risk factors in chronic kidney disease: AGEs, total homocysteine and metabolites, and the C-reactive protein. *Kidney Int* 2004; **66**:338–47.

20. Schwedhelm E, Boger RH. The role of asymmetric and symmetric dimethylarginines in renal disease. *Nat Rev Nephrol* 2011;**7**:275–85.

21. Ridker PM, Danielson E, Fonseca FA, *et al.* Rosuvastatin to prevent vascular events in men and women with elevated C-reactive protein. *N Engl J Med* 2008; **359**:2195–207.

22. Fellstrom BC, Jardine AG, Schmieder RE, *et al.* Rosuvastatin and cardiovascular events in patients undergoing hemodialysis. *N Engl J Med* 2009; **360**:1395–407.

23. Lonn E, Yusuf S, Arnold MJ, *et al.* Homocysteine lowering with folic acid and B vitamins in vascular disease. *N Engl J Med* 2006;**354**:1567–77.

24. Heinz J, Kropf S, Domrose U, *et al.* B vitamins and the risk of total mortality and cardiovascular disease in end-stage renal disease: results of a randomized controlled trial. *Circulation* 2010;**121**: 1432–8.

25. Qin X, Huo Y, Langman CB, *et al.* Folic acid therapy and cardiovascular disease in ESRD or advanced chronic kidney disease: a meta-analysis. *Clin J Am Soc Nephrol* 2011;**6**:482–8.

26. Levin A. Clinical epidemiology of cardiovascular disease in chronic kidney disease prior to dialysis. *Semin Dial* 2003; **16**:101–5.

27. Amann K. Media calcification and intima calcification are distinct entities in chronic kidney disease. *Clin J Am Soc Nephrol* 2008;**3**:1599–605.

28. Toussaint ND, Kerr PG. Vascular calcification and arterial stiffness in chronic kidney disease: implications and management. *Nephrology (Carlton)* 2007; **12**:500–9.

29. Cozzolino M, Brandenburg V. Warfarin: to use or not to use in chronic kidney disease patients? *J Nephrol* 2010;**23**: 648–52.

30. Pilz S, Tomaschitz A, Drechsler C, *et al.* Vitamin D deficiency and heart disease. *Kidney International Supplements* 2011;**1**: 111–5.

31. Pignone M, Alberts MJ, Colwell JA, *et al.* Aspirin for primary prevention of cardiovascular events in people with diabetes: a position statement of the

American Diabetes Association, a scientific statement of the American Heart Association, and an expert consensus document of the American College of Cardiology Foundation. *Diabetes Care* 2010;**33**:1395–402.

32. Jardine MJ, Ninomiya T, Perkovic V, *et al*. Aspirin is beneficial in hypertensive patients with chronic kidney disease: a post-hoc subgroup analysis of a randomized controlled trial. *J Am Coll Cardiol* 2010;**56**: 956–65.

33. Luscher TF, Creager MA, Beckman JA, *et al*. Diabetes and vascular disease: pathophysiology, clinical consequences, and medical therapy: Part II. *Circulation* 2003;**108**:1655–61.

34. Baigent C, Keech A, Kearney PM, *et al*. Efficacy and safety of cholesterol-lowering treatment: prospective meta-analysis of data from 90,056 participants in 14 randomised trials of statins. *Lancet* 2005;**366**:1267–78.

35. Collins R, Armitage J, Parish S, *et al*. MRC/BHF Heart Protection Study of cholesterol-lowering with simvastatin in 5963 people with diabetes: a randomised placebo-controlled trial. *Lancet* 2003; **361**:2005–16.

36. Keech A, Simes RJ, Barter P, *et al*. Effects of long-term fenofibrate therapy on cardiovascular events in 9795 people with type 2 diabetes mellitus (the FIELD study): randomised controlled trial. *Lancet* 2005;**366**:1849–61.

37. Ginsberg HN, Elam MB, Lovato LC, *et al*. Effects of combination lipid therapy in type 2 diabetes mellitus. *N Engl J Med* 2010;**362**:1563–74.

38. Kalantar-Zadeh K, Block G, Humphreys MH, *et al*. Reverse epidemiology of cardiovascular risk factors in maintenance dialysis patients. *Kidney Int* 2003;**63**:793–808.

39. Lewington S, Clarke R, Qizilbash N, *et al*. Age-specific relevance of usual blood pressure to vascular mortality: a meta-analysis of individual data for one million adults in 61 prospective studies. *Lancet* 2002;**360**:1903–13.

40. Patel A, MacMahon S, Chalmers J, *et al*. Effects of a fixed combination of perindopril and indapamide on macrovascular and microvascular outcomes in patients with type 2 diabetes mellitus (the ADVANCE trial): a randomised controlled trial. *Lancet* 2007; **370**:829–40.

41. Califf RM, Lokhnygina Y, Velazquez EJ, *et al*. Usefulness of beta blockers in high-risk patients after myocardial infarction in conjunction with captopril and/or valsartan (from the VALsartan In Acute Myocardial Infarction [VALIANT] trial). *Am J Cardiol* 2009;**104**:151–7.

42. Cushman WC, Evans GW, Byington RP, *et al*. Effects of intensive blood-pressure control in type 2 diabetes mellitus. *N Engl J Med* 2010;**362**:1575–85.

43. Nilsson PM, Cifkova R, Treatment of hypertension in patients with type 2 diabetes mellitus. *European Society of Hypertension Scientific Newsletter: Update on Hypertension Management* 2011;**12**:No. 1R.

44. Selvin E, Marinopoulos S, Berkenblit G, *et al*. Meta-analysis: glycosylated hemoglobin and cardiovascular disease in diabetes mellitus. *Ann Intern Med* 2004; **141**:421–31.

45. Ray KK, Seshasai SR, Wijesuriya S, *et al*. Effect of intensive control of glucose on cardiovascular outcomes and death in patients with diabetes mellitus: a meta-analysis of randomised controlled trials. *Lancet* 2009;**373**:1765–72.

46. Skyler JS, Bergenstal R, Bonow RO, *et al*. Intensive glycemic control and the prevention of cardiovascular events: implications of the ACCORD, ADVANCE,

and VA diabetes trials: a position statement of the American Diabetes Association and a scientific statement of the American College of Cardiology Foundation and the American Heart Association. *Diabetes Care* 2009;**32**:187–92.

47. Ovalle F. Cardiovascular implications of antihyperglycemic therapies for type 2 diabetes. *Clin Ther* 2011;**33**:393–407.

48. USRDS. *2011 USRDS Annual Data Report: atlas of end-stage renal disease in the united states.* NIH, 2011:322.

49. Hage FG, Venkataraman R, Zoghbi GJ, *et al*. The scope of coronary heart disease in patients with chronic kidney disease. *J Am Coll Cardiol* 2009;**53**:2129–40.

50. Abboud H, Henrich WL. Clinical practice. Stage IV chronic kidney disease. *N Engl J Med* 2010;**362**:56–65.

51. Locatelli F, Aljama P, Canaud B, *et al*. Target haemoglobin to aim for with erythropoiesis-stimulating agents: a position statement by ERBP following publication of the Trial to reduce cardiovascular events with Aranesp therapy (TREAT) study. *Nephrol Dial Transplant* 2010;**25**:2846–50.

52. KDIGO clinical practice guideline for the diagnosis, evaluation, prevention, and treatment of Chronic Kidney Disease-Mineral and Bone Disorder (CKD-MBD). *Kidney Int Suppl* 2009;S1–130.

53. Sobel BE. Coronary revascularization in patients with type 2 diabetes and results of the BARI 2D trial. *Coron Artery Dis* 2010;**21**:189–98.

54. Hyvarinen M, Tuomilehto J, Mahonen M, *et al*. Hyperglycemia and incidence of ischemic and hemorrhagic stroke-comparison between fasting and 2-hour glucose criteria. *Stroke* 2009;**40**: 1633–7.

55. Melton LJ, 3rd, Macken KM, Palumbo PJ, *et al*. Incidence and prevalence of clinical peripheral vascular disease in a population-based cohort of diabetic patients. *Diabetes Care* 1980;**3**:650–4.

56. O'Hare AM, Bacchetti P, Segal M, *et al*. Factors associated with future amputation among patients undergoing hemodialysis: results from the Dialysis Morbidity and Mortality Study Waves 3 and 4. *Am J Kidney Dis* 2003;**41**:162–70.

57. Jude EB, Eleftheriadou I, Tentolouris N. Peripheral arterial disease in diabetes—a review. *Diabet Med* 2010;**27**:4–14.

58. Wolf G, Muller N, Busch M, *et al*. Diabetic foot syndrome and renal function in type 1 and 2 diabetes mellitus show close association. *Nephrol Dial Transplant* 2009;**24**:1896–901.

Statin therapy in patients with diabetic nephropathy

Christoph Wanner

University of Würzburg, Würzburg, Germany

> **Key points**
>
> - Meta-analyses have proven the principle that the relative risk reduction achieved by a certain absolute reduction in low-density lipoprotein (LDL) cholesterol is uniform independent of baseline LDL cholesterol values.
> - Therapy with statins reduces risk of major atherosclerotic events, at least in the early stages in patients with diabetic nephropathy.
> - In contrast, in later stages of the disease, two prospective, randomized, placebo-controlled trials in patients undergoing hemodialysis did not show a significant benefit of statins.
> - Some of the early benefits of statins may be independent of their LDL-lowering effects and due to pleiotropic mechanisms (e.g., reduction in inflammation).
> - By these mechanisms, statins may even slow the progression of diabetic nephropathy, as has been shown in certain trails.

Diabetes mellitus and chronic kidney disease (CKD) commonly occur together, and both are associated with an increased risk of vascular disease [1]. Cardiovascular events are a frequent cause of morbidity and mortality in this population. Both conditions are characterized by dyslipidemia, with raised levels of triglycerides and reduced levels of high-density lipoprotein (HDL) cholesterol but relatively preserved levels of LDL cholesterol. These lipid abnormalities seem particularly suited to being treated with fibric acid derivatives, which alter levels of triglycerides and HDL cholesterol more than they do levels of LDL cholesterol, the main target of statins. However statins have been investigated widely and lowering LDL cholesterol with statin-based therapies reduces risk of major atherosclerotic events, in

Diabetes and Kidney Disease, First Edition. Edited by Gunter Wolf.
© 2013 John Wiley & Sons, Ltd. Published 2013 by John Wiley & Sons, Ltd.

patients with CKD including those with diabetes [2, 3].

Patients receiving hemodialysis for chronic renal failure are at increased risk of cardiovascular events [4] as well. Previous studies in different patient populations showed that lowering LDL cholesterol with statin therapy reduces the incidence rate of cardiovascular events, with a greater benefit achieved in persons at high or very high risk. Although in earlier stages of CKD or in renal transplant recipients cholesterol lowering appears effective, this does not seem to be the case in later stages, such as in patients on dialysis. Two prospective, randomized, placebo-controlled trials in patients undergoing hemodialysis did not show a significant benefit of statins [5, 6]. In 2778 participants of the AURORA study (A Study to Evaluate the Use of Rosuvastatin in Subjects on Regular Hemodialysis: An Assessment of Survival and Cardiovascular Events), the administration of rosuvastatin (10 mg per day) during a median follow-up of 3.8 years did not reduce the primary end point of combined cardiovascular events. Similarly, in the 4D study (Die Deutsche Diabetes Dialyse Study), despite effective lowering of LDL cholesterol (38 mg/dL, 0.9 mmol/L, 42%), atorvastatin did not improve the incidence rate of the primary end point in 1255 hemodialysis patients with type 2 diabetes mellitus [5].

Macrovascular risk and atherogenic dyslipidemia

So-called atherogenic dyslipidemia is characterized by elevated triglycerides (TGs) and low HDL cholesterol, which are also predictors for cardiovascular disease (CVD), independent of LDL cholesterol. The Prospective Cardiovascular Münster (PROCAM) study assessed the non-LDL cholesterol-related dyslipidemia risk of myocardial infarction (MI) in 823 men with a first MI compared with 823 MI-free controls matched for sex, age, smoking, diabetes mellitus, blood pressure, and LDL cholesterol. Overall, the odds of MI in men with low HDL cholesterol (<1.15 mmol/L) were 2.6 times those of men with high HDL cholesterol ($\geq$1.15 mmol/L), and the odds of MI in men with high TGs ($\geq$ 1.71 mmol/L) were 1.4 times those of men with lower TG. If LDL cholesterol was <2.58 mmol/L, relative MI odds attributed to low HDL cholesterol increased to 3.4, whereas relative odds attributed to high TG increased to 2.6; men in this LDL category with low HDL cholesterol and/or high TG displayed an MI odds ratio of 5.0. MI risk associated with low HDL cholesterol and/or high TGs is substantial, particularly if LDL cholesterol is low [7].

In a recent meta-analysis of 29 prospective studies including 262 525 subjects of whom 10 158 were coronary heart disease (CHD) cases, the OR for coronary risk was 1.72 (95% CI 1.56–1.90) when individuals in the highest TG tertile were compared with those in the lowest tertile of usual log-TG values (corresponding to >178 versus <115 mg/dL), adjusted for major conventional CV risk factors including age, sex, smoking history, LDL cholesterol, and blood pressure [8].

Diabetic microvascular risk

Atherogenic dyslipidemia is also implicated in the pathogenesis of diabetic microvascular disease [9]. Elevated levels of TGs and TG-rich very low-density lipoprotein also appear to be closely involved in driving the progression of albuminuria [10]. In the United Kingdom Prospective Diabetes Study (UKPDS), elevated TGs were independently associated with incident microalbuminuria (HR 1.13, 95% CI 1.07–1.19, $p < 0.0001$) and macroalbuminuria (1.19, 95% CI 1.11–1.27, $p < 0.0001$) [11]. These data add to other findings that hypertriglyceridemia was a predictive factor for the development and progression of renal complications [12] and the need for future renal replacement therapy [13,

14]. Individuals with diabetes and without nephropathy have higher HDL cholesterol levels than those with nephropathy, suggesting the possibility that higher HDL cholesterol levels may be protective against the development of albuminuria [15–17].

A body of evidence supports the benefits of statin therapy in reducing the rate of decline in renal function. Meta-analysis of 27 studies involving 39 704 subjects showed that statin treatment significantly reduced the rate of decline in estimated glomerular filtration rate (eGFR) [1.22 (95% CI 0.44–2.00) mL/min/1.73 m^2 per year slower than with placebo, $p = 0.002$], equivalent to approximately 76% reduction [18]. Evidence from large prospective studies suggests that statins may reduce the rate of kidney function loss in subjects with or at risk of CVD. In the HPS (Heart Protection Study), treatment with simvastatin (40 mg/day) was associated with a significantly smaller decline in the eGFR in patients at high risk of CVD ($p = 0.0003$), and this effect was more marked among patients with diabetes [19]. The GREek Atorvastatin and Coronary heart disease Evaluation (GREACE) study also showed a modest improvement (12%) in kidney function over 4 years in 800 patients treated with atorvastatin, compared with a decrease by 4% in placebo patients [20]. Furthermore, combined analysis of three large prospective studies (WOSCOPS, CARE, and LIPID) showed that treatment with pravastatin reduced the adjusted rate of renal function loss by 8% and the risk of renal failure. In patients with CKD stages 2 and 3 at baseline, pravastatin reduced the adjusted rate of renal function loss by about 34%, although the absolute reduction in rate of loss was small [21]. The TNT (Treating to New Targets) study

showed that statin-related improvement in eGFR was significantly greater in patients treated with atorvastatin 80 mg than 10 mg daily [22]. Experimental evidence suggests that statins may alter the renal response to dyslipidemia via effects on inflammatory responses and endothelial function [23].

Preliminary analysis of SHARP (Study of Heart and Renal Protection) does not show a benefit of combination therapy of simvastatin/ezetimibe on progression of renal disease and incidence of end-stage renal disease.

Regarding proteinuria, analysis of 15 randomized trials in 1384 patients that evaluated the change in proteinuria or albuminuria, stratified by baseline urinary protein excretion, showed that statin treatment reduced albuminuria by 47% (95% CI 26–67%) and 48% (95% CI 25–71%) in people with baseline albuminuria ≥300 mg/dL and 30–299 mg/dL, respectively, but did not affect albuminuria when baseline levels were <30 mg/dL. However, the strength of these findings was limited by the quality, size, or design of the studies included in the analysis [24].

Multifactorial interventions

Current standards of care for primary and secondary CVD prevention emphasize the importance of multifactorial intervention to achieve recommended targets for LDL cholesterol which are often not met [25–30]. In the STENO-2 study intensive multifactorial intervention significantly reduced CV events during a mean of 7.8 years post-treatment follow-up (HR 0.47, 95% CI 0.24–0.73, $p = 0.008$) and CV mortality during a mean of 5.5 years (HR 0.43, 95% CI 0.19–0.94, $p = 0.04$), but failed to prevent the development or progression of microvascular disease in up to 50% of patients [31, 32].

Several studies indicate that significant CVD risk persists after treatment with statins [33–43]. Three recent meta-analyses of the Cholesterol

103

Treatment Trialists (CTT) collaborators including 90056 and 170000 subjects (18686 with diabetes) from 14 and 26 randomized trials reported that for each mmol/L lowering of LDL cholesterol statin therapy was effective in reducing the risk for major vascular events by 21%. Despite this, the residual risk of major vascular events over a 5-year period remained at 14% of patients experiencing a CV event [3, 44, 45]. Achieving new targets of 70mg/dL LDL cholesterol patients are left with a high residual risk [46, 47].

In patients with type 2 diabetes mellitus, nephropathy and/or established CVD atherogenic dyslipidemia, characterized by elevated TGs and a low plasma concentration of HDL cholesterol, often with elevated non-HDL cholesterol, is prevalent [48–50]. About two-thirds of statin-treated patients with CHD risk equivalents and well-controlled LDL cholesterol levels have low HDL cholesterol levels (<40mg/dL in men and <50mg/dL in women) [51]. Elevated TGs (>150mg/dL) is also common, affecting about 50% of adults with prior CVD [50].

Lifestyle modification such as traditional Mediterranean diets, dietary sodium, and exercise are cornerstones in the prevention and treatment of CVD, type 2 diabetes mellitus, the metabolic syndrome, and most likely also in patients with incipient diabetic nephropathy. Data to support pharmacologic intensification of blood glucose and blood pressure control are less than conclusive. In the Action in Diabetes and Vascular Disease: Preterax and Diamicron Modified Release Controlled Evaluation (ADVANCE) trial [52], intensive glycemic control versus conventional control reduced the incidence of combined microvascular and major macrovascular events by 10%, mainly due to a decrease in nephropathy (reduction in relative risk (RR) 21%, $p = 0.01$). ADVANCE also showed that intensive blood pressure lowering did not reduce the overall risk of microvascular events (RR reduction 9%, $p = 0.16$) [53]. Interim analysis of the ACCORD (Action to Control Cardiovascular Risk in Diabetes) study showed that intensive glycemic control (lowering HbA1c to a median of 6.4% versus 7.5% with conventional control) increased mortality (by 22%, $p = 0.04$) after a mean of 3.5 years of follow-up [54].

Although statins are effective in reducing non-HDL cholesterol and apolipoprotein B, effects on raising HDL cholesterol and lowering TG tend to be less impressive and dependent on dose and lipid phenotype. Although further reduction of LDL cholesterol can be achieved with inhibitors of cholesterol absorption, such as ezetimibe, other lipid-modifying therapies are usually needed for treatment of higher TG concentrations and low HDL cholesterol. Current treatment guidelines therefore recommend the addition of either a fibrate, niacin, or omega-3 fatty acids to achieve non-HDL targets in patients with atherogenic dyslipidemia and at high risk of CVD [25–30].

The ACCORD lipid trial [54] randomized 5518 high-risk type 2 diabetes patients at target for LDL cholesterol (~100mg/dL or ~2.6mmol/L at baseline decreasing to ~80mg/dL or ~2.0mmol/L on simvastatin, mean dose 22mg/day) to fenofibrate or placebo. Fenofibrate treatment lowered TG by 22% from baseline versus 8.7% with simvastatin alone, and raised HDL cholesterol by 8.4% versus 6.0% with simvastatin alone. The study failed to demonstrate a benefit for a composite of cardiovascular death, nonfatal MI, or non-fatal stroke. Fenofibrate significantly reduced the incidence of both microalbuminuria ($p = 0.01$) and macroalbuminuria ($p = 0.03$) versus simvastatin alone. Predefined subgroup analysis highlighted a group of patients with baseline TG levels ≥204mg/dL (2.3mmol/L) and HDL cholesterol levels ≤34 mg/dL (0.88 mmol/L) who received simvastatin alone. This group suffered 70% more primary end points than those without this lipid profile (17.3% versus 10.1%). Adding fenofibrate to simvastatin resulted in a 31% reduction in events (from 17.3% to 12.4%, absolute risk reduction 4.9%). The conclusion from ACCORD Lipid is that the extension of fibrate treatment is not appropriate with respect to cardiovascular outcomes. Unlike statins, it appears that fibrates lower cardiovascular events mainly in patients who have abnormal lipid levels at baseline, especially elevated TG and low levels of HDL cholesterol (i.e., atherogenic dyslipidemia) [55–58]. A conservative estimate of the percentage of type 2 diabetes patients with atherogenic dyslipidemia (TG ≥ 204 mg/dL and HDL cholesterol ≤34 mg/dL) is likely to be between 10% and 15%. The implication from ACCORD Lipid is that not all patients with type 2 diabetes benefit from dyslipidemia management beyond LDL cholesterol [59]. Combination treatment with fenofibrate-simvastatin was safe and well tolerated in the total study population, with no excess myopathy versus simvastatin monotherapy.

Improvements in CVD outcomes are now challenged by the impact of global epidemics of obesity, metabolic syndrome, and diabetes. Highlighting atherogenic dyslipidemia as a key modifiable factor contributing to residual macrovascular risk in statin-treated patients implicates this in the pathogenesis of microvascular residual risk in diabetes patients. Considering the evidence, the following actions should be addressed: (1) increase awareness of the extent and importance of residual vascular risk among the clinical community; (2) understand by research factors which contribute to the residual vascular risk remaining in dyslipidemic patients; (3) lifestyle modification is an important first step for reducing residual vascular risk; the strong potential of nutrition and exercise is not well appreciated and underutilized;

(4) optimal therapeutic intervention aimed at achievement of all lipid targets with the addition of niacin or a fibrate, or possibly omega-3-fatty acids for optimal statin therapy; (5) earlier intervention in the natural history of atherosclerosis, with lifestyle therapy and drug treatment as appropriate; and (6) multifactorial intervention involving lifestyle modification, combination therapy targeting all lipid goals, and tight control of blood pressure and glycemia as the optimal approach to reducing residual vascular risk in dyslipidemic patients. A recent position paper from two major ongoing studies, AIM-HIGH and HPS2-THRIVE, provides crucial information regarding the use of combination lipid-altering treatments in the future.

In the general population, meta-analyses of prospective trials of statins have revealed an approximately 25% reduction in cardiovascular events per 39 mg/dL (1 mmol/L) decrease in LDL cholesterol [2, 3, 44, 45]. Notably, these analyses have proven the principle that the relative risk reduction achieved by a certain absolute reduction in LDL cholesterol is uniform across all strata of baseline LDL cholesterol values.

In 2005, to the surprise of many, the results of the 4D study demonstrated that lowering LDL cholesterol with atorvastatin (20 mg/day) in 1255 hemodialysis patients with type 2 diabetes did not produce statistically significant reductions in the primary outcome measure [5]. Four years later, AURORA (A Study to Evaluate the Use of Rosuvastatin in Subjects on Regular Hemodialysis: An Assessment of Survival and Cardiovascular Events) 2 was hoped to provide clarification of whether LDL lowering with rosuvastatin (10 mg/day) would offer any benefit to 2776 hemodialysis patients [6]. Like 4D, the main results of AURORA were negative. In 2011 The Study of Heart and Renal Protection (SHARP) added new hope to the treatment expectations [60] similarly to the results in the Assessment of Lescol in Renal Transplant (ALERT) [61].

Die Deutsche Diabetes Dialyse Studie

The 4D study [5] was motivated by the recommendation regarding statin treatment in patients with type 2 diabetes on maintenance hemodialysis in the original 2003 KDOQI diabetes guideline [62]. In brief, 4 weeks of treatment with 20 mg/day of atorvastatin caused a reduction in the median level of LDL cholesterol by 42% among patients receiving atorvastatin, and among those receiving placebo it was reduced by 1.3%. During a median follow-up period of 4 years, 469 patients (37%) reached the primary end point, of whom 226 were assigned to atorvastatin and 243 to placebo (relative risk, 0.92; 95% CI 0.77–1.10; $p = 0.37$). Atorvastatin had no significant effect on the individual components of the primary end point, except that the relative risk of fatal stroke among those receiving the drug was 2.03 (95% confidence interval, 1.05–3.93; $p = 0.04$). Atorvastatin reduced the rate of all cardiac events combined (relative risk, 0.82; 95% confidence interval, 0.68–0.99; $p = 0.03$, nominally significant) but not all cerebrovascular events combined (relative risk, 1.12; 95% confidence interval, 0.81–1.55; $p = 0.49$) or total mortality (relative risk, 0.93; 95% confidence interval, 0.79–1.08; $p = 0.33$).

However, absolute reductions in LDL cholesterol produced by a given dose of a statin are larger at high than at low pretreatment concentrations. Accordingly, statin trials commonly show higher relative reductions in cardiovascular events at high baseline LDL cholesterol. We therefore hypothesized that the cardiovascular benefit of atorvastatin was greater at higher baseline LDL cholesterol in 4D. Furthermore, we aimed to determine the effect of baseline LDL cholesterol on the incidence rate of future cardiovascular events. In particular, we intended to assess whether the association between baseline LDL cholesterol and adverse outcomes differed between the treatment groups, as it has been demonstrated in previous studies. In this *post hoc* analysis of the 4D trial [63], we found that fatal and non-fatal cardiac events were significantly reduced if the pretreatment LDL cholesterol was >145 mg/dL. Although *post hoc* analyses provide a different look at the data from the previous studies, they must be viewed as hypothesis generating, and, therefore, do not alter the main message of the guideline update, which is based on the primary prespecified outcomes from these clinical trials.

AURORA

Concerns that the results of 4D were attributable to the futility of a single intervention in such high-risk patients inspired AURORA [6]. AURORA, a clinical trial that randomized 2776 patients on hemodialysis to rosuvastatin 10 mg a day and placebo. Only 26% of the patients in AURORA had diabetes. As found in 4D, AURORA reported no significant effect of statin therapy on the primary cardiovascular outcome that included cardiac death or non-fatal myocardial infarction and fatal or non-fatal stroke, either in the overall study population or in the subgroup of patients with diabetes. After 3 months, the mean reduction in LDL cholesterol levels was 43% in patients receiving rosuvastatin, from a mean baseline level of 100 mg/ dL (2.6 mmol/L). During a median follow-up period of 3.8 years, 396 patients in the rosuvastatin group and 408 patients in the placebo group reached the primary end point (9.2 and 9.5 events per 100 patient-years, respectively; hazard ratio for the combined end point in the rosuvastatin group versus the placebo group,

0.96; 95% CI 0.84–1.11; $p = 0.59$). Rosuvastatin had no effect on individual components of the primary end point. There was also no significant effect on all-cause mortality (13.5 versus 14.0 events per 100 patient-years; hazard ratio 0.96; 95% CI 0.86–1.07; $p = 0.51$).

Recently, Holdaas et al. [64] in a *post hoc* analysis of AURORA focused on a subgroup of 731 hemodialysis patients who had diabetes. In this analysis rosuvastatin significantly reduced the rates of cardiac events combined [cardiac death and non-fatal myocardial infarction (MI)] by 32% (HR 0.68; 95% CI 0.51–0.90). Analyzing the original AURORA primary end point (death from cardiovascular causes, non-fatal MI, or non-fatal stroke) in AURORA-diabetes, patients showed a larger, albeit non-significant, 16% RR reduction (HR 0.84; 95% CI 0.65–1.07). For comparison, an 8% non-significant RR reduction for the primary end point (HR 0.92; 95% CI 0.77–1.1) was observed in the 4D study. Holdaas et al. [64] built the rationale of their analysis on the results of a secondary end point of the 4D study (all cardiac events combined) with a nominal significant reduction by 18% (RR 0.82; 95% CI 0.68–0.99). This is similar to the 22% relative reduction in MI or coronary death (HR 0.78; 95% CI 0.69–0.87) obtained in the Cholesterol Treatment Trialists (CTT) meta-analysis six of 18 686 people with diabetes from 14 randomized statin trials. In assessing an anti-atherosclerotic therapy, it would be most logical to examine an end point including non-fatal events such as coronary revascularization and/or ischemic stroke, which are clearly affected by LDL lowering. It would even be more logical in a population such as dialysis patients, in whom there remains uncertainty about the relative contributions of structural heart disease and coronary disease to cardiac death. Thus, it seems reasonable to have chosen both cardiac and cerebrovascular events to be represented within the primary end point. One might vote for picking out

hemorrhagic strokes from the primary end point and also non-atherosclerotic cardiac events. In AURORA, the risk for non-fatal stroke was not significantly higher in the active arm, and the effect of treatment, although not significantly different by subgroup of baseline diabetic status, was shifted toward benefit in patients with diabetes (12.6% versus 15.1%). So, in hindsight, if one wanted to go in search of a significant benefit, it would be interesting to investigate cardiac events in patients with diabetes. Interpretation of any *post hoc* analysis should be treated with caution and is at best hypothesis generating rather than hypothesis testing. An interesting observation was that rosuvastatin affected cardiac events but not stroke. The evidence from the general population (CTT meta-analysis) is that lipid lowering significantly reduces the risk for development of several different manifestations of atherosclerosis (coronary disease, ischemic stroke, coronary revascularizations) and that the significant effects on a combination of these vascular end points are consistent in patients with mildly to moderately reduced GFR and in those with normal GFR (CTT webfigure 10). Therefore, one would expect that ischemic stroke would be reduced by LDL cholesterol lowering, but Holdaas et al. [64] do not include this in their *post hoc* analysis. It is possible that, as for 4D, the increased rate of stroke observed in the main results is just chance, but its lack of inclusion here is surprising. Holdaas et al. suggest that end point choice is arbitrary. Rather, it has been defined as follows: "The primary variable should be the variable capable of providing the most clinically relevant and convincing evidence directly related to the primary objective of the trial." I admit that choosing the appropriate outcome measures in clinical trials is difficult, and even more difficult and with certain variability is the outcome adjudication. Meta-analysis data from 170 000 participants in large-scale statin trials found statins to reduce the risk for ischemic strokes by 16% (HR 0.84; 95% CI 5–26). In SHARP, LDL cholesterol was lowered by an average of 33 mg/dL, which produced a reduction of 19% in total stroke (HR 0.81; 95% CI 0.66–0.99), driven by a 28% reduction in ischemic stroke. There was an excess of hemorrhagic stroke (HR 1.21; 95% CI 0.78–1.86). AURORA-diabetes showed an excess of hemorrhagic stroke as well (HR 5.21;95% CI 1.17–23.3), but the result is not in keeping with the 4D study (eight versus five hemorrhagic strokes in placebo versus active), which included more patients with diabetes and followed them for longer. Is this a concern, and should this discourage the use of statins in dialysis patients? A recent meta-analysis suggested that statins might increase the risk for hemorrhagic stroke, but this increase is of the order of 20%, and because the risk for ischemic stroke in most populations is substantially higher, the absolute effect on all stroke is beneficial. Nevertheless, the small number of events (two versus 12) in this analysis means that this result should be interpreted with caution. The evidence would be stronger if all of the available evidence were included in a meta-analysis of the individual data from AURORA, 4D and the dialysis patients in SHARP. This might have enough events to assess reliably the effects of statin therapy in patients both with and without diabetes on coronary events as well as stroke.

SHARP

The SHARP trial [60] randomized 9270 participants ≥40 years old with CKD (mean eGFR of 27 mL/min/1.73 m²) to receive simvastatin 20 mg plus ezetimibe 10 mg daily or placebo, and followed them for 5 years. Thirty-three percent of the patients (n = 3023) were receiving maintenance dialysis at randomization and 23% (n = 2094) of the participants had diabetes, with equal proportions in the simvastatin plus ezetimibe and placebo groups. Allocation to ezetimibe/simvastatin yielded an average

LDL cholesterol difference of 0.85 mmol/L (with about two-thirds compliance) during a median follow-up of 4.9 years, and produced a 17% proportional reduction in major atherosclerotic events [526 (11.3%) ezetimibe/simvastatin versus 619 (13.4%); RR 0.83, 95% CI 0.74–0.94; log rank p = 0.0022]. There was a non-significant reduction in non-fatal myocardial infarction or coronary death [213 (4.6%) versus 230 (5.0%); RR 0.92, 95% CI 0.76–1.11; p = 0.37], and significant reductions in non-hemorrhagic stroke [131 (2.8%) versus 174 (3.8%); RR 0.75, 95% CI 0.60–0.94; p = 0.01] and revascularization procedures [284 (6.1%) versus 352 (7.6%); RR 0.79, 95% CI 0.68–0.93; p = 0.0036]. Among the patients with CKD not treated by dialysis at randomization (n = 6247), treatment with simvastatin plus ezetimibe did not reduce the frequency of doubling of the baseline serum creatinine concentration or progression to end-stage renal disease. Although the study was not powered to reliably estimate the effect of treatment on primary outcomes among clinical subgroups, the proportional effect on major atherosclerotic events did not appear to differ between those with or without diabetes.

ALERT

The ALERT trial [61] examined the effect of statin therapy on cardiovascular risk reduction in 2102 patients with functioning kidney transplants who were followed for 5–6 years. Fluvastatin therapy (40–80 mg/day), compared with placebo, was associated with a significant 35% relative reduction in the risk of cardiac death or definite non-fatal myocardial infarction, HR = 0.65 (95% CI 0.48–0.88). The study included a prespecified analysis for a subset of 396 patients with diabetes, of whom 197 were randomized to fluvastatin and 199 to placebo. In this subset, the benefit was similar in magnitude as in the overall cohort, but was not statistically significant, HR = 0.71 (95% CI

0.41–1.21), suggesting limitations of under-powering due to small sample size. Given these limitations and the lack of a significant interaction between diabetes and treatment assignment for the primary outcome, the Work Group based its recommendation for statin treatment in kidney transplant patients on the overall results from the ALERT study.

Accordingly, the evidence that treatment with statin or statin/ezetimibe combination improves health outcomes is based primarily on prevention of CVD events. There is no evidence from these trials that such treatment improves kidney disease outcomes, including doubling of serum creatinine or progression to end stage renal disease.

The original 2003 Kidney Disease Outcomes Quality Initiative (KDOQI) recommendations were based largely on four *post hoc* analyses [62] that reported results of lipid-lowering therapy for a subpopulation of patients with CKD and diabetes compared with placebo. The recent 2012 KDOQI diabetes guideline [65] summarizes the four randomized controlled trials and recommended using LDL cholesterol-lowering medicines, such as statins or statin/ezetimibe combination, to reduce risk of major atherosclerotic events in patients with diabetes and CKD, including those who have received a kidney transplant. Based on these data the recent KDOQI guidelines do not recommend initiating statin therapy in patients with diabetes who are treated by dialysis.

Possible rationale of guideline statements

The SHARP trial [60] indicated that risk for the primary outcome of major atherosclerotic events other than death was reduced by simvastatin/ezitimibe combination among a wide range of patients with CKD. Yet, the "subgroup" of over 3000 patients on dialysis did not show a statistically significant reduction in risk of the primary outcome. The SHARP investigators advocate that this group is still likely to benefit because of lack of statistical heterogeneity. However, even as a subgroup, this is still the largest trial of LDL cholesterol lowering conducted to date in patients on dialysis. Taking into account the 4D and AURORA trials along with the SHARP data, overall evidence to support a favorable effect of initiating LDL cholesterol-lowering treatment on atherosclerotic events in dialysis patients is lacking. Moreover, since most of the clinical CVD events experienced by hemodialysis patients with diabetes are vascular deaths, for which statins provide little or no benefit as illustrated in the SHARP trial [60].

A recent meta-analysis concluded that the available evidence continues to support the recommendation that statin therapy not be initiated in dialysis patients, especially with diabetes. Whether previously treated patients should be continued on statin therapy once they commence dialysis, or not, has not been studied, and, as such, data are insufficient to provide guidance for this group.

With the exception of SHARP, data to support recommendations for LDL cholesterol lowering come from *post hoc* subgroup analyses of clinical trials that included CKD patients with and without diabetes. Nevertheless, a growing body of evidence demonstrates a clear benefit of statin therapy on clinical CVD events among patients with diabetes and across a wide range of CKD stages, perhaps with the exception of those on dialysis.

Of note, the results of the AdDIT trial (Adolescent type 1 diabetes mellitus cardio-renal Intervention Trial) are awaited, and will provide data on the effectiveness of atorvastatin and quinalapril to prevent cardiovascular and kidney complications in adolescents with type 1 diabetes.

Special considerations

Reduced dosing of statins is generally recommended for patients with advanced CKD. On the other hand, increased dosing of statin therapy may be beneficial in some patients with diabetes and CKD. The TNT trial [66] reported a benefit for secondary prevention of major cardiovascular events from treatment with atorvastatin 80 mg/day compared with atorvastatin 10 mg/day in 546 patients with diabetes and CKD and pre-existing coronary artery disease over 5 years of follow-up. The risk of stroke was 4.8% (13/273) for the higher dose, compared with 7.3% (20/271) for the lower dose. There was no reduction in all-cause mortality. Higher statin doses, however, are associated with an increased risk of myopathy particularly among patients with reduced kidney function, signifying that treatment regimens require modification in advanced CKD. Therefore, reliance less on higher dosing of statins and more on combination therapy to reduce LDL cholesterol is an attractive strategy. The SHARP trial [60] addressed this issue by using lower dose simvastatin (20 mg/day) and adding the cholesterol absorption inhibitor ezetimibe (10 mg/day) to achieve an average LDL cholesterol reduction of about 1 mmol/L. Of note, the US FDA issued a Safety Announcement in June 2011 that recommends limited use of the highest approved dose of simvastatin (80 mg) because of increased risk of myopathy. Simvastatin 80 mg should be used only in patients who have been taking this dose for 12 months or more without evidence of muscle injury. Simvastatin 80 mg should not be started in new patients, including patients already taking lower doses of the drug. In addition to these new limitations, the FDA requires changes to the simvastatin label to add new contraindications (concurrent ciclosporin or gemfibrozil use) and dose limitations for use with other medicines such as calcium channel blockers or amiodarone. Further information can be obtained at the FDA website (fda.gov/Drugs/DrugSafety).

Perspectives

The best treatment efforts to reduce LDL cholesterol are saving substantial numbers of lives. However, type 2 diabetes mellitus patients with chronic kidney disease still experience progression of CVD. Even with intensifying statin therapy, residual cardiovascular risk remains, and atherogenic dyslipidemia is an important driver of this so-called residual risk in early stages of kidney disease. New strategies evaluate the role of intensive combination lipid treatment for the entire type 2 diabetic population above eGFR of 60 mL/min/1.73 m^2. The link between dyslipidemia treatment and diabetic retinopathy, nephropathy, and neuropathy is an emerging new field and microvascular complications are targets for new treatments.

References

1. Booth GL, Kapral MK, Fung K, Tu JV. Recent trends in cardiovascular complications among men and women with and without diabetes. *Diabetes Care* 2006;**29**:32–7.
2. Kearney PM, Blackwell L, Collins R, Keech A, Simes J, Peto R, Armitage J, Baigent C. Cholesterol Treatment Trialists' (CTT) Collaborators: Efficacy of cholesterol-lowering therapy in 18,686 people with diabetes in 14 randomised trials of statins: A meta-analysis. *Lancet* 2008;**371**:117–25.
3. Baigent C, Blackwell L, Emberson J, *et al.*, Cholesterol Treatment Trialists' (CTT) Collaborators: Efficacy and safety of more intensive lowering of LDL cholesterol: A meta-analysis of data from 170,000 participants in 26 randomised trials. *Lancet* 2010;**376**:1670–81.

4. Foley RN, Parfrey PS, Sarnak MJ. Clinical epidemiology of cardiovascular disease in chronic renal disease. *Am J Kidney Dis* 1998;**32**:112–19.

5. Wanner C, Krane V, März W, *et al.*, German Diabetes and Dialysis Study Investigators: Atorvastatin in patients with type 2 diabetes mellitus undergoing hemodialysis. *N Engl J Med* 2005;**353**:238–48.

6. Fellstrom BC, Jardine AG, Schmieder RE, *et al.*, AURORA Study Group: Rosuvastatin and cardiovascular events in patients undergoing hemodialysis. *N Engl J Med* 2009;**360**:1395–407.

7. Assmann G, Cullen P, Schulte H. Non-LDL-related dyslipidaemia and coronary risk: a case–control study. *Diab Vasc Dis Res* 2010;**7**:204–12.

8. Sarwar N, Danesh J, Eiriksdottir G, *et al.* Triglycerides and the risk of coronary heart disease: 10,158 incident cases among 262,525 participants in 29 Western prospective studies. *Circulation* 2007;**115**:450–8.

9. Jenkins AJ, Rowley KG, Lyons TJ, *et al.* Lipoproteins and diabetic microvascular complications. *Curr Pharm Des* 2004;**10**:3395–18.

10. Caramori ML, Fioretto P, Mauer M. The need for early predictors of diabetic nephropathy risk: is albumin excretion rate sufficient? *Diabetes* 2000;**49**:1399–408.

11. Retnakaran R, Cull CA, Thorne KI, *et al.*, UKPDS Study Group. Risk factors for renal dysfunction in type 2 diabetes: U.K. Prospective Diabetes Study 74. *Diabetes* 2006;**55**:1832–39.

12. Hadjadj S, Duly-Bouhanick B, Bekherraz A, *et al.* Serum triglycerides are a predictive factor for the development and the progression of renal and retinal complications in patients with type 1 diabetes. *Diabetes Metab* 2004;**30**:43–51.

13. Cusick M, Chew EY, Hoogwerf B, *et al*, Early Treatment Diabetic Retinopathy Study Research Group. Risk factors for renal replacement therapy in the Early Treatment Diabetic Retinopathy Study (ETDRS). ETDRS 26. *Kidney Int* 2004;**66**:1173–9.

14. Smulders Y, Rakic M, Stehouwer C, *et al.* Determinants of progression of microalbuminuria in patients with NIDDM: a prospective study. *Diabetes Care* 1997;**20**:999–1005.

15. Chaturvedi N, Fuller JH, Taskinen M-R, EURODIAB PCS Group. Differing associations of lipid and lipoprotein disturbances with the macrovascular and microvascular complications of type 1 diabetes. *Diabetes Care* 2001;**24**:2071–7.

16. Jenkins AJ, Lyons TJ, Zheng D, *et al*, Klein RL, DCCT/EDIC Research Group. Lipoproteins in the DCCT/EDIC Research Group: associations with diabetic nephropathy. *Kidney Int* 2003;**64**:817–28.

17. Molitch ME, Rupp D, Carnethon M. Higher levels of HDL cholesterol are associated with a decreased likelihood of albuminuria in patients with long-standing type 1 diabetes. *Diabetes Care* 2006;**29**:78–82.

18. Sandhu S, Wiebe N, Fried LF, Tonelli M. Statins for improving renal outcomes: a meta-analysis. *J Am Soc Nephrol* 2006;**17**:2006–16.

19. HPS Collaborative Group. MRC/BHF Heart Protection Study of cholesterol-lowering with simvastatin in 5963 people with diabetes: a randomised placebo-controlled trial. *Lancet* 2003;**361**:2005–16.

20. Athyros VG, Mikhailidis DP, Papageorgiou AA, *et al.* The effect of statins versus untreated dyslipidaemia on renal function in patients with coronary heart disease. A subgroup analysis of the Greek atorvastatin and coronary heart disease

evaluation (GREACE) study. *J Clin Pathol* 2004;**57**:728–34.

21. Tonelli M, Isles C, Craven T, *et al*. Effect of pravstatin on rate of kidney function loss in people with or at risk for coronary disease. *Circulation* 2005;**112**:171–8.

22. Shepherd J, Kastelein JJ, Bittner V, *et al*., Treating to New Targets Investigators. Effect of intensive lipid lowering with atorvastatin on renal function in patients with coronary heart disease: the Treating to New Targets (TNT) study. *Clin J Am Soc Nephrol* 2007;**2**:1131–9.

23. Campese VM, Park J. HMG-CoA reductase inhibitors and the kidney. *Kidney Int* 2007;**71**:1215–22.

24. Douglas K, O'Malley PG, Jackson JL. Meta-analysis: the effect of statins on albuminuria. *Ann Intern Med* 2006;**145**:117–24.

25. National Cholesterol Education Program (NCEP) Expert Panel on Detection, Evaluation, and Treatment of High Blood Cholesterol in Adults (Adult Treatment Panel III). Third Report of the National Cholesterol Education Program (NCEP) Expert Panel on Detection, Evaluation, and Treatment of High Blood Cholesterol in Adults (Adult Treatment Panel III). Final report. *Circulation* 2002;**106**:3143–421.

26. American Diabetes Association. Standards of medical care in diabetes-2008. *Diabetes Care* 2008;**31**(Suppl 1):S12–S54.

27. Smith SC Jr, Allen J, Blair SN, *et al*. AHA/ACC guidelines for secondary prevention for patients with coronary and other atherosclerotic vascular disease: 2006 update: endorsed by the National Heart, Lung, and Blood Institute. *Circulation* 2006;**113**:2363–72.

28. Buse JB, Ginsberg HN, Bakris GL, *et al*., American Diabetes Association. Primary prevention of cardiovascular diseases in people with diabetes mellitus. A Scientific Statement from the American Heart Association and the American Diabetes Association. *Circulation* 2007;**115**:114–26.

29. Fourth Joint Task Force of the European Society of Cardiology and Other Societies on Cardiovascular Disease Prevention in Clinical Practice (constituted by representatives of nine societies and by invited experts). Graham I, Atar D, Borch-Johnsen K, *et al*. European guidelines on cardiovascular disease prevention in clinical practice: executive summary. *Eur Heart J* 2007;**28**:2375–414.

30. Rydén L, Standl E, Bartnik M, *et al*., Task Force on Diabetes and Cardiovascular Diseases of the European Society of Cardiology (ESC): European Association for the Study of Diabetes (EASD). Guidelines on diabetes, pre-diabetes, and cardiovascular disease: executive summary. The Task Force on Diabetes and Cardiovascular Diseases of the European Society of Cardiology (ESC) and of the European Association for the Study of Diabetes (EASD). *Eur Heart J* 2007;**28**:88–136.

31. Gaede P, Vedel P, Larsen N, *et al*. Multifactorial intervention and cardiovascular disease in patients with type 2 diabetes. *N Engl J Med*. 2003;**348**:383–93.

32. Gaede P, Lund-Andersen H, Parving HH, Pedersen O. Effect of a multifactorial intervention on mortality in type 2 diabetes. *N Engl J Med* 2008;**358**:580–591.

33. Randomised trial of cholesterol lowering in 4444 patients with coronary heart disease: the Scandinavian Simvastatin Survival Study (4S). *Lancet* 1994;**344**:1383–9.

34. Sacks FM, Pfeffer MA, Moye LA, *et al*. The effect of pravastatin on coronary events after myocardial infarction in patients with average cholesterol levels. *N Engl J Med* 1996;**335**:1001–9.

35. The Long-term Intervention with Pravastatin in Ischaemic Disease (LIPID) Study Group. Prevention of cardiovascular events and death with pravastatin in patients with coronary heart disease and a broad range of initial cholesterol levels. N Engl J Med 1998;**339**:1349–57.

36. Heart Protection Study Collaborative Group. MRC/BHF Heart Protection Study of cholesterol lowering with simvastatin in 20 536 high-risk individuals: a randomised placebo-controlled trial. Lancet 2002;**360**:7–22.

37. Shepherd J, Blauw GJ, Murphy MB, et al., Westerndorp RG, PROSPER study group. Pravastatin in elderly individuals at risk of vascular disease (PROSPER): a randomised controlled trial. Lancet 2002;**360**:1623–30.

38. Sever PSS, Dahlöf B, Poulter N, et al., ASCOT Investigators. Prevention of coronary and stroke events with atorvastatin in hypertensive patients who have average or lower-than-average cholesterol concentrations, in the Anglo-Scandinavian Cardiac Outcomes Trial-Lipid Lowering Arm (ASCOT-LLA): a multicentre randomised controlled trial. Lancet 2003;**361**:1149–58.

39. The ALLHAT Officers and Coordinators for the ALLHAT Collaborative Research Group. Major outcomes in moderately hypercholesterolemic, hypertensive patients randomized to pravastatin vs usual care: the Antihypertensive and Lipid-Lowering Treatment to Prevent Heart Attack (ALLHAT-LLT). JAMA 2002;**288**:2998–3007.

40. Knopp RH, D'Emden M, Smilde JG, Pocock SJ. Efficacy and safety of atorvastatin in the prevention of cardiovascular end points in subjects with type 2 diabetes. The Atorvastatin Study for Prevention of Coronary Heart Disease Endpoints in Non-Insulin-Dependent Diabetes Mellitus (ASPEN). Diabetes Care 2006;**29**:1478–85.

41. Shepherd J, Cobbe SM, Ford I, et al. Prevention of coronary heart disease with pravastatin in men with hypercholesterolemia. N Engl J Med 1995;**333**:1301–7.

42. Downs JR, Clearfield M, Weis S, et al. Primary prevention of acute coronary events with lovastatin in men and women with average cholesterol levels: results of AFCAPS/TexCAPS. Air Force/Texas Coronary Atherosclerosis Prevention Study. JAMA 1998;**279**:1615–22.

43. Colhoun HM, Betteridge DJ, Durrington PN, et al., CARDS Investigators. Primary prevention of cardiovascular disease with atorvastatin in type 2 diabetes in the Collaborative Atorvastatin Diabetes Study (CARDS): multicentre randomised placebo-controlled trial. Lancet 2004;**364**:685–96.

44. Baigent C, Keech A, Kearney PM, et al., Cholesterol Treatment Trialists' (CTT) Collaborators. Efficacy and safety of cholesterol-lowering treatment: prospective meta-analysis of data from 90 056 participants in 14 randomised trials of statins. Lancet 2005;**366**: 1267–78.

45. Cholesterol Treatment Trialists' (CTT) Collaborators, Kearney PM, Blackwell PM, Collins R, et al. Efficacy of cholesterol-lowering therapy in 18,686 people with diabetes in 14 randomised trials of statins: a meta-analysis. Lancet 2008;**371**:117–25.

46. LaRosa JC, Grundy SM, Waters DD, et al., Treating to New Targets (TNT) Investigators. Intensive lipid lowering with atorvastatin in patients with stable coronary disease. N Engl J Med 2005;**352**:1425–35.

47. Cannon CP, Braunwald E, McCabe *et al.*, Pravastatin or Atorvastatin Evaluation and Infection Therapy-Thrombolysis in Myocardial Infarction-22 Investigators. Intensive versus moderate lipid lowering with statins after acute coronary syndromes. *N Engl J Med* 2004; **350**: 1495–504.

48. Yusuf S, Hawken S, Ounpuu S, *et al.*, INTERHEART Study Investigators. Effect of potentially modifiable risk factors associated with myocardial infarction in 52 countries (the INTERHEART study): case-control study. *Lancet* 2004; **364**:937–52.

49. Austin MA, King MC, Vranizan KM, Krauss RM. Atherogenic lipoprotein phenotype. A proposed genetic marker for coronary heart disease risk. *Circulation* 1990;**82**:495–506.

50. Ninomiya JK, L'Italien G, Criqui MH, *et al.* Association of the metabolic syndrome with history of myocardial infarction and stroke in the Third National Health and Nutrition Examination Survey. *Circulation* 2004;**109**:42–6.

51. Alsheikh-Ali AA, Lin J-L, Abourjaily P, *et al.* Prevalence of low high-density lipoprotein cholesterol in patients with documented coronary heart disease or risk equivalent and controlled low-density lipoprotein cholesterol. *Am J Cardiol* 2007;**100**:1499–501.

52. The Advance Collaborative Group. Intensive blood glucose control and vascular outcomes in patients with type 2 diabetes. *N Engl J Med* 2008;**358**: 2560–72.

53. ADVANCE Collaborative Group; Patel A, MacMahon S, Chalmers J, *et al.* Effects of a fixed combination of perindopril and indapamide on macrovascular and microvascular outcomes in patients with type 2 diabetes mellitus (the ADVANCE trial): a randomised controlled trial. *Lancet* 2007;**370**:829–40.

54. The Action to Control Cardiovascular Risk in Diabetes Study Group. Effects of intensive glucose lowering in type 2 diabetes. *N Engl J Med* 2008;**358**: 2545–59.

55. Manninen V, Tenkanen L, Koskinen P, *et al.* Joint effects of serum triglyceride and LDL cholesterol and HDL cholesterol concentrations on coronary heart disease risk in the Helsinki Heart Study. Implications for treatment. *Circulation* 1992;**85**;37–45.

56. Robins SJ, Collins D, Wittes JT, *et al* for the VA-HIT Study Group. Relation of gemfibrozil treatment and lipid levels with major coronary events. *JAMA* 2001;**285**:1585–91.

57. The BIP Study Group. Secondary prevention by raising HDL cholesterol and reducing triglycerides in patients with coronary artery disease. The Bezafibrate Infarction Prevention (BIP) study. *Circulation* 2000;**102**: 21–7.

58. Scott R, O'Brien R, Fulcher G, *et al.* The effects of fenofibrate treatment on cardiovascular disease risk in 9795 people with type 2 diabetes and various components of the metabolic syndrome: the FIELD study. *Diabetes Care* 2009; **32**:493–8.

59. The ACCORD Study Group. Effects of combination lipid therapy in type 2 diabetes mellitus. *N Eng J Med* 2010;**362**: 1563–74.

60. Baigent C, Landray MJ, Reith C, *et al.*, on behalf of the SHARP Investigators. The effects of lowering LDL cholesterol with simvastatin plus ezetimibe in patients with chronic kidney disease (Study of Heart and Renal Protection): a randomised placebo-controlled trial. *Lancet* 2011;**377**:2181–92.

61. Holdaas H, Fellström B, Jardine AG, *et al.*, Assessment of LEscol in Renal Transplantation (ALERT) Study Investigators. Effect of fluvastatin on cardiac outcomes in renal transplant recipients: a multicentre, randomised, placebo-controlled trial. *Lancet* 2003;**361**:2024–31.

62. Kidney Disease Outcomes Quality Initiative (KDOQI) Group, KDOQI clinical practice guidelines for management of dyslipidemias in patients with kidney disease. *Am J Kidney Dis* 2003;**41** (Suppl 3):S1–91.

63. März W, Genser B, Drechsler C, *et al.*, German Diabetes and Dialysis Study Investigators. Atorvastatin and low-density lipoprotein cholesterol in type 2 diabetes mellitus patients on hemodialysis. *Clin J Am Soc Nephrol* 2011;**6**:1316–25.

64. Holdaas H, Holme I, Schmieder RE, *et al.*, on behalf of the AURORA study group: Rosuvastatin in diabetic hemodialysis patients. *J Am Soc Nephrol* 2011;**22**:1335–41.

65. Shepherd J, Kastelein JJ, Bittner V, *et al.*, TNT (Treating to New Targets) Investigators. Intensive lipid lowering with atorvastatin in patients with coronary heart disease and chronic kidney disease: the TNT (Treating to New Targets) study. *J Am Coll Cardiol* 2008;**51**:1448–54.

66. Kidney Disease Outcomes Quality Initiative (K/DOQI) Guidelines for managing dyslipidemias. *Am J Kidney Dis* 2012 (in press).

Chapter 9

Diabetes mellitus, bone and kidney

Thomas Neumann and Gabriele Lehmann

Jena University Hospital, Jena, Germany

Key points

- Fracture risk is increased in patients with type 1 and type 2 diabetes.
- Impaired bone quality leads to reduced bone strength.
- Prevention of falls is a major requirement in diabetes.
- Bone remodeling is linked with energy metabolism by osteocalcin.
- Alterations in bone turnover are a common complication of renal failure.

- Renal osteodystrophy increases fracture risk.
- Forms of renal osteodystrophy can be diagnosed correctly only by bone biopsy.
- Bone turnover markers and bone mineral density measurements are not able to differentiate forms and severity of renal osteodystrophy.
- Therapeutic options of renal osteodystrophy are limited.

Introduction

Osteoporosis is a systemic skeletal disease characterized by low bone mass and micro-architectural deterioration of bone tissue, with subsequent increase in bone fragility and susceptibility to fracture [1]. In the year 2000, 9 million osteoporotic fractures were estimated to occur worldwide, of which 1.6 million involved the hip, 1.7 million the forearm, and 1.4 million the vertebrae [2]. The peak number of hip fractures occurred between the ages of 75 and 79 years in both men and women. Osteoporotic fractures accounted for a total loss of disability-adjusted life years (DALYs) of 5.8 million [2].

Patients with diabetes have multiple skeletal disorders, including osteoporosis with increased fracture risk, Charcot's disease, and diffuse idiopathic skeletal hyperostosis (DISH) [3]. Occurrence of osteoporosis in patients with diabetes may pose a further burden of disease.

Diabetes and Kidney Disease, First Edition. Edited by Gunter Wolf.
© 2013 John Wiley & Sons, Ltd. Published 2013 by John Wiley & Sons, Ltd.

To provide optimal bone health care to patients with diabetes, awareness of the epidemiology, consideration of pathophysiological mechanisms, careful clinical assessment, and appropriate prevention or treatment of skeletal diseases are pivotal.

Osteoporosis in type 1 and type 2 diabetes

For type 1 diabetes mellitus, the prevalence of osteopenia and osteoporosis determined by dual X-ray absorptiometry (DXA) varies. Osteopenia is found in about 50–60% and osteoporosis in 14–20% of patients [4]. It must be considered whether the onset of diabetes occurred within childhood—in a growing skeleton—or after adolescence and therefore after achieving peak bone mass. Bone mineral loss occurs during the first few years after onset of diabetes. Several studies have shown that children and young adults (older than 20 years) with type 1 diabetes mellitus have a lower bone mineral density (BMD) than matched controls [4]. The interference of diabetes onset and formation of peak bone mass may result in insufficient skeletal mineralization and have a negative impact on the skeleton at later times. Indeed, a recent study has shown that patients with disease onset in adolescence had lower hip strength at later times when diabetes had started earlier [5]. Many studies have investigated BMD in adult patients with type 1 diabetes mellitus, but with heterogeneous results. The majority of the studies have described a lower BMD at the lumbar spine or femoral neck—or both sites—in this patients group [4]. Most studies have reported no association between BMD and glycemic control via glycosylated hemoglobin (HbA1c) levels [6, 7].

Using the BMD–fracture risk relationship for postmenopausal women according to Marshall et al. [8], a younger cohort with type 1 diabetes mellitus would have an estimated fracture risk of 1.3–2.3 at the lumbar spine and 1.4–2.6 at the femoral neck [4]. In a meta-analysis of epidemiologic fracture data in type 1 diabetes mellitus, however, the observed fracture risk was clearly higher than that expected using the BMD-based estimation [9]. For hip fractures, for example, the observed risk was 6.94 (3.25–14.78). Several studies indicate an association among diabetic complications, such as retinopathy, peripheral neuropathy, and nephropathy, as well as peripheral vascular complications with BMD or fractures [10]. One might speculate that patients with retinopathy or neuropathy have low physical activity and therefore less musculoskeletal interactions. Despite the fact that several studies have described a differential BMD for men and women, the fracture risk is probably the same [11].

Concerning type 2 diabetes mellitus, this condition usually starts in patients who have already reached their peak bone mass, and typically the onset of disease is less abrupt. The largest study on BMD and fracture incidence in type 2 diabetes mellitus is the Rotterdam Study (483 women and 309 men; mean age 74 years) [12]. This study has evidenced an increased fracture risk in patients with diabetes compared with 5863 controls without diabetes (hazard ratio 1.33; 95% CI 1.00–1.77), although the BMD at the lumbar spine and proximal femur were higher. Patients with treated diabetes were at increased risk of fractures, but the diabetes medications were not mentioned. Janghorbani et al. [11] have published a meta-analysis of 12 studies indicating a summary relative risk of 1.7 (95% CI 1.3–2.2) for hip fractures. The risk of hip fractures was slightly higher in men, but statistically not significant.

The inverse association between BMD and fracture risk in patients with type 2 diabetes mellitus has led to a substantial body of research. Retrospective cohort studies on patients with type 2 diabetes mellitus have revealed that even the Fracture Risk Algorithm (FRAX) score underestimated the fracture risk in this cohort [13]. Although the BMD at the femoral neck is an accepted diagnostic instrument for predicting hip fractures, bone strength is related to body size and bone size, independently of BMD. Body size determines the forces during falls, and bone size determines the bone structural strength. In a prospective study design it could be demonstrated that a calculated composite score, which integrates femoral neck size and body size with bone density, was inversely associated with hip fractures [14]. A recently published prospective study in type 2 diabetes mellitus has revealed that—after adjusting for various covariates—patients have lower composite strength indices in spite of higher BMD at the femoral neck [15]. This may easily result in impaired resistance to fracture forces relative to load.

Falls and fracture risk

Falls are a major extraskeletal risk for fractures. About one-third of community-dwelling people older than 65 years fall at least once a year, with one of 10 falls causing a serious injury [16]. Major risk factors for accidental fall are previous falls, balance impairment, and decreased muscle strength [16]. Pijpers *et al.* [17] have found that recurrent falls occur more frequently in patients with diabetes than in controls (30.6 versus 19.4%, $p = 0.017$). Factors explaining the increased incidence of falls were a greater number of medicines used, higher level of body pain, poorer self-perceived health, lower level of physical activity, more limitations in activities of daily life, and cognitive impairment. Polypharmacy is another major risk factor of incident falls in patients with type 2 diabetes mellitus [18].

Hypoglycemia is a well-known risk factor of incident falls. If patients with type 2 diabetes mellitus use insulin, then the risk of falls increases dramatically in patients with HBA1c <6% compared with those with HBA1c >8% (OR 4.36, 95% CI 1.32–14.46) [19]. Interest-

ingly, in patients with type 2 diabetes mellitus who do not use insulin, there is no association between low HBA1c and risk of falls. In the same study, reduced peripheral nerve function (determined by peroneal nerve response amplitude at the popliteal fossa) and reduced visual function (determined by contrast sensitivity) were both independently associated with the risk of falls. Furthermore, impairment of renal function, as measured by blood levels of cystatin-c, was associated with falls.

Vitamin D deficiency is another well-known risk factor for falls. In addition to its importance in skeletal health by regulation of calcium and phosphorus homeostasis, vitamin D has direct effects on muscle strength. Many studies have found decreased 25-OH vitamin D levels in patients with type 1 diabetes mellitus and type 2 diabetes mellitus—more pronounced in type 2 diabetes mellitus—when compared with non-diabetic controls [20].

Proposed mechanisms underlying the increased fracture risk in diabetes

Animal and clinical data suggest that insulin has an anabolic role in bone. Whereas low insulin levels characterize type 1 diabetes mellitus, in type 2 diabetes mellitus insulin levels are actually increased due to insulin resistance. Concentrations of insulin-like growth factor-I (IGF-I), another anabolic hormone, are decreased in type 1 diabetes mellitus and decreased or normal in type 2 diabetes mellitus [21]. Mice lacking insulin receptors that mediate insulin- and IGF-I signaling had impaired bone formation and low bone turnover [22]. Human data support the "insulin deficiency" hypothesis, as intensive insulin therapy has been shown to exert positive effects on bone metabolism over the course of 7 years [23].

Concerning type 1 diabetes mellitus, it is still unclear whether the autoimmune process itself is involved in impaired bone metabolism, given that autoimmunity is characterized by the presence of activated T cells and an osteoclastogenic cytokine microenvironment. However, animal data suggest that the increase in the number of osteoclasts is not associated with an upregulation of receptor for activation of NF-κB ligand (RANKL) expression in the bone of rats with streptozotocin-induced diabetes [24].

Both type 1 diabetes mellitus and type 2 diabetes mellitus diabetes are characterized by hyperglycemia. Hyperglycemia may have several adverse effects on bone metabolism, including non-enzymatic glycosylation of various bone proteins, hypercalciuria caused by glycosuria, and various interactions of hyperglycemia with the parathyroid hormone (PTH)/vitamin D system. The positive effects of obesity on BMD might counteract some of the detrimental effects of hyperglycemia. Both, osteoblasts and adipocytes are derived from mesenchymal stem cells. Soluble factors that are released from adipocytes have recently emerged as crucial mediators in bone metabolism. High levels of leptin are predictive of low risk of fractures, whereas high levels of adiponectin are predictive of a higher risk of vertebral fractures, but only in men [25]. Animal experiments suggest that the effects of leptin on the skeleton are divergent depending on the site of action. By serotonin-mediated stimulation of the central nervous system sympathetic output, leptin suppresses osteoblast proliferation. In contrast, leptin may partially prevent ovariectomy-induced bone loss in rats, if administrated peripherally [26].

Animal studies confirm that bone strength is impaired in both types of diabetes [27, 28]. Increased formation of advanced glycation end products (AGEs) by non-enzymatic glycosylation is associated with diabetes and leads to damage of the extracellular matrix, tissue stiffening, and accelerated sclerosis in arteries [29]. An increase in AGE formation in diabetic bone may result in the reduction of bone strength independently of BMD [30]. Increased serum or urine level of AGEs is independently associated with prevalent or incident fractures in type 2 diabetes mellitus [31, 32]. AGE accumulation not only impairs material properties of the bone matrix, but also inhibits bone formation by increased osteoblast apoptosis [33].

Specific influence of diabetes drugs on fracture risk

As already mentioned, insulin treatment may increase the risk of fracture in type 2 diabetes mellitus when compared with non-insulin-treated patients. However, most patients with type 2 diabetes mellitus on insulin treatment have longstanding disease and mostly a higher prevalence of diabetic complications and comorbidities, and these may independently or additionally interfere with the fracture risk. In patients with longer duration of insulin treatment, for example, there was no significant association with bone fracture [34].

Metformin shows a direct osteogenic effect *in vitro* by stimulating the proliferation and differentiation of osteoblast-like cell lines, leading to the hypothesis that it might be protective against fractures. Although only limited clinical data are available, metformin treatment has been shown to be associated with reduced fracture risk in one study [35]. The same study has also shown a reduction of fracture risk in patients with type 2 diabetes mellitus on sulfonylureas.

Thiazolidinediones (TZDs) are antidiabetic drugs that mediate insulin sensitivity by binding to the peroxisome proliferator-activated receptor γ (PPAR-γ). Activation of PPAR-γ by TZDs suppresses several key osteogenic transcription factors, and induces a shift in mesenchymal stem cell specification from osteogenesis to adipogenesis. This shift results in increased bone marrow adiposity. Randomized clinical trials with TZDs have shown an increased fracture risk in women with type 2 diabetes mellitus. The cumulative fracture incidence in ADOPT (Analysis from A Diabetes

Outcome Progression Trial) with rosiglitazone was 15.1% after 5 years of treatment compared with 7.3% for metformin [36]. In a retrospective cohort study, women older than 65 years appeared to be at the greatest risk of fracture on TZD treatment [37]. Concerning the risk of fracture in men, the data are conflicting with no increased fracture risk in clinical trials and the opposite results in observational studies [37].

Cross-talk between bone remodeling and energy metabolism

Within the last few years some fascinating studies have been published on the interplay between the skeleton and energy metabolism. Bone remodeling is an active process that requires a large amount of energy; therefore, the hypothesis was generated that the same hormones may regulate bone and energy metabolism [38]. Earlier in this chapter we have mentioned the importance of leptin and adiponectin, two adipocyte-derived hormones that can regulate bone mass by signaling on osteoblasts. Recent insights into the role of bone in energy metabolism as a feedback loop have emerged from several animal studies. Insulin signaling in bone has been suggested to be necessary for whole-body glucose homeostasis. Mice lacking the insulin receptor on osteoblasts display glucose intolerance [39]. Insulin signaling mediates inhibition of osteoprotegerin formation in osteoblasts and therefore decreases osteoclast activity [40]. Osteoblasts secrete osteocalcin, a small molecule present in blood and stored in the bone matrix. Post-translational vitamin K-dependent γ-carboxylation is essential for the protein to acquire a high affinity for mineral ions and incorporate these into hydroxyapatite crystals. Conversely, undercarboxylated osteocalcin is more susceptible to release into the systemic circulation. Furthermore, osteoclasts may release undercarboxylated osteocalcin into the circulation by acidifying the bone extracellular matrix

and by protein decarboxylation. Insulin action on osteoblasts determines the release of osteocalcin, as demonstrated in insulin receptor mutant mice that had a lower level of systemic total and undercarboxylated osteocalcin [39]. Lee and colleagues [41] have demonstrated in rodent genetic models that undercarboxylated osteocalcin affects insulin production by the β-cells of the pancreas and insulin sensitivity in peripheral tissues. In general, patients with type 1 diabetes mellitus and type 2 diabetes mellitus have lower levels of total osteocalcin [42]. Some studies report an increase in osteocalcin level during improvement of glycemic control in diabetes [42]. Despite emerging evidence of regulation of energy metabolism by bone-derived osteocalcin, the exact mechanisms of action on different tissues—including the β-cells of the pancreas—remain unknown.

Kidney and bone: renal osteodystrophy

Epidemiology

Renal insufficiency due to diabetic nephropathy is similar to renal insufficiency due to other underlying conditions followed by disturbances in bone metabolism. Alterations in bone turnover occur at early insufficiency stages and are not associated with clinical manifestations. They continue throughout the course of the disease, finally affecting all patients who reach end-stage renal disease [43] and persist in a large extent after renal transplantation [44]. Apart from increased cardiovascular morbidity rate and mortality, fractures are a frequent complication of patients on long-term hemodialysis. The annual fracture rate of a patient on long-term hemodialysis is 10–25 per 100 patient-years. These fractures may not be apparent. After the occurrence of so-called major fractures, the annual mortality rate rises to 60% and represents a threefold increase compared with patients without fracture [45].

Pathophysiology

Depending on the activity of bone remodeling, high turnover and low turnover bone diseases can be distinguished. Regarding the complex pathogenesis of the more frequent high-turnover bone disease, secondary hyperparathyroidism due to the disordered mineral metabolism, it is generally believed that two principles are true: first, the increase in PTH due to the phosphate retention, known as the trade-off hypothesis, aiming to retain normophosphatemia [46] and deficiency of 25-hydroxy vitamin D in early stages, and, second, the development of a calcitriol deficiency as a consequence of the reduced activity of the 1-α-hydroxylase in the advanced stages of chronic renal insufficiency [47]. Calcitriol constitutes an important differentiation factor for osteoclasts [48] and for osteoblasts [49]. The molecular characterization of the calcium-sensing receptor and its expression in different organs has further enriched pathogenetic comprehension. Because of localization on the parathyroid gland, the relation between serum calcium level and PTH is explainable. A stimulation of this receptor can inhibit the synthesis and excretion of PTH by the parathyroid gland [50]. Further clarification is due to the better knowledge of the links between the fibroblast growth factor (FGF) 23 and regulation of phosphate homeostasis and development of vascular and soft-tissue calcification. Dialysis patients may show a link between high FGF 23 levels and increased mortality. For healthy patients, this association has not yet been proven [51].

For development of the two forms of low-turnover bone disease—osteomalacia and adynamic bone disease—aluminum overload with accumulation in bone and aluminum-induced PTH hyposecretion was first held causally responsible [52]. After a reduction in the application of aluminum-containing phosphate binders and the use of aluminum-free dialysis water, the incidence of osteomalacia clearly declined [53]; in contrast, the incidence of the adynamic bone disease was rising [54]. The possible reasons for the development of a low turnover are numerous and besides calcitriol deficiency [55] include hyperphosphatemia [56], metabolic acidosis [57], elevated circulating interleukin 1 and tumor necrosis factor α levels [58], and also a deficiency in estrogen and testosterone. Age, diabetes mellitus, and malnutrition each independent risk factors for an adynamic bone disease [59].

Diagnostic procedures: bone turnover markers, bone mineral density, bone biopsy

To consider the turnover of an individual patient, the knowledge of the PTH value is not sufficient [60]. In addition to the analytical variability, the particular PTH value is influenced by the comorbidity—notably in concurrence with diabetes [61]—the type of dialysis [62], the extent of aluminum load [44], and of the skeletal resistance to PTH [63]. This requires considering the cellular and enzymatic markers of bone remodeling by renal osteodystrophy (ROD). The "ideal" bone remodeling marker should be bone specific and should show a good correlation with bone histology [64]. For most bone remodeling markers, the second stipulation has still to be proven [65].

Bone formation markers

Bone-specific alkaline phosphatase
Bone-specific alkaline phosphatase is produced by osteoblasts in the early period of osteoblastic differentiation. It is not affected by increased renal function [66] and thus can be used to characterize bone formation. A study based on histomorphometric classification of ROD alkaline phosphatase and bone-specific alkaline phosphatase showed significant correlations with the osteoid surface and osteoblast-covered

surface in patients with high turnover treated by hemodialysis [67]. Furthermore, high levels of alkaline phosphatase were found to be associated with fracture incidence, and cardiovascular and overall mortality [68].

Osteocalcin (bone γ-carboxylglutamic acid-containing protein)

This vitamin K-dependent enzyme is produced and secreted by osteoblasts and influences bone mineralization. Osteocalcin is the most abundant non-collagenous protein in the skeleton and a marker of late osteoblast differentiation and bone formation. Because osteocalcin accumulates in patients with impaired renal function, its use as a bone formation marker has a limited significance.

Bone resorption markers

Serum cross-linked telopeptide of type 1 collagen

Cross-linked telopeptide of type 1 collagen (NTX) is a collagen breakdown parameter; it is an organ and process-specific bone resorption marker. However, accumulation in renal insufficiency and urinary excretion complicate interpretation in patients with decreased renal function. Nevertheless, it has been reported to be a useful marker to distinguish high and low bone turnover [69].

Tartrate-resistant acid phosphatase

Serum type 5b tartrate-resistant acid phosphatase (TRAP 5b) is exclusively secreted from activated osteoclasts [70]. TRAP 5b describes the number of osteoclasts and their activity. It is possible that the correlation of TRAP 5b and histological parameters of bone resorption is higher than for PTH [71].

In summary, however, all bone resorption and formation markers alone or in combination with PTH have failed to discriminate reliably between high and low bone turnover, and for clinical and therapeutic decisions

they cannot replace bone biopsy. At present, a routine determination of bone resorption markers is not recommended. The evidence of this recommendation is graded as 2C (KDIGO, Kidney Disease: Improving Global Outcomes).

In contrast, because considerably higher or lower values have a predictive value in regard to bone turnover, periodic measurements of PTH or bone-specific alkaline phosphatase should be taken for evaluation (evidence level 2B).

Bone mineral density

Measurement of BMD is widely used in the general population to evaluate fracture risk. Mostly, dual-energy X-ray absorptiometry (DXA) is used. This method captures overall BMD without distinguishing between cortical and trabecular bone. For patients with osteoporosis, a direct correlation between DXA-measured BMD and fracture risk has been proven. For this group of patients, the value of the BMD measurement is uncontested [72]. Thanks to the increasing availability of DXA, patients with impaired renal function have been examined; however, the significance of a singular mineral density measurement concerning fracture risk, turnover, or ROD type has not been sufficiently validated [73].

A reduction in bone mineral density has also been described several times for patients with secondary renal hyperparathyroidism [74]. The reported results were thought not consistent and the examined patients were not comparable.

Several authors [75, 76] have described the development of the mineral density after renal transplantation as a reduction of the mineral density at the lumbar spine for the first year and for the second year an increase in bone mineral density.

Although the use of bisphosphonates in renal osteodystrophy for reducing the fracture risk has been controversially discussed [77], after therapy with bisphosphonates a reduction in bone mass loss in the first months after renal transplantation has been shown [78].

According to current knowledge, it is recommended to discontinue routine measurements of bone density for patients in stated 3–5D of chronic renal disease because the bone density in this collective neither predicts the fracture risk nor the type of renal osteodystrophy (evidence level 2B).

Classification of renal osteodystrophy by bone biopsy

For differentiating from osteoporosis, bone changes by renal failure are classified under "renal osteodystrophy" [79]. Despite the improvements in diagnostic imaging and laboratory diagnostics, histological evaluation of the bone is today essential for the exact classification. However, iliac crest biopsy is an invasive diagnostic procedure; moreover, it is time-consuming, expensive, and not ubiquitously available.

Indications for bone biopsy according to KDIGO 2009 [79]:
• unexplained fractures
• persistent bone pain
• unexplained hypercalcemia
• unexplained hypophosphatemia
• potential aluminum toxicity
• rendering an initial result before therapy with bisphosphonates in patients with documented disturbances, associated with renal insufficiency, of the bone and mineral balance (without indicating any evidence).

The histopathologic spectrum comprises "high turnover" osteitis fibrosa and mixed uremic osteodystrophy, and "low turnover" adynamic bone disease and osteomalacia.

Osteitis fibrosa

The leading histologic symptom is a deep, tunneling and trabeculae-perforating osteoclasia with consecutive endosteal and marrow fibrosis. The number of osteoclasts is elevated. Those cells typically have several nuclei and prominent nucleoli. The activated osteoblasts are often multilayered. Because of the overproduction of bone matrix, volume and surface osteoidosis develops; the osteoid produced is arranged irregularly. With tetracycline marking, increased mineralization activity and an increased mineral apposition rate can be visualized.

Mixed uremic osteodystrophy

Apart from the symptoms of osteitis fibrosa, this shows a significant increase in osteoid surface due to a disturbed mineralization. The variability of both components is very important.

Osteomalacia

Because of the mineralization defect and the increased accumulation of non-mineralized bone matrix, volume and surface osteoidosis dominates. The rate of active bone remodeling entities is low; the bone volume is not reduced.

Adynamic bone disease

This is characterized by a veritable lack of active bone remodeling cells with consecutive decrease in bone remodeling. The bone volume is often reduced.

Therapeutic options

According to the new consideration of chronic kidney disease-mineral and bone disorder as a systematic disease, prevention of cardiovascular events and fractures, and a reduction in morbidity and mortality can be formulated as objectives of the therapy [79].

Concerning to the KDIGO recommendations, phosphate binders, calcitriol, active vitamin D analogues and calcimimetics are applied exclusively or in combination. Serum calcium, serum phosphate, and the PTH values could be used as control parameters for therapy initiation and adaption. For interpreting the PTH value, it is not the absolute amount which is important but its development in the course of disease. For patients in stages 3–5D of a chronic renal disease with serious hyperparathyroidism, without response to medical treatment, a parathyroidectomy is still recommended (evidence level 2B).

The application of specific osteotropic pharmaceuticals as bisphosphonates, such as denosumab, strontium ranelat and teriparatid, for those in whom the fracture inhibiting effects in the therapy of osteoporosis are proven cannot be recommended for patients from stage 3 of a chronic renal disease with laboratory findings which indicate a perturbation associated with renal insufficiency of mineral and bone balance. The data currently available are controversial. Multicenter, randomized, double-blind studies which show fracture prevention have not been carried out. If such treatment is carried out, a bone biopsy before therapy initiation is advised.

References

1. Consensus development conference: prophylaxis and treatment of osteoporosis. *Am J Med* 1991;**90**: 107–10.
2. Johnell O, Kanis JA. An estimate of the worldwide prevalence and disability associated with osteoporotic fractures. *Osteoporos Int* 2006;**17**:1726–33.
3. Schwartz AV. Diabetes mellitus: does it affect bone? *Calcif Tissue Int* 2003;**73**:515–9.
4. Hofbauer LC, Brueck CC, Singh SK, Dobnig H. Osteoporosis in patients with diabetes mellitus. *J Bone Miner Res* 2007;**22**:1317–28.
5. Maser RE, Kolm P, Modlesky CM, *et al.* Hip strength in adults with type 1 diabetes is associated with age at onset of diabetes. *J Clin Densitom* 2012;**15**: 78–85.
6. Neumann T, Samann A, Lodes S, *et al.* Glycaemic control is positively associated with prevalent fractures but not with bone mineral density in patients with Type 1 diabetes. *Diabet Med* 2011;**28**: 872–5.
7. Lopez-Ibarra PJ, Pastor MM, Escobar-Jimenez F, *et al.* Bone mineral density at time of clinical diagnosis of adult-onset type 1 diabetes mellitus. *Endocr Pract* 2001;**7**:346–51.
8. Marshall D, Johnell O, Wedel H. Meta-analysis of how well measures of bone mineral density predict occurrence of osteoporotic fractures. *BMJ* 1996;**312**:1254–9.
9. Vestergaard P. Discrepancies in bone mineral density and fracture risk in patients with type 1 and type 2 diabetes—a meta-analysis. *Osteoporos Int* 2007;**18**:427–44.
10. Miao J, Brismar K, Nyren O, *et al.* Elevated hip fracture risk in type 1 diabetic patients: a population-based cohort study in Sweden. *Diabetes Care* 2005;**28**:2850–5.
11. Janghorbani M, Van Dam RM, Willett WC, Hu FB. Systematic review of type 1 and type 2 diabetes mellitus and risk of fracture. *Am J Epidemiol* 2007;**166**: 495–505.
12. de Liefde I, van der Klift M, de Laet CE, *et al.* Bone mineral density and fracture risk in type-2 diabetes mellitus: the Rotterdam Study. *Osteoporos Int* 2005;**16**: 1713–20.
13. Schwartz AV, Vittinghoff E, Bauer DC, *et al.* Association of BMD and FRAX score with risk of fracture in older adults with type 2 diabetes. *JAMA* 2011;**305**:2184–92.

14. Karlamangla AS, Barrett-Connor E, Young J, Greendale GA. Hip fracture risk assessment using composite indices of femoral neck strength: the Rancho Bernardo study. *Osteoporos Int* 2004;**15**: 62–70.

15. Ishii S, Cauley JA, Crandall CJ, Srikanthan P, *et al*. Diabetes and femoral neck strength: findings from the Hip Strength Across the Menopausal Transition Study. *J Clin Endocrinol Metab* 2012;**97**:190–7.

16. Tinetti ME, Kumar C. The patient who falls: "It's always a trade-off". *JAMA* 2010;**303**:258–66.

17. Pijpers E, Ferreira I, de Jongh RT, *et al*. Older individuals with diabetes have an increased risk of recurrent falls: analysis of potential mediating factors: the Longitudinal Ageing Study Amsterdam. *Age Ageing* 2012;**41**:358–65.

18. Huang ES, Karter AJ, Danielson KK, *et al*. The association between the number of prescription medications and incident falls in a multi-ethnic population of adult type-2 diabetes patients: the diabetes and aging study. *J Gen Intern Med* 2010;**25**: 141–6.

19. Schwartz AV, Vittinghoff E, Sellmeyer DE, *et al*. Diabetes-related complications, glycemic control, and falls in older adults. *Diabetes Care* 2008;**31**:391–6.

20. Di Cesar DJ, Ploutz-Snyder R, Weinstock RS, Moses AM. Vitamin D deficiency is more common in type 2 than in type 1 diabetes. *Diabetes Care* 2006;**29**:174.

21. Thrailkill KM. Insulin-like growth factor-I in diabetes mellitus: its physiology, metabolic effects, and potential clinical utility. *Diabetes Technol Ther* 2000;**2**: 69–80.

22. Ogata N, Chikazu D, Kubota N, *et al*. Insulin receptor substrate-1 in osteoblast is indispensable for maintaining bone turnover. *J Clin Invest* 2000;**105**:935–43.

23. Campos Pastor MM, Lopez-Ibarra PJ, Escobar-Jimenez F, *et al*. Intensive insulin therapy and bone mineral density in type 1 diabetes mellitus: a prospective study. *Osteoporos Int* 2000;**11**:455–9.

24. Hie M, Tsukamoto I. Increased expression of the receptor for activation of NF-kappaB and decreased runt-related transcription factor 2 expression in bone of rats with streptozotocin-induced diabetes. *Int J Mol Med* 2010;**26**:611–8.

25. Biver E, Salliot C, Combescure C, Gossec L, *et al*. Influence of adipokines and ghrelin on bone mineral density and fracture risk: a systematic review and meta-analysis. *J Clin Endocrinol Metab* 2011;**96**:2703–13.

26. Burguera B, Hofbauer LC, Thomas T, *et al*. Leptin reduces ovariectomy-induced bone loss in rats. *Endocrinology* 2001;**142**: 3546–53.

27. Silva MJ, Brodt MD, Lynch MA, *et al*. Type 1 diabetes in young rats leads to progressive trabecular bone loss, cessation of cortical bone growth, and diminished whole bone strength and fatigue life. *J Bone Miner Res* 2009;**24**:1618–27.

28. Kawashima Y, Fritton JC, Yakar S, *et al*. Type 2 diabetic mice demonstrate slender long bones with increased fragility secondary to increased osteoclastogenesis. *Bone* 2009, 44648–55.

29. Monnier VM, Sell DR, Dai Z, *et al*. The role of the amadori product in the complications of diabetes. *Ann N Y Acad Sci* 2008;**1126**:81–8.

30. Saito M, Marumo K. Collagen cross-links as a determinant of bone quality: a possible explanation for bone fragility in aging, osteoporosis, and diabetes mellitus. *Osteoporos Int* 2010;**21**:195–214.

31. Yamamoto M, Yamaguchi T, Yamauchi M, *et al*. Serum pentosidine levels are positively associated with the presence of vertebral fractures in postmenopausal

women with type 2 diabetes. *J Clin Endocrinol Metab* 2008;**93**:1013–9.

32. Schwartz AV, Garnero P, Hillier TA, *et al.* Pentosidine and increased fracture risk in older adults with type 2 diabetes. *J Clin Endocrinol Metab* 2009;**94**:2380–6.

33. Alikhani M, Alikhani Z, Boyd C, *et al.* Advanced glycation end products stimulate osteoblast apoptosis via the MAP kinase and cytosolic apoptotic pathways. *Bone* 2007;**40**:345–53.

34. Monami M, Cresci B, Colombini A, *et al.* Bone fractures and hypoglycemic treatment in type 2 diabetic patients: a case-control study. *Diabetes Care* 2008; **31**:199–203.

35. Vestergaard P, Rejnmark L, Mosekilde L. Relative fracture risk in patients with diabetes mellitus, and the impact of insulin and oral antidiabetic medication on relative fracture risk. *Diabetologia* 2005;**48**:1292–9.

36. Kahn SE, Zinman B, Lachin JM, *et al.* Rosiglitazone-associated fractures in type 2 diabetes: an Analysis from A Diabetes Outcome Progression Trial (ADOPT). *Diabetes Care* 2008;**31**:845–51.

37. Habib ZA, Havstad SL, Wells K, *et al.* Thiazolidinedione use and the longitudinal risk of fractures in patients with type 2 diabetes mellitus. *J Clin Endocrinol Metab* 2010;**95**:592–600.

38. Karsenty G. Convergence between bone and energy homeostases: leptin regulation of bone mass. *Cell Metab* 2006; **4**:341–8.

39. Ferron M, Wei J, Yoshizawa T, *et al.* Insulin signaling in osteoblasts integrates bone remodeling and energy metabolism. *Cell* 2010;**142**:296–308.

40. Fulzele K, Riddle RC, DiGirolamo DJ, *et al.* Insulin receptor signaling in osteoblasts regulates postnatal bone acquisition and body composition. *Cell* 2010;**142**:309–19.

41. Lee NK, Sowa H, Hinoi E, *et al.* Endocrine regulation of energy metabolism by the skeleton. *Cell* 2007;**130**:456–69.

42. Motyl KJ, McCabe LR, Schwartz AV. Bone and glucose metabolism: a two-way street. *Arch Biochem Biophys* 2010;**503**: 2–10.

43. Torres A, Lorenzo V, Hernandez D, *et al.* Bone disease in predialysis, hemodialysis, and CAPD patients: evidence of a better bone response to PTH. *Kidney Int* 1995; **47**:1434–42.

44. Dumoulin G, Hory B, Nguyen NU, *et al.* No trend toward a spontaneous improvement of hyperparathyroidism and high bone turnover in normocalcemic long-term renal transplant recipients. *Am J Kidney Dis* 1997;**29**:746–53.

45. Jadoul M, Albert JM, Akiba T, *et al.* Incidence and risk factors for hip or other bone fractures among hemodialysis patients in the Dialysis Outcomes and Practice Patterns Study. *Kidney Int* 2006;**70**:1358–66.

46. Slatopolsky E, Gradowska L, Kashemsant C, *et al.* The control of phosphate excretion in uremia. *J Clin Invest* 1966;**45**:672–7.

47. Llach F, Velasquez Forero F. Secondary hyperparathyroidism in chronic renal failure: pathogenic and clinical aspects. *Am J Kidney Dis* 2001;**38**(Suppl 5): S20–33.

48. Suda T, Takahashi N, Martin TJ. Modulation of osteoclast differentiation. *Endocr Rev* 1992;**13**:66–80.

49. Owen TA, Aronow MS, Barone LM, *et al.* Pleiotropic effects of vitamin D on osteoblast gene expression are related to the proliferative and differentiated state of the bone cell phenotype: dependency upon basal levels of gene expression, duration of exposure, and bone matrix competency in normal rat osteoblast

cultures. *Endocrinology* 1991;**128**: 1496–504.

50. Cummings SR, Black DM, Nevitt MC, *et al.* Bone density at various sites for prediction of hip fractures. The Study of Osteoporotic Fractures Research Group. *Lancet* 1993;**341**:72–5.

51. Gutierrez OM, Mannstadt M, Isakova T, *et al.* Fibroblast growth factor 23 and mortality among patients undergoing hemodialysis. *N Engl J Med* 2008;**359**:584–92.

52. Diaz Lopez JB, Jorgetti V, Caorsi H, *et al.* Epidemiology of renal osteodystrophy in Iberoamerica. *Nephrol Dial Transplant* 1998;**13**(Suppl 3):41–5.

53. Moriniere P, Cohen-Solal M, Belbrik S, *et al.* Disappearance of aluminic bone disease in a long term asymptomatic dialysis population restricting A1(OH)3 intake: emergence of an idiopathic adynamic bone disease not related to aluminum. *Nephron* 1989;**53**:93–101.

54. Spasovski GB, Bervoets AR, Behets GJ, *et al.* Spectrum of renal bone disease in end-stage renal failure patients not yet on dialysis. *Nephrol Dial Transplant* 2003; **18**:1159–66.

55. Massry SG, Stein R, Garty J, *et al.* Skeletal resistance to the calcemic action of parathyroid hormone in uremia: role of 1,25 (OH)2 D3. *Kidney Int* 1976;**9**:467–74.

56. Ritz E, Malluche HH, Krempien B, *et al.* Pathogenesis of renal osteodystrophy: roles of phosphate and skeletal resistance to PTH. *Adv Exp Med Biol* 1978;**103**: 423–36.

57. Bushinsky DA, Frick KK. The effects of acid on bone. *Curr Opin Nephrol Hypertens.* 2000l;**9**:369–79.

58. Kaneki H, Guo R, Chen D, *et al.* Tumor necrosis factor promotes Runx2 degradation through up-regulation of Smurf1 and Smurf2 in osteoblasts. *J Biol Chem* **281**:4326–33.

59. Malluche HH, Monier-Faugere MC. Risk of adynamic bone disease in dialyzed patients. *Kidney Int Suppl* 1992;**38**: S62–7.

60. Wang M, Hercz G, Sherrard DJ, *et al.* Relationship between intact 1–84 parathyroid hormone and bone histomorphometric parameters in dialysis patients without aluminum toxicity. *Am J Kidney Dis* 1995;**26**:836–44.

61. Panuccio V, Mallamaci F, Tripepi G, *et al.* Low parathyroid hormone and pentosidine in hemodialysis patients. *Am J Kidney Dis* 2002;**40**:810–5.

62. Salusky IB, Ramirez JA, Oppenheim W, *et al.* Biochemical markers of renal osteodystrophy in pediatric patients undergoing CAPD/CCPD. *Kidney Int* 1994;**45**:253–8.

63. Urena P, Ferreira A, Morieux C, *et al.* PTH/PTHrP receptor mRNA is down-regulated in epiphyseal cartilage growth plate of uraemic rats. *Nephrol Dial Transplant* 1996;**11**:2008–16.

64. Hutchison AJ, Whitehouse RW, Boulton HF, *et al.* Correlation of bone histology with parathyroid hormone, vitamin D3, and radiology in end-stage renal disease. *Kidney Int* 1993;**44**:1071–7.

65. Ferreira MA. Diagnosis of renal osteodystrophy: when and how to use biochemical markers and non-invasive methods; when bone biopsy is needed. *Nephrol Dial Transplant* 2000;**15**(Suppl 5): 8–14.

66. Ueda M, Inaba M, Okuno S, *et al.* Serum BAP as the clinically useful marker for predicting BMD reduction in diabetic hemodialysis patients with low PTH. Life sciences. 2005;**77**:1130–9.

67. Lehmann G, Ott U, Kaemmerer D, *et al.* Bone histomorphometry and biochemical markers of bone turnover in patients with chronic kidney disease Stages 3–5. *Clin Nephrol* 2008;**70**:296–305.

68. Regidor DL, Kovesdy CP, Mehrotra R, *et al*. Serum alkaline phosphatase predicts mortality among maintenance hemodialysis patients. *J Am Soc Nephrol* 2008;**19**:2193–203.

69. Asci G, Basci A, Shah SV, *et al*. Carbamylated low-density lipoprotein induces proliferation and increases adhesion molecule expression of human coronary artery smooth muscle cells. *Nephrology* 2008;**13**:480–6.

70. Yamada S, Inaba M, Kurajoh M, *et al*. Utility of serum tartrate-resistant acid phosphatase (TRACP5b) as a bone resorption marker in patients with chronic kidney disease: independence from renal dysfunction. *Clin Endocrinol* 2008;**69**:189–96.

71. Chu P, Chao TY, Lin YF, *et al*. Correlation between histomorphometric parameters of bone resorption and serum type 5b tartrate-resistant acid phosphatase in uremic patients on maintenance hemodialysis. *Am J Kidney Dis* 2003;**41**:1052–9.

72. Dawson-Hughes B, Tosteson AN, *et al*. Implications of absolute fracture risk assessment for osteoporosis practice guidelines in the USA. *Osteoporos Int* 2008;**19**:449–58.

73. Gerakis A, Hadjidakis D, Kokkinakis E, *et al*. Correlation of bone mineral density with the histological findings of renal osteodystrophy in patients on hemodialysis. *J Nephrol*. 2000;**13**: 437–43.

74. Asaka M, Iida H, Entani C, *et al*. Total and regional bone mineral density by dual photon absorptiometry in patients on maintenance hemodialysis. *Clin Nephrol* 1992;**38**:149–53.

75. Bubenicek P, Sotornik I, Vitko S, Teplan V. Early bone mineral density loss after renal transplantation and pre-transplant PTH: a prospective study. *Kidney Blood Press Res* 2008;**31**:196–202.

76. Mikuls TR, Julian BA, Bartolucci A, Saag KG. Bone mineral density changes within six months of renal transplantation. *Transplantation* 2003;**75**:49–54.

77. Grotz W, Nagel C, Poeschel D, *et al*. Effect of ibandronate on bone loss and renal function after kidney transplantation. *J Am Soc Nephrol* 2001; **12**:1530–7.

78. Cunningham J. Posttransplantation bone disease. *Transplantation* 2005,**79**: 629–34.

79. Moe S, Drueke T, Cunningham J, *et al*. Definition, evaluation, and classification of renal osteodystrophy: a position statement from Kidney Disease: Improving Global Outcomes (KDIGO). *Kidney Int* 2006;J**69**:1945–53.

Diabetes, pregnancy and the kidney

Helmut Kleinwechter[1] and Ute Schäfer-Graf[2]

[1] Diabetes Center and Diabetes Education Center, Kiel, Germany
[2] St. Joseph Hospital, Berlin, Germany,

Key points

- Incipient or early stages of nephropathy are no longer a contraindication for pregnancy in women with diabetes mellitus, and pregnancy does not aggravate kidney function postpartum in women with normal serum creatinine.
- The main risks during pregnancy are pre-eclampsia, intrauterine growth reduction, and preterm delivery.
- These complications may be reduced by strict metabolic control with glycosylated hemoglobin <7% prior to pregnancy and intensive antihypertensive treatment with angiotensin-converting enzyme inhibitors until pregnancy is established.
- In women with type 1 diabetes, early antihypertensive treatment during pregnancy in normotensive cases with microalbuminuria and low-dose aspirin starting before 16 weeks' gestation might further improve outcome by reduction of severe complications.
- In women with type 2 diabetes normalization or reduction of overweight/obesity before pregnancy, replacing oral antidiabetic drugs or GLP-1 analogues with insulin and evaluation of concomitant drugs is mandatory.
- Women with advanced stages of nephropathy need careful counseling from specialists in diabetology, nutrition, obstetrics, nephrology, transplantation, cardiology, and neonatology.
- A baby take-home rate of 90–95% in pregnancies of women with nephropathy is attainable in a specialized care network setting.

Diabetic nephropathy is one of the most frequent microvascular complications of type 1 diabetes and type 2 diabetes. Outside pregnancy, diabetic nephropathy is defined by internationally accepted criteria and classification of its stages [1–3]. During pregnancy this approach is less clear because pregnancy-specific complications like pre-eclampsia are characterized by proteinuria and hypertension. So, differentiation of diabetic nephropathy from complications during pregnancy could be difficult.

Diabetes and Kidney Disease, First Edition. Edited by Gunter Wolf.
© 2013 John Wiley & Sons, Ltd. Published 2013 by John Wiley & Sons, Ltd.

Historical perspective

Twenty to 30 years ago, a women with overt diabetic nephropathy was advised not to become pregnant due to the risk of severe, life-threatening health problems induced by pregnancy. Manifest diabetic nephropathy with increased serum creatinine, decreased glomerular filtration rate (GFR), and proteinuria had been considered medical contraindications for pregnancy. Manifest nephropathy with reduced kidney function showed serious, sometimes life-threatening, risks for the mother (e.g., acute renal failure in the course of severe pre-eclampsia) and the fetus (e.g., intrauterine fetal death). To date, the lowest rates of perinatal mortality in pregnancies from type 1 diabetic women have been reported from specialized clinical centers [4,5]. Outpatient management by experienced teams does not impair neonatal outcome compared with hospital care [6]. With regard to the mother's risk, reports from Finland with 972 births of women with type 1 diabetes during 1975–1997 showed a more than 100-fold increase in maternal mortality rate compared with the general population (0.51% versus 0.0047%) [7].

For quality management, all pregnancies of women with known diabetes should be registered with standardized parameters to compare the pregnancy outcome on an international basis. Today, in centers with specialized care for pregnant women with diabetic nephropathy, perinatal mortality is about 5% [8]. However, this is still 10 times higher than in the general population in industrial countries. The main reason is preterm delivery, often preceded by pre-eclampsia. With the wide distribution of urine albumin measurement, a more differentiated picture appeared for the courses and results of pregnant diabetic women [9].

Health aims

The St. Vincent declaration, published by the European sections of WHO and IDF in 1989, intended to bring the outcome of pregnancies with diabetes to the level of the background population within 5 years [10]. This aim was not fulfilled until 1994. In 1999, a new aim was set by WHO Europe to improve the outcome by approximately one-third until the year 2020 [11]. The various structures of health care available in different countries make comparison of pregnancy complications and associated outcomes difficult.

Physiological adaptations in normal pregnancy

During pregnancy, there are some profound physiologic adaptations to kidney function such as lower serum creatinine and lower uric acid levels as well as increase in glomerular filtration rate (GFR). This should be considered when interpreting laboratory results. Specific reference values for diabetic pregnant women for serum creatinine and GFR have not been established. Furthermore, there are decisive parameters of cardiovascular risk change during pregnancy: blood pressure is lower and blood lipids are higher.

Prevalence and diagnosis of diabetic nephropathy in pregnant women

Of patients with type 1 diabetes, 12.6–54% will develop clinically relevant nephropathy after 7.3–18 years of diabetes duration [12–14]. In a population-based cross-sectional analysis nephropathy was found in 3% of women with type 1 diabetes [15]. Therefore, diabetic nephropathy is a function of diabetes duration. When type 1 diabetes becomes manifest during childhood or adolescence, the probability of overt nephropathy rises in the reproductive years.

Notwithstanding, 10 years after diagnosis the prevalence rate is 25% for microalbuminuria, 5% for macroalbuminuria, and 0.8% for increased serum creatinine, but the frequent delay in diagnosis of type 2 diabetes has to be kept in mind when counseling patients [16]. A large cohort study covered a 40% prevalence of microalbuminuria [17]. Data on diabetic nephropathy and pregnancies in type 2 diabetes show 1.4% overt nephropathy in Japan [18], and 13% microalbuminuria and 0% macroalbuminuria in Denmark [19]. Thus, nephropathy is of clinical relevance in pregnancies predominantly for women with type 1 diabetes. It should be mentioned that even leading clinical centers have seen only a few pregnant women with type 1 diabetes and advanced nephropathy (<5 per year) because of rare occurrence [20–22].

How can nephropathy be diagnosed in pregnancy? For pregnant women it may be difficult to collect a 24-hour urine specimen. The evidence for alternative measurements from spontaneous urine specimens is good. The mean average value from twice repeated measurements of normoalbuminuria in spontaneous urine (collected at arbitrary times during the day) showed a high correlation in women with type 1 diabetes [23] with mean average albuminuria results from two 24-hour urine sample collections (sensitivity 83%, specificity 100%, positive predictive value 100%, negative predictive value 97%). The results for random urine samples are reported as the albumin–creatinine ratio.

It is well accepted that albuminuria is suitable as a warning system for the development of nephropathy early in the course of diabetes. Today there is evidence that microalbuminuria can also be detected at a considerable percentage in the non-diabetic general population. The prevalence of microalbuminuria in patients with arterial hypertension (without diabetes) has been reported to be 7% in Groningen, the Netherlands, (macroalbuminuria 0.2%), and 8% in the US population [24]. In recent times, albuminuria also applies as a predictor for the development of renal insufficiency or cardiovascular complications in patients without diabetes.

Measurement of albuminuria may be affected by
• exercise [25]
• urine infections, fever
• excessive protein content in meals
• elevated blood pressure
• decompensation of diabetes control.

When serum creatinine is measured today, an estimated GFR is automatically given on the basis of the serum creatinine, age, sex, and race according to the Modification of Diet in Renal Disease formula. This estimate is not accurate in pregnancy [26]. So measurement of 24-hour urine creatinine clearance (CrCl) in the (first) assessment of diabetic nephropathy during pregnancy is preferable.

In the long run, pregnancies or the number of births have no adverse influence on the development or progression of diabetic nephropathy in type 1 diabetes [27,28]. Therefore, women under optimal metabolic control and no signs of incipient or overt nephropathy or other microvascular complications may become pregnant without concern and do not need to restrict the number of their children. The decrease in CrCl in diabetic nephropathy was 3.2 mL/min/year after pregnancy compared with 3.4 mL/min/year in women who were not pregnant, and was not significantly different [22].

Besides the generally recognized risk factors for the development of diabetic nephropathy [29], one study in women with type 1 diabetes showed evidence that using oral hormonal contraceptives versus not-using led to macroalbuminuria after a median follow-up of 20.7 years (range 1–24 years) in 18% versus 2%, adjusted relative risk 8.9 (95% CI 1.79–44.36, $p = 0.008$) [30].

Nephropathy stages 1a and 1b are associated with increased risk of pre-eclampsia. Microalbuminuria versus normoalbuminuria is the best predictor for pre-eclampsia (58% versus 7%) [31]. Additional self-measurement of blood pressure or 24-hour blood pressure profiles did not improve predictive value. However, a Spanish group demonstrated that self-monitoring of blood pressure may be useful in normotensive pregnant women with type 1 diabetes in contrast to non-diabetic women [32]. A systolic blood pressure during night-time >105 mmHg in the 24-hour profile during the second trimester was the best predictor for pregnancy-induced hypertension: sensitivity 85%, specificity 92%, positive predictive value 87%, negative predictive value 95%, relative risk 6.1.

The frequency of preterm births is increased at the level of microalbuminuria: normoalbuminuria 35%, microalbuminuria 62%, overt nephropathy 91% [33]. This was also confirmed for the rate of small for gestational age (SGA) newborns: Normoalbuminuria 2%, microalbuminuria 4%, overt nephropathy 45%; in this study the rates of pre-eclampsia were as follows: normoalbuminuria 6%, microalbuminuria 42%, overt nephropathy 64%. In pregnant women with type 1 diabetes and microalbuminuria, cases of so-called transitory nephrotic syndrome have been described with protein excretion >3 g/day in the third trimester without change in kidney function parameters—postpartum protein excretion returned to normal [34].

In a Danish study two cohorts of pregnant women with microalbuminuria were compared after intensifying the antihypertensive management strategy [35]. In the second cohort, the women received methyldopa with a target of blood pressure <140/90 mmHg start-ing before 20 weeks of pregnancy. The frequency of preterm birth could be reduced significantly from 23% to 0% accompanied by a clinically meaningful (but not significant) reduction in pre-eclampsia from 42% to 20%. The progression of diabetic nephropathy (established with progression of albuminuria) versus no progression was also associated with a significantly higher rate of preterm birth (OR 7.7; 95% CI 1.3–46.9) [36].

To date, to our knowledge, the largest population-based investigation in women with type 1 diabetes has come from Denmark [37]. All pregnancies of Danish women were included in a register of the Danish Diabetes Association were prospectively entered in 1993–1999 (n = 1215). The women delivered in eight centers; in total 846 pregnancies with normoalbuminuria (n = 762) versus microalbuminuria (n = 84) and without antihypertensive therapy in early pregnancy were analyzed.

Prevalence of microalbuminuria was 10% in the first trimester, the median diabetes duration was 11 years, and the median glycosylated hemoglobin (HbA1c) in the third trimester was 6.6%. The prevalence of pre-eclampsia and preterm delivery were 40% and 13%, respectively, both significantly higher in the microalbuminuria group than in the normoalbuminuria group (12% and 6%). In the general Danish population, pre-eclampsia is found in 2.6%. After adjustment for confounders, significant predictors for pre-eclampsia were microalbuminuria (OR 4.0; 95% CI 2.2–7.2), nulliparity (OR 3.1; 95% CI 1.9–5.1), and HbA1c in the third trimester (OR 1.3; 95% CI 1.1–1.5 per 1% absolute increase). In the multivariate analysis, only HbA1c, but not microalbuminuria, was predictive of delivery before 34 weeks of pregnancy, and pre-eclampsia increased the risk threefold.

Advanced stages of nephropathy are associated with high fetal and neonatal risks. This affects premature birth (30%) [21], fetal growth restriction, intrauterine death [38], and perinatal/neonatal mortality. In a follow-up study, 22% of liveborn children were re-examined after an average 4.5 years (range 0.4–10 years); children of mothers with overt nephropathy more often showed a delay in psychomotor development, classified as severe in 11% [21].

Further prognostically meaningful data for the mother should be taken into account for risk evaluation and counseling besides increased rates of induction and cesarean sections. Thirty-five percent of mothers with nephropathy died on average 16 years after pregnancy (range 3–28 years), and 19% reached the kidney failure stage [22]. In a review of published series, 45% of women with a mildly decreased GFR of 60–89 mL/min went to the final stage of renal disease by 12 years postpartum [39]. Kimmerle *et al.* [21] reported a rate of 11% maternal deaths, and 22% for women started on dialysis. In another study the SGA frequency was 24% [40]; of these, 57% of the children were born prior to 37 weeks. All children were transferred to neonatal intensive care, and the perinatal/neonatal mortality was 10%. In a further cohort, every tenth woman with advanced nephropathy developed massive proteinuria, and had to start dialysis after preterm delivery [20]. Pregnancies in diabetic women during hemodialysis or continuous ambulant peritoneal dialysis (CAPD) are very rare [41].

Frequencies of fetal growth retardation and premature births were higher in women with nephropathy than after renal transplant. Pregnancies in women with type 1 diabetes after kidney transplant [41–43] or combined kidney and pancreas transplant have been reported [44,45]. After kidney transplant the rate of premature birth <34 weeks was about 35%, the frequency of malformations was about 5.4%. After combined transplant (37 women, 53 pregnancies) the mean duration of gestation was 34 weeks and mean birth weight was 2130 g; 75% of the women developed hypertension (33% pre-eclampsia); and the outcome shows 80% live births in 52% of cesarean sections, and in 17% of the cases transplant loss was seen within 2 years [46].

In contrast to earlier recommendations, women should not wait at least 2 years after transplant before planning a pregnancy, a period of 1 year might be sufficient [47]. Since the primarily reduced fertility improves after kidney transplant, reliable contraception is recommended in the first year after transplant [48]. The most important reasons are a diminution of immunosuppressive medication, decrease in renal rejection risk, and stabilization of kidney function. A recently published meta-analysis reported the results of 4706 pregnancies for 3570 recipients of a kidney transplant. The general live-birth rate was 73.5%, abortion occurred in 14%, pre-eclampsia in 27%, and 56.9% of the women were delivered by a cesarean section [49].

Women should be counseled about the huge benefit of exact and extensive evaluation and treatment of diabetes complications and accompanying diseases at the time of planning a pregnancy. Her partner should participate in the discussion. One should reckon that a larger number of women with established nephropathy are already pregnant when they present at the first visit.

The following aspects should be analyzed:
- periconceptional HbA1c in target <7%
- supplementation of folic acid started
- severe hypoglycemia in the last year
- sufficient diabetes education
- psychosocial situation, kind of work
- retinopathy stage; fundus hypertonicus
- autonomic neuropathy

- clinical signs of macroangiopathy
- anemia
- sufficient management of hypertension; hypertensive heart disease
- quantification of proteinuria
- signs of secondary renal hyperparathyroidism; osteoporosis
- compensation for metabolic acidosis be effective
- signs of thyroidal dysfunction; thyroid peroxidase antibodies provable

Pregnant women should be informed about the following topics:

- diabetic nephropathy is not a contraindication *per se* for pregnancy
- risk is increased when serum creatinine is 1.5 mg/dL (1.33 µmol/L) or higher, GFR is less than 60–75 mL/min per 1.73 m^2 measured with CrCl, and blood pressure is ≥140/90 mmHg with multiple medication and intensive support
- pregnancy should be avoided in advanced hypertensive heart disease with reduced left ventricular function, and after myocardial infarction or stroke
- women with stage 4 or 5 nephropathy should be informed about the options of improved course of pregnancy after renal transplant from a nephrologist and a specialist in transplant medicine
- while planning a pregnancy and during pregnancy albuminuria should be evaluated repeatedly to estimate pre-eclampsia risk
- women with type 1 diabetes on oral contraceptives should be observed carefully for increase in albumin excretion
- women with nephropathy and arterial hypertension before 20 weeks of gestation should be managed to a target <140/90 mmHg
- in normotensive women with microalbuminuria management with methyldopa might reduce very preterm birth <34 weeks
- prescription of low-dose aspirin should be decided in individual high-risk cases for pre-eclampsia; aspirin is then started before 16 weeks.

Management of women with diabetic nephropathy during pregnancy

The treatment and support of pregnant women with diabetic nephropathy is complex and should be guided by established recommendations and guidelines based on actual and weighted evidence [39]. Before conception, HbA1c should be stabilized at <7% for at least 3 months; the blood pressure target is <140/90 mmHg, and women should start with 800 µg of folic acid supplementation per day after stopping contraception.

Medical nutritional therapy

Normal weight women may choose their daily calories and quantity of carbohydrates according to their personal needs. Women with type 2 diabetes are often overweight or obese, thus calorie restriction before and during pregnancy is important. Daily calories should not be less than 1600–1800 kcal. To rule out hypocaloric food, occasional urine ketone monitoring is helpful. All pregnant women receive information on preferable weight gain ranges and weight targets based on the Institute of Medicine (IOM) guidelines [50]. Women should weigh themselves without clothes once weekly at home and document the results.

Evidence for counseling regarding daily protein intake is weak. In the early stages of nephropathy with microalbuminuria, restriction of daily protein is not recommended. With advanced nephropathy (stage 2 and higher) restriction of daily protein intake should be weighed against the risk of loss of muscle mass of the pregnant women and undernutrition of the fetus. Daily intake of 1.1 g of protein per kg body weight should be achieved [39]; a protein intake of about 10% of total daily calories is currently recommended for adults. The daily intake of protein should not be less than 60 g per day. A daily amount of protein <0.6 g/kg body weight increases the risk of deficiency in essential amino acids [1].

Iron need not be supplemented unless hemoglobin is <11.0 g/dL in the first trimester and <10.5 g/dL in the second trimester, and the blood count shows evidence of iron deficiency. In cases of severe anemia of renal origin, discussion with the nephrologist is mandatory to decide if starting erythropoietin is advisable.

Insulin

Insulin is given as intensified conventional therapy or as a continuous subcutaneous insulin infusion. Women with type 2 diabetes on oral antidiabetic agents should preconceptionlly switch to insulin. Human insulin is the medication of first choice. Insulin analogues do not offer advantages with respect to pregnancy outcome. Women with preconceptional therapy with the short-acting insulin analogue aspart or the long-acting insulin detemir may continue during pregnancy, since randomized studies with aspart and detemir have proved their safety in pregnancy [51–54].

Women with type 1 diabetes and nephropathy usually have longer diabetes duration. Therefore, it is important to re-evaluate further micro- and macrovascular complications during pregnancy. Often hypoglycemia requiring help from another person and hypoglycemia unawareness underlying by autonomous neuropathy are found. Lower targets for blood glucose and HbA1c in pregnancy should be weighed against the risk of hypoglycemia in the mother.

Arterial hypertension

Because of their nephroprotective effect, impeding influences on profibrogene, and proinflammatory effect of angiotensin II, diabetic patients in general take angiotensin-converting enzyme inhibitors and AT1-blockers as the therapy of choice. The drugs can reduce or stabilize excess albuminuria. During pregnancy there is clear evidence that the drugs have fetotoxic effects, whereas their teratogenity is somewhat controversial [55]. The latest results show that hypertension *per se*—independently of the kind of drugs used—is associated with malformations, which has also been confirmed in hypertensive women without therapy [56]. However, for safety reasons a shift to methyldopa is recommended preconceptionally, if necessary in combination with metoprolol and calcium channel blockers like nifedipine. Experience from centers for diabetes and pregnancy show that continuing diuretic therapy started before pregnancy is without further risk. During pregnancy, starting diuretic therapy has to considered very carefully since reduced intravasal blood volume may cause decreased placental blood flow and undersupply of the fetus. The blood pressure target should be 110–129 mmHg systolic and 65–79 mmHg diastolic whenever possible.

Dyslipidemia, smoking

During pregnancy lipid-lowering drugs like statins, fibrates, nicotinic acid, and ezetimibe must be stopped because they are not approved in pregnancy or show increased fetal risk. If dyslipidemia has been diagnosed previously, a lipid profile at the beginning of pregnancy should be evaluated. There is no evidence that interruption of lipid-lowering therapy during pregnancy will modify cardiovascular risk. During pregnancy, blood lipids increase substantially [57]. In women with triglycerides >1000 mg/dL, therapy is indicated to reduce the risk of acute pancreatitis. Fish oil capsules and a low-fat diet are of advantage to attain n-3 fatty acid intakes of 3–9 g/day. Therapeutic options as secondary strategies are medium-chain triglycerides, total parenteral nutrition, fibrates, and extended release niacin. It is essential to stop cigarette smoking as soon as possible.

Exercise

Pregnant women with diabetic nephropathy should be advised to take regular exercise. Brisk walking of at least 3×30 minutes per week is advisable and easily feasible. Medical and obstetric contraindications have to be taken into account. There is no clear evidence to what extent exercise could improve metabolic control, but women definitely profit from better physical fitness in the third trimester and intrapartum.

Acute diabetes-specific complications

Hypoglycemia

Severe hypoglycemia requiring help from another person is seen predominantly in women with type 1 diabetes until 20 weeks of gestation [58]. If nephropathy accelerates with increasing deterioration of kidney function, the daily insulin demand may decrease because of reduced renal insulin clearance.

Diabetic ketoacidosis

During pregnancy diabetic ketoacidosis is a rare and life-threatening complication. It may occur in women on insulin pump therapy, e.g., when the insulin catheter is unintentionally disconnected. Admission to hospital is mandatory. The absolute level of blood glucose does not reflect the stage of metabolic acidosis. Ketoacidosis is confirmed by further laboratory investigation such as β-OH-butyrate in blood, arterial pH, and base excess.

Pre-eclampsia

Pre-eclampsia is a common pregnancy-specific disorder characterized by elevated arterial blood pressure and excess proteinuria with onset after the 20th week of pregnancy. If elevated blood pressure shows no concomitant proteinuria, it is defined as gestational or pregnancy-induced hypertension. Elevated arterial blood pressure before 20 weeks of pregnancy is defined as chronic arterial hypertension. If chronic arterial hypertension or another underlying disease with hypertension or proteinuria is followed by pre-eclampsia, the term is superimposed pre-eclampsia. Pre-eclampsia is differentiated into mild and severe forms. Pre-eclampsia is an important cause of maternal and fetal morbidity and mortality worldwide, affecting 5–8% of pregnancies [59]. The risk of developing pre-eclampsia during pregnancy is substantially higher in diabetic women and affects all types of diabetes. Hypertension and proteinuria may persist up to 6 weeks after pregnancy, and about 10–15% of pre-eclampsia first occurs after pregnancy [60], accompanied by typical symptoms.

The etiology of the disease is multifactorial and still not completely explained. In cases of severe pre-eclampsia delivery is effective, often life-saving treatment. The majority of the cases of pre-eclampsia show abnormal maternal uterine vascular remodeling by fetal trophoblast cells (extravillous cytotrophoblasts). The cytotrophoblasts move from the fetal compartment into the mother's compartment, that is endometrium and myometrium, via interstitial invasion. Some of the trophoblasts enter the wall of the maternal uterine spiral arteries and replace the endothelial vessel cells, becoming endovascular cytotrophoblasts. As a consequence, spiral arteries shift from resistance vessels to compliance vessels with increasing blood flow into placental blood spaces. In the placenta of pre-eclamptic women, interstitial invasion of cytotrophoblast cells is incomplete and shallow, remaining in the basal plate attached to anchoring villi. Endovascular invasion fails, and the spiral arteries remain resistant and "stiff." To restore placental blood flow, systemic blood pressure is increased. Pre-eclampsia is associated with endothelial dysfunction and cardiovascular risk later in life [61].

Analysis of all 650 000 pregnancies in Germany in 2006 showed that gestational diabetes, preconceptional overweight/obesity, and excessive weight gain during pregnancy are associated with a significant pre-eclampsia risk. The same has been found in women with social deprivation and increased psychosocial stress [62]. A Dutch analysis of all 364 pregnancies in the year 1999/2000 in women with type 1 diabetes showed a rate of pre-eclampsia of 12.7%, corresponding to a 12-fold increased risk compared with the general population of 197 000 pregnancies [63]. A study from England found an increased rate of pre-eclampsia in pregnant women with type 1 diabetes and vascular complications (OR 3.5; 95% CI 1.28–9.53) as well as an increased frequency of fetal growth reduction (OR 6.0; 95% CI 1.54–23.33) [64].

A Swedish study confirmed a fourfold increased prevalence of pre-eclampsia compared with the general population at a rate of 20.6%. The authors demonstrated that insufficient metabolic control (high HbA1c) early in pregnancy in women with normoalbuminuria led to higher risk of pre-eclampsia [65]. An investigation from Finland of 683 consecutive, non-selected pregnancies of type 1 diabetic women without nephropathy compared with 854 matched controls reached the same conclusion [66]. The rate of 12.8% versus 2.7% for pre-eclampsia was significantly higher (OR 5.2; 95% CI 3.3–8.4). The adjusted odds ratio for pre-eclampsia was 1.6 (95% CI 1.3–2.0) for each 1% absolute increment in the HbA1c value at 4–14 weeks of gestation (median 7 weeks) and 0.6 (95% CI 0.5–0.8) for each 1% decrement achieved during the first half of pregnancy.

Meanwhile the influence of pre-eclampsia on the later risk of renal disease has been investigated. In a meta-analysis with a mean follow-up time of 7.1 years, 273 women with pre-eclampsia were compared with 333 women without pre-eclampsia [67]. The rate of microalbuminuria was 31% versus 7%. The results were confirmed in Helsinki, Finland, in 203 women with type 1 diabetes from the years 1996–1998 and a mean follow-up of 11 years [68]. Women who had pre-eclampsia during pregnancy developed diabetic nephropathy in 41.9% versus 8.9% ($p < 0.001$). Furthermore, the women had a higher prevalence of coronary heart disease (12.2% versus 2.2%, $p = 0.03$).

Diagnostic criteria of pre-eclampsia

• Arterial hypertension >140 mmHg systolic and/or >90 mmHg diastolic, first established after 20 weeks of gestation, minimum two elevated measurements at least 6 hours apart during bed rest.
• Proteinuria >300 mg/day or 2+ protein in at least two consecutive urine samples.

Severe pre-eclampsia is defined if in addition one, or more, of the following criteria is present [69]:

• blood pressure ≥160 mmHg systolic and/or ≥110 mmHg diastolic, minimum of two elevated measurements at least 6 hours apart during bed rest
• proteinuria >5 g/day or 3+ protein or greater in 2 random urine samples at least 4 h apart
• oliguria (<500 mL/24 hours)
• cerebral or visual disturbances
• pulmonary edema or cyanosis
• epigastric or right upper-quadrant pain
• impaired liver function
• thrombocytopenia
• fetal growth restriction.

A specific variant of severe pre-eclampsia is HELLP syndrome. Abdominal pain is clinically important, and diagnosis is confirmed with blood analysis.

The acronym HELLP stands for
- **h**emolysis
- **e**levated **l**iver enzymes
- **l**ow **p**latelet count (thrombocytopenia)

Eclampsia is characterized by seizures and status epilepticus with risk of intracerebral hemorrhage followed by permanent neurologic deficit or exitus letalis.

Different strategies for prevention of pre-eclampsia have been examined. All attempts to decrease oxidative stress by supplementation of vitamin C and vitamin E have been unsuccessful [70,71]. In 1998 the often cited work of Caritis *et al.* [72] was published, who examined in a randomized, double-blind, placebo-controlled study the effect of low-dose aspirin (60 mg) to prevent pre-eclampsia in pregnant women at high risk. The complete study population comprised 2539 women and involved 471 preconceptional insulin-treated diabetic women as the high-risk group. Neither the incidence of pre-eclampsia nor perinatal outcome was improved significantly. Although later observational studies showed positive results, a general recommendation on prophylactic aspirin was held back until two meta-analysis in 2007 proved a reduction in the incidence of pre-eclampsia of about 20%, independently of when aspirin had been started during pregnancy [73,74].

Starting aspirin after 16 weeks of gestation showed no decrease in pre-eclampsia (10.3% versus 10.5%). All studies with aspirin starting before 16 weeks were limited to pregnant women with moderate or high risk. As a result of the meta-analysis, the authors stated that low-dose aspirin started before 16 weeks could reduce the occurrence of pre-eclampsia by more than a half. There are various opinions on the length of time aspirin should be taken during pregnancy. Whereas some authors recommend aspirin up to delivery, others remove aspirin some weeks before delivery to minimize bleeding risk. Therefore, decisions should be made on a case-by-case basis.

Future perspectives

The prognosis of diabetic pregnancies is improved by optimal metabolic control during childhood and adolescence. Today, immediately after diabetes diagnosis in type 1 diabetes intensive conventional insulin therapy or CSII is started at all ages. With this strategy, early stages of nephropathy with microalbuminuria and arterial hypertension could be primarily prevented. In type 2 diabetes, it is important to reduce obesity before pregnancy and manage hypertension to target. If there is already a diagnosis of nephropathy, one should achieve strict metabolic control prior to pregnancy with HbA1c levels <7% and intensive antihypertensive treatment to a target of <140/90 mmHg with ACE inhibitors until pregnancy is confirmed. Early use of low-dose aspirin is promising for lowering the risk of pre-eclampsia. Women with advanced stages of nephropathy with a GFR <60 mL/min/1.73 m^2 or difficulties with management of hypertension should be referred to a center experienced in diabetic renal disease and pregnancy offering complete diagnostic and therapeutic equipment in close cooperation with an obstetric and neonatology department.

References

1. Rüster C, Sämann A, Wolf G. Nieren und Diabetes. *Dtsch Med Wschr* 2008;**133**: 1848–52.
2. Gross J, De Azevedo M, Silveiro S, *et al.* Diabetic Nephropathy: Diagnosis, Prevention, and Treatment. *Diabetes Care* 2005;**28**:176–88.
3. Matthaei S, Forst T, Ritzel R, *et al.* Diabetische Nephropathie beim Diabetes Typ 2. *Thieme-Refresher Diabetologie* 2011; **2**:R13–R24.
4. Johnstone F, Lindsay R, Steel J. Type 1 Diabetes and pregnancy. trends in birth weight over 40 years at a single

clinic. *Obstet Gynecol* 2006; **107**: 1297–302.

5. Mølsted-Pedersen L, Kuhl L. Obstetrical management in diabetic pregnancy: the Copenhagen experience. *Diabetologia* 1986; **29**:13–16.

6. Vääräsmäki M, Hartikainen, A, Anttila M, Pirttiaho H. Out-patient management does not impair outcome of pregnancy in women with type 1 diabetes. *Diab Res Clin Pract* 2000; **47**:111–17.

7. Leinonen P, Hiilesmaa V, Kaaja R, Teramo K. Maternal mortality in type 1 diabetes. *Diabetes Care* 2001; **24**:1501–2.

8. Matthiesen E, Damm P. Diabetic vascular complications in pregnancy: nephropathy. In: Hod M (ed.) *Textbook of diabetes and pregnancy*, 2nd edn. London: Informa Healthcare, 2008, pp. 330–2.

9. Mogensen C, Klebe J. Microalbuminuria and diabetic pregnancy. In: Mogensen C (ed.) *The kidney and hypertension in diabetes mellitus*. Boston, MA: Kluwer Academic Publishers, 1998, pp. 455–62.

10. World Health Organization (Europe) an International Diabetes Federation (Europe). Diabetes care and research in Europe: the St. Vincent Declaration. *Diab Med* 1990;**7**:260.

11. World Health Organization Europa. *GESUNDHEIT21—Gesundheit für alle im 21. Jahrhundert.* Copenhagen: WHO Regionalbüro für Europa, 1999, 70.

12. Parving H, Hommel E, Mathiesen E, *et al.* Prevalence of microalbuminuria, arterial hypertension, retinopathy and neuropathy in patients with insulin dependent diabetes. *BMJ* 1988;**296**: 156–60.

13. Chaturvedi N, Bandinelli S, Mangili R, *et al.* Microalbuminuria in type 1 diabetes: rates, risk factors and glycemic threshold. *Kidney Int* 2001;**60**:219–27.

14. Hovind P, Tarnow L, Rossing P, *et al.* Predictors for the development of microalbuminuria and macroalbuminuria in patients with type 1 diabetes: inception cohort study. *BMJ* 2004; **328**:1105–10.

15. Conell F. Epidemiologic approaches to the identification of problems in diabetes care. *Diabetes Care* 1985; **8**(Suppl 1):82–6.

16. Adler A, Stevens R, Manley S, *et al.* Development and progression of nephropathy in type 2 diabetes: the United Kingdom Prospective Diabetes Study (UKPDS 64). *Kidney Int* 2003;**63**: 225–32.

17. Parving H, Lewis J, Ravid M, *et al.* Prevalence and risk factors for microalbuminuria in a referred cohort of type II diabetic patients: a global perspective. *Kidney Int* 2006;**69**:2057–63.

18. Omory Y, Minei S, Testuo T. Current status of pregnancy in diabetic women: a comparison in IDDM and NIDDM mothers. *Diabetes Res Clin Pract* 1994;**24**: S273–78.

19. Clausen T, Mathiesen E, Ekbom P, *et al.* Poor Pregnancy Outcome in Women With Type 2 Diabetes. *Diabetes Care* 2005;**28**:323–8.

20. Hopp H, Vollert W, Ebert A, *et al.* Diabetische Retinopathie und Nephropathie–Komplikationen während der Schwangerschaft und Geburt. *Geburtsh Frauenheilk* 1995;**55**:275–9.

21. Kimmerle R, Zaß R, Cupisti S, *et al.* Pregnancies in women with diabetic nephropathy: long-term outcome for mother and child. *Diabetologia* 1995;**38**:227–35.

22. Rossing K, Jacobsen P, Hommel E, *et al.* Pregnancy and progression of diabetic nephropathy. *Diabetologia* 2002;**45**: 36–41.

23. Justesen T, Petersen J, Ekbom P, *et al.* Albumin-to-creatinine ratio in random urine samples might replace 24-h urine collections in screening for micro- and

marcoalbuminuria in pregnant woman with type 1 diabetes. *Diabetes Care* 2006; **29**:924–5.

24. Chatzikyrkou C, Haller H, Menne J. Albuminurie. Prognostischer Marker oder therapeutisches Ziel? *Internist* 2012;**53**: 38–44.

25. Kornhauser C, Malacara J, Macías-Cervnates M, *et al.* Effect of exercise intensity on microalbuminuria in adolescents with type 1 diabetes mellitus. *Diab Med* 2011;**29**:70–3.

26. Smith M, Moran P, Ward M, *et al.* Assessment of glomerular filtration rate during pregnancy using the MDRD formula. *BJOG* 2008;**115**:109–12.

27. DCCT Research Group. Effect of pregnancy on microvascular complications in the diabetes control and complications trial. *Diabetes Care* 2000;**23**:1084–91.

28. Vérier-Mine O, Chaturvedi N, Webb D, *et al.* The EURODIAB Prospective Complications Study. Is pregnancy a risk factor for microvascular complications? *Diabet Med* 2005;**22**:1503–9.

29. Gross J, De Azevedo M, Silveiro S, *et al.* Diabetic nephropathy: diagnosis, prevention, and treatment. *Diabetes Care* 2005;**28**:176–88.

30. Ahmed S, Hovind P, Parving H, *et al.* Oral contraceptives, angiotensin-dependent renal vasoconstriction, and risk of diabetic nephropathy. *Diabetes Care* 2005;**28**:1988–94.

31. Ekboom P, Damm P, Nørgaard K, *et al.* Urinary albumin excretion and 24-hour blood pressure as predictors of pre-eclampsia in Type I diabetes. *Diabetologia* 2000;**43**:927–31.

32. Flores L, Levy I, Aguilera E, *et al.* Usefulness of ambulatory blood pressure monitoring in pregnant women with type 1 diabetes. *Diabetes Care* 1999;**22**:1507–11.

33. Ekboom P, Damm P, Feldt-Rasmussen B, *et al.* Pregnancy Outcome in type 1 diabetic women with microalbuminuria. *Diabetes Care* 2001;**24**:1739–44.

34. Biesenbach G, Zazgornik J. Incidence of transient nephrotic syndrome during pregnancy in diabetic women with and without pre-existing microalbuminuria. *BMJ* 1989;**299**:366–7.

35. Nielsen R, Müller, C Damm P, *et al.* Reduced prevalence of early delivery in women with Type 1 diabetes and microalbuminuria—possible effect of early antihypertensive treatment during pregnancy. *Diab Med* 2006;**23**: 426–31.

36. Lepercq J, Coste J, Theau A, *et al.* Factors associated with preterm delivery in women with type 1 diabetes: a cohort study. *Diabetes Care* 2004;**27**:2824–8.

37. Jensen D, Damm P, Ovesen P, *et al.* Microalbuminuria, preeclampsia and preterm delivery in pregnant women with type 1 diabetes—results from a nation-wide Danish Study. *Diabetes Care* 2010;**33**:90–4.

38. Lauenborg J, Mathiesen E, Ovesen P, *et al.* Audit on Stillbirths in women with pregestational type 1 diabetes. *Diabetes Care* 2003;**26**:1385–9.

39. Kitzmiller J, Block J, Brown F, *et al.* Managing preexisting diabetes for pregnancy. summary of evidence and consensus recommendations for care. *Diabetes Care* 2008;**31**:1060–79.

40. Dunne F, Chowdhury T, Hartland A, *et al.* Pregnancy outcome in women with insulin-dependent diabetes mellitus complicated by nephropathy. *Q J Med* 1999; **92**:451–4.

41. Rizzoni G, Ehrich J, Broyer M. Successful pregnancies in women on renal replacement therapy: report from the EDTA Registry. *Nephrol Dialysis Transpl* 1992;**7**:279–87.

42. Tagatz G, Arnold N, Goetz F, *et al.* Pregnancy in a juvenile diabetic after transplantation (class T diabetes mellitus). *Diabetes* 1975;**24**:497–501.

43. Vinicor F, Golichowski A, Filo R, *et al.* Pregnancy following renal transplantation in a patient with insulin-dependent diabetes mellitus. *Diabetes Care* 1984;**7**:280–4.

44. Barrou B, Gruessner A, Sutherland D, *et al.* Pregnancy after pancreas transplantation in the cyclosporine era: report from the International Pancreas Transplant Registry. *Transplantation* 1998; **65**:524–7.

45. Baltzer J, Kürzl R, Schramm T, *et al.* Schwangerschaften bei Frauen nach Nieren- bzw. Pankreastransplantation. *Geburtsh Frauenheilk* 1989;**49**:769–75.

46. McKay D, Josephson M. Pregnancy in recipients of Solid organs—effects on mother and child. *N Engl J Med* 2006; **354**:1281–93.

47. Davison J. Dialysis, transplantation and pregnancy. *Am J Kidney Dis* 1991;**27**: 127–32.

48. Davison J. Bailey D. Pregnancy following renal transplantation. *J Obstet Gynaecol Res* 2003;**29**:227–33.

49. Deshpande N, James N, Kucirka L, *et al.* Pregnancy outcomes in kidney transplant recipients: a systematic review and meta-analysis. *Am J Transplant* 2011; **11**:2388–404.

50. Institut of Medicine (IOM). *Weight gain during pregnancy: reexamining the guidelines.* Washington, DC: The National Academies Press, 2009.

51. Mathiesen E, Kinsley B, Amiel S, *et al.* Maternal glycemic control and hypoglycemia in type 1 diabetic pregnancy. A randomized trial of insulin aspart versus human insulin in 322 pregnant women. *Diabetes Care* 2007;**30**: 771–6.

52. Hod M, Damm P, Kaaja R, *et al.* Fetal and perinatal outcomes in type 1 diabetes pregnancy: a randomized study comparing insulin aspart with human insulin in 322 subjects. *Am J Obstet Gynecol* 2008;**198**:186.e1–7.

53. Mathiesen M; Damm P, Hod M, *et al.* Maternal efficacy and safety outcomes in a randomized trial comparing insulin detemir with NPH insulin in 310 pregnant women with type 1 diabetes. *Annual meeting of the American Diabetes Association (ADA)* 2011, Abstract Number 0061-LB.

54. Hod M, McCance D, Ivanisevic M, *et al.* Perinatal Outcomes in a Randomized Trial Comparing Insulin Detemir with NPH Insulin in 310 Pregnant Women with Type 1 Diabetes. *Annual meeting of the American Diabetes Association (ADA)* 2011, Abstract Number 0062-LB.

55. Cooper W, Hernandez-Diaz S, Arbogast P, *et al.* Major Congenital Malformations after First-Trimester Exposure to ACE Inhibitors. *N Engl J Med* 2006;**354**:2443–551.

56. Li D, Yang C, Andrade S, *et al.* Maternal exposure to angiotensin converting enzyme inhibitors in the first trimester and risk of malformations in offspring: a retrospective cohort study. *BMJ* 2011; **343**:d5931.

57. Wiznitzer A, Mayer A, Novack V, *et al.* Association of lipid levels during gestation with preeclampsia and gestational diabetes mellitus: a population-based study. *Am J Obstet Gynecol* 2009;**201**:1.e1–1.e8.

58. García-Peterson A, Gich I, Amini S, *et al.* Insulin requirements throughout pregnancy in women with type 1 diabetes mellitus: three changes of direction. *Diabetologia* 2010;**53**:446–51.

59. Pennington K, Schlitt J, Jackson D, *et al.* Preeclampsia: multiple approaches for a

multifactorial disease. *Dis Model Mech* 2012;**5**:9–18.

60. Al-Safi Z, Imudia A, Filetti L, *et al.* Delayed Postpartum Preeclampsia and Eclampsia. *Obstet Gynecol* 2011;**118**: 1102–7.

61. Ray J, Vermeulen M, Schull M, *et al.* Cardivascular health after maternal placental syndromes (CHAMPS): population-based retrospective cohort study. *Lancet* 2005;**366**:1797–803.

62. Schneider S, Freerksen N, Maul H, *et al.* Risk groups and maternal-neonatal complications of preeclampsia—Current results from the national German Perinatal Quality Registry. *J Perinat Med* 2011;**39**:257–65.

63. Evers I, de Valk H, Visser G. Risk of complications of pregnancy in women with type 1 diabetes: nationwide prospective study in the Netherlands. *BMJ* 2004;**328**:915–18.

64. Howarth C, Gazis A, James D. Association of Type 1 diabetes mellitus, maternal vascular disease and complications of pregnancy. *Diab Med* 2007;**24**:1229–34.

65. Hanson U, Persson B. Epidemiology of pregnancy-induced hypertension and preeclampsia in Type 1 (insulin-dependent) diabetic pregnancies in Sweden. *Acta Obstet Gynecol Scand* 1998; **77**:620–4.

66. Hiilesma V, Suhonen L, Teramo K. Glycaemic control is associated with pre-eclampsia but not with pregnancy-induced hypertension in women with type I diabetes mellitus. *Diabetologia* 2000;**43**:1534–9.

67. McDonald S, Han Z, Walsh M, *et al.* Kidney disease after preeclampsia: a systematic review and meta-analysis. *Am J Kidney Dis* 2010;**55**:1026–39.

68. Gordin D, Hiilesma V, Fagerudd J, *et al.* Pre-eclampsia but not pregnancy-induced hypertension is a risk factor for diabetic nephropathy in type 1 diabetic women. *Diabetologia* 2007;**50**:516–22.

69. ACOG-American Collge of Obstetricians and Gynecologists practice bulletin. Diagnosis and management of preeclampsia and eclampsia. *Int J Gynaecol Obstet* 2002;**77**:67–75.

70. Poston L, Briley A, Seed P, *et al.* Vitamin C and Vitamin E in pregnant women at risk for pre-eclampsia (VIP trial): randomised placebo-controlled trial. *Lancet* 2006;**367**:1145–54.

71. Rumbold A, Crowther C, Haslam R, *et al.* Vitamin C and E and the Risks of Preeclampsia and Perinatal Complications. *N Engl J Med* 2006; **354**:1796–806.

72. Caritis S, Sibai B, Hauth J, *et al.* Low-dose aspirin to prevent preeclampsia in women at high risk. *N Engl J Med* 1998;**338**:701–5.

73. Askie L, Duley L, Henderson-Smart D, *et al.* Anti-platelet agents for prevention of pre-eclampsia: a meta-analysis of individual patients. *Lancet* 2007;**369**: 1791–8.

74. Duley L, Henderson-Smart D, Meher S, *et al.* Antiplatelet agents for preventing pre-eclampsia and its complications. *Cochrane Database Syst Rev* 2007; (2):CD004659.

Diabetic nephropathy in children

Kai D Nüsken and Jörg Dötsch

University Hospital of Cologne, Cologne, Germany

Key points

- The development of diabetic nephropathy begins at the onset of diabetes.
- There is a substantial prevalence of clinically manifest diabetic nephropathy in children and adolescents.
- In young adults with type 1 diabetes, the prevalence of manifest diabetic nephropathy (macroalbuminuria without or with renal failure) is 10%.
- Main risk factors are the duration of diabetes, poor glycemic control, adolescent-onset diabetes (puberty), and hypertension.
- Regular screening for microalbuminuria is mandatory and allows early detection of diabetic nephropathy.
- In case of albuminuria, nephrological work-up in children and adolescents includes history, family history, physical examination, ultrasound of the kidneys and urinary tract, microscopic examination of the urine, albumin, immunoglobulin G and α-1-microglobulin in spot urine, 24-hour urine collection carried out separately day and night for total protein quantification, and at least a blood count and determination of serum electrolytes, creatinine for calculation of glomerular filtration rate, BUN, albumin, total protein, C3 complement and C4 complement.
- Progression of clinically manifest diabetic nephropathy can be retarded, stopped, or even reversed by good glycemic control as well as adequate antiproteinuric and antihypertensive treatment.
- Angiotensin converting enzyme inhibitors or angiotensin II receptor type 1 blockers are the first-choice drugs for therapy.

Diabetes mellitus is one of the most frequent chronic diseases in childhood and adolescence. Type 1 diabetes is most common and accounts for at least two-thirds of all cases, and type 2 for about one-sixth of all cases [1]. As type 1 diabetes is diagnosed early, the development of diabetic nephropathy is well understood. However, although early diagnosis and improved treatment has resulted in declining incidence of macroalbuminuria [2], the long-term

Diabetes and Kidney Disease, First Edition. Edited by Gunter Wolf.
© 2013 John Wiley & Sons, Ltd. Published 2013 by John Wiley & Sons, Ltd.

prognosis of childhood- and adolescent-onset type 1 diabetes is still poor. Ten percent to 30% of patients show microalbuminuria about 15 years after diagnosis, and 20–40% of patients with microalbuminuria will develop macroalbuminuria over the next 5–10 years [2–5]. The prevalence of clinically manifest diabetic nephropathy is about 1% in children and adolescents and, even more important, about 10% in young adults [4, 5]. Macroalbuminuria is a precondition for declining renal function due to diabetic nephropathy. When renal function declines [glomerular filtration rate (GFR) <60 mL/min/1.73 m²], there is a high risk for end-stage renal disease (ESRD) requiring renal replacement therapy. The main risk factors are duration of diabetes, poor glycemic control, adolescent-onset diabetes, and hypertension. Regular screening for microalbuminuria is mandatory and allows early detection of diabetic nephropathy [6]. In case of albuminuria, nephrological work-up in children and adolescents should include consultation of a pediatric nephrologist. Progression of clinically manifest diabetic nephropathy can be retarded, stopped, or even reversed by good glycemic control as well as adequate antiproteinuric and antihypertensive treatment [6]. As there are tremendous differences between adults compared with children and adolescents, different standards of care have to be applied [7].

Prevalence of diabetic nephropathy in children and adolescents

As the majority of cases are due to type 1 diabetes, a diagnostic advantage of most children and adolescents is the manifestation of diabetes with significant symptoms. Therefore, the development of diabetic nephropathy is well understood in type 1 diabetes. The prevalence of albuminuria is substantial in children and adolescents, but alarming in young adults with onset of diabetes in childhood or adolescence.

In a prospective study performed in Germany and Austria, 3.3% out of 27 805 patients (median age 16.3 years, range 12.5–22.2 years) with type 1 diabetes mellitus showed microalbuminuria and 0.3% showed macroalbuminuria [8] according to the guidelines of the American Diabetes Association [6]. The prevalence of ESRD requiring dialysis or renal transplantation was 0.7% (203 out of 27 805 patients) [8]. A longitudinal study assessing patients aged 17–25 years with a medium diabetes duration of 10 years, and a follow-up assessment 11 years later in Oxford described a rise in micro- and macrovascular complications in patients from 3% to 37% [4]. The prevalence of microalbuminuria was 6–21% at follow-up; macroalbuminuria was detected in 8–11%, and dialysis in 2% of patients [4, 5].

Type 2 diabetes is still relatively rare in children and adolescents, but the prevalence is rising concomitantly with the rising prevalence of adiposity [1]. With respect to diabetic nephropathy, children with type 2 diabetes have a much higher risk than children with type 1 diabetes. Type 2 diabetes is diagnosed later as it manifests slower, and chronic kidney disease (CKD) may already have developed in the prediabetic state. Additionally, patients may have comorbidities from the spectrum of the metabolic syndrome which may induce kidney damage, particularly hypertension [9]. Among young adults, there is a considerable number of patients with decreased GFR but normal urinary albumin excretion, including patients with type 2 diabetes and type 1 diabetes.

As there are rare cases of declining renal function without microalbuminuria in diabetic children and adolescents, annual measurements of serum creatinine and calculation of GFR in addition to the urine screening after at least 5 years of diabetes duration are recommended [9, 10]. Whether CKD was due to diabetic nephropathy in the studies mentioned above, however, is unclear because renal biopsies were not performed. Nevertheless, as signs of diabetic glomerulopathy in kidney biopsies can be present without micro- or macroalbuminuria, low GFR may be due to diabetic nephropathy even in the absence of albuminuria [11].

The main risk factors are duration of diabetes, poor glycemic control, adolescent-onset diabetes, puberty, and hypertension [12, 13]. Additional risk factors may be a family history of essential hypertension or cardiovascular disease, smoking, adiposity, and dyslipidemia [14, 15]. Microalbuminuria is the first sign of diabetic nephropathy in almost all patients and a strong risk factor for the development of macroalbuminuria. As microalbuminuria does often appear without hypertension, blood pressure measurements are not sufficient to recognize diabetic nephropathy [16]. However, hypertension may become manifest because of diabetic nephropathy as early as in the micoalbuminuric state and is a risk factor for accelerated disease progression [17, 7]. The importance of good glycemic control for the prevention of vascular complications of diabetes in children, adolescents, and young adults has been clearly shown [18]. At an glycosylated hemoglobin (HbA1c) above 9.6%, the risk of clinically manifest nephropathy increases substantially [19]. Intensive treatment may yield better results than conventional therapy [12]. However, the mode of therapy is no risk factor itself, as optimized conventional therapy achieves equal glycemic control [20]. Adiposity is a vascular risk factor *per se* [21], even more so in the presence of diabetes [15]. Important special aspects in adolescents and young adults are puberty and transition to adult care. During puberty, malcompliance is strongly promoted, and the risk for short- and long-term complications is increased. There are also patients who do not take enough self-responsibility

when transferred to adult medicine and are therefore unable to cope adequately with the less intense care.

In almost all diabetic patients, the finding of an increased albumin-to-creatinine ratio will be the first sign of nephropathy. After confirming the diagnosis by repeating the measurement in a sample of first morning spot urine sample, the question is whether albuminuria is due to a typical diabetic glomerular microangiopathy or for another reason [22]. In pediatric nephrology, urinary protein excretion over $100\,mg/m^2/24$ hour is classified as proteinuria. Moderate proteinuria is present when the urinary protein concentration is $>100\,mg/m^2/24$ hour and $<1000\,mg/m^2/24$ hour, nephrotic range proteinuria (gross proteinuria) is present at a urinary protein concentration of $\geq1000\,mg/m^2/24$ hour. It is important to distinguish between different types of proteinuria. Prerenal (overflow) proteinuria is extremely rare in children and adolescents, as it primarily results from the overproduction of immunoglobulin light chains due to plasma cell dyscrasia in older adults. However, performing serum electrophoresis in a pediatric patient with proteinuria should be discussed in individual cases to exclude gammopathy. Renal proteinuria is found in the majority of all cases and is subdivided into glomerular and tubular proteinuria. Finally, glomerular proteinuria is further subdivided into selective and unselective. Urinary albumin is the main marker of glomerular protein loss. Urinary immunoglobulin (IgG) is an additional marker for glomerular protein loss. Selective glomerular proteinuria is present if albumin is excreted exclusively, unselective glomerular proteinuria if the proportion of IgG is significant. α-1-Microglobulin is the main marker for tubular protein loss. In all cases of diabetic patients in which the albumin-to-creatinine ratio is elevated consistently, urinary proteins should be differentiated to classify the type of proteinuria exactly.

Urinary protein may be elevated due to exercise ("orthostatic"), stress, infection (especially urinary tract), fever, hypertension, and significant hyperglycemia. Therefore, these conditions have to be ruled out before further diagnostic investigation. As exercise is a very common benign cause for proteinuria, complete bladder emptying just before bedtime and examination of the first morning spot urine sample is recommended to avoid false-positive results. A 24-hour urine collection carried out separately day and night is a more accurate option, of course, but not recommended for screening because of the great effort. For the diagnosis of orthostatic proteinuria, it is mandatory that protein excretion during resting periods is absolutely normal, but consistently increased after periods in the upright position or exercise.

Most important nephrological differential diagnoses are nephritis or nephrosis. Nephritis typically is associated with either microscopic or gross hematuria, including dysmorphic erythrocytes and red cell casts in the urine sediment, hypertension, and renal failure. Moderate to heavy proteinuria is also present. Renal failure may result in retention of water, edemas, hyperkalemia, acidosis, hyperphosphatemia, uremia, and further disorders. Heavy proteinuria may result in hypoalbuminemia (<25 mg/dL) and additional edemas. Nephrosis is associated with gross proteinuria and hypoalbuminemia (<25 mg/dL). Edema and hypercholesterolemia are often present. Both nephritis and nephrosis result from glomerular disease. The most important forms of glomerulonephritis which typically cause nephritis are postinfectious (e.g., streptococcal infection), para-infectious, IgA nephritis, Henoch–Schoenlein nephritis, lupus nephritis, and some forms of vasculitis. The most important

forms typically causing nephrosis are minimal change glomerulopathy, focal segmental glomerulosclerosis (FSGS), and membranoproliferative glomerulonephritis. Family history should be done to check for hereditary nephritis, especially Alport syndrome and hereditary FSGS.

Because of these differential diagnoses, a pediatric nephrologist should be involved at initial diagnosis of proteinuria/albuminuria. A standard nephrological "proteinuria work-up" includes history, family history, physical examination, ultrasound of the kidneys and urinary tract, microscopic examination of the urine, albumin, IgG, and α-1-microglobulin in spot urine, 24-hour urine collection carried out separately day and night for total protein quantification, and at least a blood count and determination of serum electrolytes, creatinine, urea, albumin, total protein, C3 complement, and C4 complement. GFR should be calculated (see Diagnostics, below).

Practical approach in patient care

Diagnostics

In all children and adolescents with diabetes, at least annual screening for albuminuria is mandatory for early detection of diabetic nephropathy, which is a CKD. Furthermore, blood pressure measurements at every visit are essential for detection of high-normal blood pressure or even hypertension. CKD according to the National Kidney Foundation [10] is defined as the presence of kidney damage or decreased renal function (reduced GFR) for at least 3 months (Table 11.1). Kidney damage means structural or functional abnormalities of the kidney, manifest by either pathological abnormalities, or abnormalities in the composition in the blood or urine (including both micro- and macroalbuminuria), or abnormalities in imaging tests. Renal function as determined by

Stages of chronic kidney disease (National Kidney Foundation – KDOQI 2009 [10])

Stage	Description	GFR (mL/min/1.73 m²)
1	Kidney damage with normal or ↑ GFR	≥90
2	Kidney damage with mild ↓ GFR	60–89
3	Moderate ↓ GFR	30–59
4	Severe ↓ GFR	15–29
5	Kidney failure	<15 (or dialysis)

Chronic kidney disease is defined as either kidney damage or GFR <60 mL/min/1.73 m² for ≥3 months. Kidney damage is defined as pathologic abnormalities or markers of damage, including abnormalities in blood or urine tests or imaging studies. GFR, glomerular filtration rate; ↑, increased; ↓, decreased.
Reproduced from National Kidney Foundation: K/DOQI clinical practice guidelines for chronic kidney disease: evaluation, classification and stratification. *Am J Kidney Dis* 2002;**39**:S46–S64.

Definitions of abnormalities in albumin excretion

Category	Spot collection (µg/mg creatinine)
Normal	<30
Microalbuminuria	30–299
Macro (clinical)-albuminuria	≥300

Reproduced from National Kidney Foundation: K/DOQI clinical practice guidelines for chronic kidney disease: evaluation, classification and stratification. *Am J Kidney Dis* 2002;**39**:S46–S64.

GFR may be concurrently increased, normal, or decreased. Decreased renal function means any GFR of <60 mL/min/1.73 m² for ≥3 months, with or without kidney damage. Previously, albuminuria was used as the main parameter to stage diabetic nephropathy [23]. Today, it is recommended to determine the degree of CKD by GFR (stages 1–5, Table 11.1) [9].

The presence and degree of albuminuria can be assessed in spot urine by measurement of the albumin-to-creatinine ratio. A dipstick test is not sufficient to detect microalbuminuria. The determination of total albumin in a 24-hour urine collection adds some accuracy compared with the albumin-to-creatinine ratio, and when carried out at day and night separately, it is possible to check for the differential diagnosis of orthostatic proteinuria. However, as 24-hour collection is much more complex and prone to errors by the patient, screening for albuminuria in previously negative patients should be carried out on spot urine samples. Microalbuminuria (Table 11.2) is diagnosed in case of urinary albumin excretion of ≥30–299 mg/24 hour or spot urine albumin-to-creatinine ratios ≥30–299 µg/mg on least at two of three occasions over a 6-month period. Macroalbuminuria (Table 11.2) is diagnosed at higher albumin excretion levels (≥300 mg/24 hour or albumin-to-creatinine ratio ≥300 µg/mg in spot urine) [9]. It is recommended to measure urinary albumin excretion at least annually in all patients from the age of 10 years with diabetes duration of 5 years or more [6]. Other authors recommend annual screening for microalbuminuria from the age of 9 years if diabetes duration is at least 5 years, and from 11 years of age if diabetes duration is at least 2 years [13]. When calculating the albumin-to-creatinine ratio, it is important to check for a urinary creatinine of at least 20 mg/dL (1.8 mmol/L) to prevent false-positive results. Calculation of the ratio is done to adjust the urinary albumin concentration to urine concentration, both of which vary considerably. Moreover, urinary albumin may be elevated due to exercise, infection, fever, hypertension, and significant hyperglycemia.

A pediatric nephrologist should be involved at least once in cases of albuminuria to exclude differential diagnoses (for proteinuria work-up see Nephrological differential diagnoses, above). A decline in calculated GFR <90 mL/min/1.73 m^2 is also an indication for immediately consulting a pediatric nephrologist to exclude other etiologies of renal failure. In the case of significant chronic renal failure <60 mL/min/1.73 m^2, a complete nephrological work-up for patients with CKD should be performed.

As high-normal blood pressure and hypertension are independent risk factors for diabetic nephropathy, it is mandatory to measure blood pressure at least at every visit [7]. However, there is not only the possibility of clinic blood pressure measurement (CBP), but also of home blood pressure measurement (HBP) and ambulatory 24-hour blood pressure monitoring (ABPM). False-positive results during CPB due to "white coat hypertension" and false-negative results due to masked hypertension are known. After verification by a second CBP, therefore, ABPM should be performed whenever possible, as it provides much more reliable and additional information. Also, HBP provides more reliable data than CBP and should be performed if ABPM is impossible [24]. Blood pressure measurements should be performed by standardized techniques with adequate blood pressure monitors and cuffs. After measurement, the blood pressure percentile should be determined. Hypertension is defined as an average systolic or diastolic blood pressure ≥95th percentile for age, sex, and height, measured on at least three different days. High-normal blood pressure according to the American Diabetes Association (ADA) is defined as an average systolic or diastolic blood pressure ≥90th but <95th percentile and should also be rated as "elevated" [7]. In case of CKD, however, there is clear evidence that target 24-hour blood pressure levels should be in the low range of normal, that is <50th percentile [25], to delay disease progression. Therefore, all blood pressure values >50th to 75th percentile in these patients are "elevated" (!). Hypertension or blood pressure rated as elevated is an

indication for immediate initiation or intensification of a strict and rigorous therapy regimen. Before initiation of treatment, hypertension due to other causes should be excluded [7, 25]. For blood pressure reference tables and recommended measurement techniques see reference [26] or http://www.nhlbi.nih.gov/guidelines/hypertension/child_tbl.pdf and http://www.nhlbi.nih.gov/health/prof/heart/hbp/hbp_ped.pdf.

With respect to renal function in children and adolescents, we suggest measuring serum creatinine and BUN at least once a year in all diabetic patients. If possible, cystatin C should also be determined. As serum creatinine does not only depend on renal function, but also on muscle mass and sex, formulas are used to calculate GFR. They allow a much more accurate estimation of GFR than creatinine alone. For calculation of GFR using creatinine and height, the new "bedside" Schwartz equation [27] or the Counahan–Barratt equation [28] are recommended. For most accurate calculation of GFR using the "CKiD" Schwartz equation, [the equation uses data from the Chronic Kidney Disease in Children (CKiD) study], serum creatinine, serum cystatin C, serum BUN, height, and gender are needed. The national kidney foundation provides an online pediatric GFR calculator which includes the three most important formulae: http://www.kidney.org/professionals/kdoqi/gfr_calculatorPed.cfm.

Therapy

The management of CKD secondary to diabetes in children and adolescents has to begin with adequate treatment of diabetes to achieve primary prevention. Intensive treatment [12] and optimized conventional therapy may be applied [20]. Age-specific glycemic goals are recommended [7]. At an HbA1c above 9.6%, the risk of clinically manifest nephropathy increases substantially [19]. Ongoing re-education of the patients is mandatory [7].

Next, adequate management of albuminuria and blood pressure control are key issues. As most of the management occurs without supervision of a health care professional, education of the patient and the parents or adult caregiver, respectively, is essential not only in the treatment of diabetes, but also in prevention and therapy of diabetic nephropathy.

Most important educational contents with respect to diabetic nephropathy are the consequences of albuminuria, hypertension, and renal failure. Education has to be adapted to the patient's age. Adults always have to be involved in the medical management of a prepubertal child. In puberty, self-identity and autonomy develop, and malcompliance is common. Therefore, the risk for short- and long-term complications is clearly increased. A main goal of medical and psychological care during this stage is to maintain compliance by ongoing education and promotion of autonomy whenever possible. The responsibility for medical care has to be gradually transferred to the adolescents, as they will not be able to take over complete management immediately. A further critical phase is the transition from pediatric to adult care. Some pediatricians tend to give intensive support to their patient. Therefore, patients sometimes do not take enough self-responsibility and are unable to cope adequately with the less intense care after transition.

In the case of microalbuminuria, treatment of all non-pregnant patients above the age of 1 year is recommended with angiotensin-converting enzyme (ACE) inhibitors or angiotensin II receptor type 1 blockers (ARBs) [7, 29, 30]. ACE inhibitors slow the progression of nephropathy in patients with type 1 diabetes, microalbuminuria, and either with [6] or without [31] hypertension. In adult patients with type 2 diabetes, ACE inhibitors or ARBs delay the development of microalbuminuria, the progression to macroalbuminuria, and the progression to ESRD [32, 33]. ARBs delay the progression from microalbuminuria to macroalbuminuria in adult patients with type 2 diabetes, microalbuminuria, and hypertension. ARBs also delay the progression of nephropathy in adult patients with type 2 diabetes, macroalbuminuria, hypertension, and renal insufficiency. If ACE inhibitors are not tolerated, they may be replaced by ARBs, or vice versa [6]. Data on ARBs in diabetic children and adolescents are scarce. One study shows safety and efficaciousness of olmesartan medoxomil in 302 hypertensive individuals aged 6–16 years, among them some patients with diabetes [34]. Therefore, ARBs probably provide an alternative in children and adolescents with significant side effects due to ACE inhibitors [35]. Usage of ACE inhibitors or ARBs requires a test of serum creatinine and potassium 1 week after introduction of the medication. Under medication, the effect of the therapy has to be checked by periodical measurement of urinary albumin and blood pressure. The aim of early therapy is to normalize urinary albumin excretion [7].

Reduction of dietary protein intake to 0.8–1.0 per kg body weight per day in diabetic patients with CKD was associated with reduced albumin excretion and improved GFR in adults. However, as children and most adolescents are still growing and dietary protein critically influences growth, dietary protein restriction in this age group should be considered with caution. Nutrient recommendations for children and adolescents with type 1 diabetes are the same as for healthy children. Micro- or macroalbuminuria without significance for blood protein levels do not alter the recommendations. In patients with diabetic nephropathy, the aim of nutrition is, equally in patients without nephropathy, to prevent critical hypoglycemia, to achieve age-specific blood glucose goals, and to ensure normal growth and development. Growth and weight have to be plotted regularly on growth and weight charts [7].

In the case of confirmed hypertension or "elevated" blood pressure according to individual criteria (see Diagnostics, above), a strict and rigorous therapy regimen should immediately be initiated or intensified [7, 25]. Initially, patients with elevated blood pressure should not add salt to their diet, they should increase exercise if they have a primarily sedentary lifestyle, and reduce weight if applicable. The individual target blood pressure should be reached within 6 months. Otherwise, drug treatment has to be started. Again, ACE inhibitors are the first-line treatment in all non-pregnant patients above 1 year of age. The target blood pressure has to be below the 90th percentile according to the ADA [7]. In diabetic children with albuminuria and elevated blood pressure, however, a target blood pressure at the 50th percentile, similar to children with CKD as a result of other causes, seems to be reasonable to prevent progression of CKD [25]. If monotherapy with an ACE inhibitor is not sufficient, additional antihypertensive treatment should be added. Drug classes frequently used include ARBs, beta-blockers, calcium channel blockers, and diuretics [26].

1. Lipton RB, Drum M, Burnet D, *et al.* Obesity at the onset of diabetes in an ethnically diverse population of children: what does it mean for epidemiologists and clinicians? *Pediatrics* 2005;**115**:e553–60.

2. Nordwall M, Bojestig M, Arnqvist HJ, Ludvigsson J, Linköping Diabetes Complications Study. Declining incidence of severe retinopathy and persisting decrease of nephropathy in an unselected population of Type 1 diabetes-the Linköping Diabetes Complications Study. *Diabetologia* 2004;**47**:1266–72.

3. Caramori ML, Fioretto P, Mauer M. The need for early predictors of diabetic

nephropathy risk: is albumin excretion rate sufficient? *Diabetes* 2000;**49**:1399–408.

4. Bryden KS, Dunger DB, Mayou RA, *et al.* Poor prognosis of young adults with type 1 diabetes: a longitudinal study. *Diabetes Care* 2003;**26**:1052–7.

5. Mattock MB, Cronin N, Cavallo-Perin P, *et al.* Plasma lipids and urinary albumin excretion rate in type diabetes: the EURODIAB IDDM complications study. *Diabet Med* 2001;**18**:59–67.

6. American Diabetes Association. Standards of medical care in diabetes—2011. *Diabetes Care* 2011;**34**(Suppl 1):S11–61.

7. Silverstein J, Klingensmith G, Copeland K, *et al.*, American Diabetes Association. Care of children and adolescents with type 1 diabetes: a statement of the American Diabetes Association. *Diabetes Care* 2005;**28**:186–212.

8. Raile K, Galler A, Hofer S, *et al.* Diabetic nephropathy in 27,805 children, adolescents, and adults with type 1 diabetes: effect of diabetes duration, A1C, hypertension, dyslipidemia, diabetes onset, and sex. *Diabetes Care* 2007;**30**:2523–8.

9. Kramer H, Molitch ME. Screening for kidney disease in adults with diabetes. *Diabetes Care* 2005;**28**:1813–16.

10. National Kidney Foundation. K/DOQI clinical practice guidelines for chronic kidney disease: evaluation, classification and stratification. *Am J Kidney Dis* 2002;**39**:S46–S64.

11. Lane PH, Steffes MW, Mauer SM. Glomerular structure in IDDM women with low glomerular filtration rate and normal urinary albumin excretion. *Diabetes* 1992;**41**:581–6.

12. Diabetes Control and Complications Trial Research Group. Effect of intensive diabetes treatment on the development and progression of long-term

complications in adolescents with insulin-dependent diabetes mellitus: Diabetes Control and Complications Trial. *J Pediatr* 1994;**125**:177–88.

13. Fröhlich-Reiterer EE, Borkenstein MH. [Microvascular and macrovascular complications in children and adolescents with type 1 diabetes mellitus]. *Wien Med Wochenschr* 2010;**160**:414–8. (In German)

14. Malcom GT, Oalmann MC, Strong JP: Risk factors for atherosclerosis in young subjects: the PDAY Study: Pathobiological Determinants of Atherosclerosis in Youth. *Ann NY Acad Sci* 1997;**817**:179–88.

15. Valerio G, Iafusco D, Zucchini S, Maffeis C, The Study-Group on Diabetes of the Italian Society of Pediatric Endocrinology and Diabetology (ISPED). Abdominal adiposity and cardiovascular risk factors in adolescents with type 1 diabetes. *Diabetes Res Clin Pract* 2012;**97**:99–104.

16. Schultz CJ, Neil HA, Dalton RN, *et al.*, Oxford Regional Prospective Study Group. Blood pressure does not rise before the onset of microalbuminuria in children followed from diagnosis of type 1 diabetes. Oxford Regional Prospective Study Group. *Diabetes Care* 2001;**24**: 555–60.

17. Mathiesen ER, Ronn B, Jensen T, *et al.* Relationship between blood pressure and urinary albumin excretion in development of microalbuminuria. *Diabetes* 1990;**39**:245–9.

18. Bojestig M, Arnqvist HJ, Hermansson G, *et al.* Declining incidence of nephropathy in insulin-dependent diabetes mellitus. *N Engl J Med* 1994;**330**:15–8.

19. Nordwall M, Arnqvist HJ, Bojestig M, Ludvigsson J. Good glycemic control remains crucial in prevention of late diabetic complications—the Linköping Diabetes Complications Study. *Pediatr Diabetes* 2009;**10**:168–76.

20. Knerr I, Hofer SE, Holterhus PM, *et al.* Prevailing therapeutic regimes and predictive factors for prandial insulin substitution in 26 687 children and adolescents with Type 1 diabetes in Germany and Austria. *Diabet Med* 2007; **24**:1478–81.

21. Juonala M, Magnussen CG, Berenson GS, *et al.* Childhood adiposity, adult adiposity, and cardiovascular risk factors. *N Engl J Med* 2011;**365**:1876–85.

22. Hogg RJ, Portman RJ, Milliner D, *et al.* Evaluation and management of proteinuria and nephrotic syndrome in children: recommendations from a pediatric nephrology panel established at the National Kidney Foundation conference on proteinuria, albuminuria, risk, assessment, detection, and elimination (PARADE). *Pediatrics* 2000; **105**:1242–9.

23. Mogensen CE. Microalbuminuria as a predictor of clinical diabetic nephropathy. *Kidney Int* 1987;**31**:673–89.

24. Wühl E, Hadtstein C, Mehls O, Schaefer F, Escape Trial Group. Home, clinic, and ambulatory blood pressure monitoring in children with chronic renal failure. *Pediatr Res* 2004;**55**:492–7.

25. ESCAPE Trial Group, Wühl E, Trivelli A, Picca S, *et al.* Strict blood-pressure control and progression of renal failure in children. *N Engl J Med* 2009 Oct 22; **361**(17):1639–50.

26. National High Blood Pressure Education Program Working Group on High Blood Pressure in Children and Adolescents. The fourth report on the diagnosis, evaluation, and treatment of high blood pressure in children and adolescents. *Pediatrics* 2004;**114**:555–76.

27. Schwartz GJ, Muñoz A, Schneider MF, Mak RH, Kaskel F, Warady BA, Furth SL. New equations to estimate GFR in

children with CKD. *J Am Soc Nephrol* 2009;**20**:629–37.

28. Counahan R, Chantler C, Ghazali S, *et al.* Estimation of glomerular filtration rate from plasma creatinine concentration in children. *Arch Dis Child* 1976;**51**:875–8.

29. Remuzzi G, Benigni A, Remuzzi A. Mechanisms of progression and regression of renal lesions of chronic nephropathies and diabetes. *J Clin Invest* 2006;**116**:288–96.

30. Wühl E, Schaefer F, Medscape. Managing kidney disease with blood-pressure control. *Nat Rev Nephrol* 2011;**7**:434–44.

31. Mathiesen ER, Hommel E, Giese J, Parving HH. Efficacy of captopril in postponing nephropathy in normotensive insulin dependent diabetic patients with microalbuminuria. *BMJ* 1991;**303**:81–7.

32. Ruggenenti P, Fassi A, Ilieva AP, *et al.*, Bergamo Nephrologic Diabetes Complications Trial (BENEDICT) Investigators. Preventing microalbuminuria in type 2 diabetes. *N Engl J Med* 2004;**351**:1941–51.

33. Lewis EJ, Hunsicker LG, Clarke WR, *et al.*, Collaborative Study Group. Renoprotective effect of the angiotensin-receptor antagonist irbesartan in patients with nephropathy due to type 2 diabetes. *N Engl J Med* 2001;**345**:851–60.

34. Hazan L, Hernández Rodriguez OA, *et al.*, Assessment of Efficacy and Safety of Olmesartan in Pediatric Hypertension Study Group. A double-blind, dose-response study of the efficacy and safety of olmesartan medoxomil in children and adolescents with hypertension. *Hypertension.* 2010;**55**:1323–30.

35. Hilgers KF, Dötsch J, Rascher W, Mann JF. Treatment strategies in patients with chronic renal disease: ACE inhibitors, angiotensin receptor antagonists, or both? *Pediatr Nephrol* 2004;**19**: 956–61.

Diabetes, the kidney and retinopathy

Hans-Peter Hammes

University of Heidelberg, Mannheim, Germany

Key points

- The incidence of diabetic retinopathy is decreasing due to the implementation of intensified therapy in clinical care.
- Diabetic retinopathy indicates increased cardiovascular risk.
- Patients with diabetic macular edema should be evaluated for concurrent nephropathy before intravitreal (focal) treatment is initiated.
- Euglycemia in type 1 diabetes and multimodal therapy in type 2 diabetes are beneficial systemic therapies to prevent incidence/progression of diabetic retinopathy.

Diabetic eye disease is seemingly easy to detect, and timely diagnosis appears helpful in protection from permanent visual loss. However, despite sophisticated diagnostic tools, and progress in the understanding of natural history and epidemiology of diabetic retinopathy, there is still considerable morbidity. Recent years have witnessed a revival and novel insights into the eye as a "window" to the vasculature in the body. The visual prognosis of a person with diabetes appears to depend on multiple components, including genetic factors, compliance, and the availability of health care. Beyond that, the awareness of health care providers about the complex interactions of factors determining microvascular complications, in particular the mutual interactions between retinal and renal compartments, is crucial for comprehensive therapy. The "renal–retinal syndrome" coined by Friedman and L'Esperance in 1979, defined "coincident kidney and eye diseases resulting from diabetic

Diabetes and Kidney Disease, First Edition. Edited by Gunter Wolf.
© 2013 John Wiley & Sons, Ltd. Published 2013 by John Wiley & Sons, Ltd.

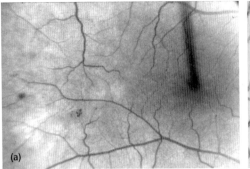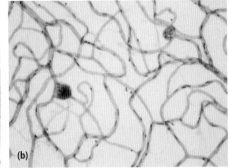

Figure 12.1 (a) Retinal fundus photography of a perimacular area with a cluster of microaneurysms. (b) Retinal digest preparation a human diabetic retina showing numerous acellular capillaries and two microaneurysms.

microvasculopathy in retinal and glomerular arterioles and capillaries" as an important diagnostic entity [1]. More than 30 years later, pathogenetic concepts, diagnostic sensitivities, and treatment modalities have changed so that this entity can be revisited. One purpose of this chapter is a joint survey of retinopathy and nephropathy.

Retinal pathology

Novel insights into the complex cellular interactions in the diabetic retina indicate that retinopathy is not an exclusive vascular disease, but that changes of the neural retina may precede and predict vascular abnormalities in the diabetic eye [2]. The implementation of sensitive diagnostic tools into research and daily practice has opened the view on retinopathy as being the result of damage to multiple different cell types in the retina. However, current grading of retinopathy is still exclusively focused on vascular changes.

The common characteristics of diabetic vascular damage are increased vascular permeability and progressive vascular occlusion. Clinically, retinopathy is divided into two distinct stages: non-proliferative and proliferative diabetic retinopathy [3]. Although only the late stage affects vision, it depends on the magnitude and velocity of the early changes.

A separate entity, termed diabetic macular edema, is defined as a condition resulting from progressive capillary dropout that causes thickening of the macula through accumulation of extracellular fluid, frequent accompanying deposition of lipoproteins, and, if the fovea is involved, vision loss. Many of the late complications start with clinically detectable vascular changes. The earliest vascular sign of diabetic retinopathy, detectable through an ophthalmoscope, or documented more permanently and objectively by (digital) fundus photography, is the microaneurysm (Figure 12.1). Clinically, it appears as a red dot >20 μm in diameter. Microaneurysms are initially hypercellular, indicating focal aberrant attempts of angiogenesis [4]. Later, they may clinically disappear because of microthrombus formation, simulating improvement. Sometimes, microaneurysms are indistinguishable from dot hemorrhages, which indicate extravasation of blood from retinal capillaries (or microaneurysms). Both microaneurysms and dot hemorrhages characterize mild non-proliferative diabetic retinopathy. Abnormal leakage of lipoproteins can precipitate around capillaries and microaneurysms. These extravasations appear as hard exudates and are yellow, sharply bounded, and of variable form and size. If these lesions cover the retinal periphery, vision remains unaffected [5].

When capillary dropout progresses into confluent avascular areas, direct or ischemic signs affect larger vessels. On the arteriolar site, microinfarcts of small arterioles disclose as "cotton-wool spots," which represent swelling of nerve fibers of the inner retina in the absence of perfusion. On the venolar site, saccular bulges ("venous beading") develop which are hypercellular in retinal digest preparations and coincide with large areas of vessel dropout. When new vessels form within the level of the retina, or microaneurysms become numerous and leaky, a severe, "preproliferative" stage of retinopathy has developed in which the risk of blinding proliferative disease is high. This second, advanced stage of retinopathy is defined by intravitreal angiogenesis, mainly originating from peripheral venules or from the optic disc. Intravitreal hemorrhages cause acute vision loss; the formation of fibrovascular tissue responding to the intravitreal discharge of inflammatory cells and its contraction is the cause of permanent vision loss through retinal detachment.

Breakdown of the blood–retinal barrier and accumulation of extracellular fluid in the macula defines diabetic macular edema. The involvement of the fovea often results in significant loss of vision. However, recent analysis also revealed that there is only a modest association between visual function as measured by acuity, and macular thickness as measured by optical coherence tomography [6].

It appears that diabetic retinopathy is more frequent in type 1 than in type 2 diabetes. The crude prevalence of any retinopathy in type 1 diabetes is 77% and 25% in type 2 diabetes according to a recent meta-analysis [7]. These figures are likely an overestimation of the current incidence and progression of retinopathy because of the implementation of glycemic and blood pressure control. Recent reanalysis of the Wisconsin Epidemiological Study of Diabetic Retinopathy (WESDR) study revealed a cumulative incidence of any retinopathy in the cohort surviving 25 years was 97%, and the cumulative rate of retinopathy progression was 83%, and the rate of progression towards the proliferative stage was 43% [8]. Of note, the yearly rate of progression over the initial 14 years of the study was similar, whereas it dropped considerably over the most recent observation period. A recent survey of 8700 type 1 diabetic patients from a large database in Germany and Austria demonstrated a cumulative proportion of any retinopathy of 84.1%, after 40 years of diabetes, and a cumulative proportion of 50.2% of advanced retinopathy [9, 10]. Other European cohorts reported a lower cumulative incidence of advanced retinopathy in type 1 diabetes (30%) [10].

Undoubtedly, the implementation of glycemic control and other measures to address the altered metabolic profile in type 1 diabetes will result in a further decrease in the incidence of diabetic retinopathy. The Diabetes Control and Complications Trial (DCCT)/Epidemiology of Diabetes Interventions and Complications results suggest that the earlier glycemia is established, the better is the retinal outcome, even when glycemic control is not maintained on the near-normal level. Comparing the two treatment groups after 30 years of diabetes, the cumulative incidence of proliferative diabetic retinopathy was 21% in the former intensive group, and 50% in the former conventional group. The latter was comparable with the 47% cumulative incidence of a population-based group of similar diabetes duration. This and the translation of Diabetic Retinopathy Study (DRS) and Early Treatment in Diabetic Retinopathy Study (ETDRS) findings into treatment of advanced retinopathy stages may also affect visual prognosis in type 1 diabetes. The implementation of panretinal laser photocoagulation increased the prevalence of eyes with proliferative diabetic retinopathy treated with photocoagulation from 55% in the 1980–1982 group to 85% in the 2005–2007 group. As a possible consequence, the prevalence of visual impairment (visual acuity <20/40 or worse in the better eye) dropped from over 15% to less than 5% in groups of similar diabetes duration when grouped for years of diabetes onset (1922–1959 versus 1975–1980). Thus, implementation of general diabetes care and specialized eye screening and laser treatment appears effective in type 1 diabetes [11].

Whether this trend extends to type 2 diabetes is unclear at present. In the WESDR study, the prevalence of any retinopathy was 50% in the 1980–1982 group, whereas in the Beaver Dam Eye Study, in 1988–1990, the prevalence was 35% [12]. More recent data from an Australian study revealed an increase in prevalence from 27% to 34% within 6 years, and preliminary data from the German DPV study reports a crude prevalence of 30% (Holl, R, *et al.*, manuscript in preparation). The proportion of patients with sight-threatening retinopathy (proliferative diabetic retinopathy and clinically significant macular edema) was similar over different onset periods. However, the numbers of patients treated for proliferative diabetic retinopathy and clinically significant macular edema (CSME) increased. As no recent estimates are published on the outcome of visual acuity in these populations, it remains uncertain whether these therapeutic effects translate into a benefit in visual outcome in type 2 diabetes. Of note, diabetic macular edema appears constant over time, at least in population-based studies such as the WESDR.

When stratifying for coincident nephropathy, it becomes clear that there is a major impact of renal disease on the progression of retinopathy to advanced stages in both type 1 and type 2 diabetes [13, 14]. This pinpoints a major task for those who treat patients with diabetes to guarantee the identification of these high-risk patients through adequate test intervals. The clinical observation that almost all patients who develop proliferative diabetic retinopathy have simultaneous nephropathy has been confirmed by numerous studies. For example, in WESDR, the odds ratio (OR) for having retinopathy in microalbuminuric patients was 3.78 for the younger and 1.8 for the older group. In a multivariate analysis, the association remained significant in the younger, but not in the older group [12]. This association is confirmed in the recent DPV study, in which the OR for severe retinopathy in microalbuminuric type 1 patients was 4.1 (95% CI 3.4–4.9) [9]. With progressive renal disease, retinopathy progression worsens to advanced sight-threatening stages. In Danish type 1 diabetic patients, the 5-year cumulative incidence of proliferative diabetic retinopathy was 74% in patients with gross proteinuria, but only 14% in patients without [15] . Similarly, the presence of gross proteinuria was associated with the 10-year incidence of proliferative diabetic retinopathy in type 1 diabetes. In the DPV study, the OR for advanced retinopathy in macroalbuminuric patients with type 1 diabetes was 8.6 (95% CI 6.4–11.5) [9].

Another problem of diabetic nephropathy is loss of renal function. There is no overview available on the association of impaired renal function in diabetes and the risk of retinopathy development and progression. From cohort studies such as the Beaver Dam Study, it is reported that the presence of chronic kidney disease (CKD) is associated with a 51% risk of developing retinopathy in a non-diabetic cohort, in which the cumulative incidence of retinopathy is 14.2% after 15 years. When CKD as defined by a glomerular filtration rate (GFR) $<60 \, mL/min/1.73 \, m^2$ was used as the entry criterion for patients to assess the prevalence of ocular pathologies, 45% were identified to have retinal pathologies, more than half of them because of diabetes, hypertension, or others. GFR less than $30 \, mL/min/1.73 \, m^2$ was associated with a threefold increased risk for retinopathy [16]. Thus, CKD may impact on retinopathy, but the present data only allow for a gross estimate compared with albuminuria and retinopathy.

CSME may strongly link to albuminuria/proteinuria in diabetic nephropathy because of the possible shared pathogenesis resulting in a generalized vascular hyperpermeability. In a small study of 40 type 2 diabetic patients, Knudsen *et al.* [17] found a significant correlation of urinary albumin excretion and transcapillary albumin escape rates with diabetic macular edema as measured by optical coherence tomography. Since generalized vascular permeability coexisted with vascular leakiness in different organs, the conclusion was that with increasing albuminuria, the impact on maculopathy would also increase. In a recent cross-sectional study in type 2 diabetes from India, multivariate regression analysis revealed a significant association of CSME with disease duration, anemia, and microalbuminuria. The study by Knudsen *et al.* [18] in North Jutland found the association of CSME and proteinuria in type 2 diabetic Caucasian patients (OR 5.18, 95% CI 1.71–15.68), but not with albuminuria. In WESDR, neither the young nor older onset groups showed any association of microalbuminuria with CSME. In contrast, gross proteinuria showed a significantly higher likelihood of association with CSME in only in the younger group (OR 2.42, 95% CI 1.20–4.88) [19].

Role of diabetic retinopathy in prediction of cardiovascular morbidity and mortality

The predictive significance of CKD and albuminuria for cardiovascular mortality is well established [19, 20]. The ease of directly visualizing parts of the vasculature through ophthalmoscopy and the opportunity for permanent documentation by digital fundus photographs have greatly stimulated research to identify and dissect the relative impact of retinal vascular pathology for prediction of cardiovascular disease (CVD) mortality [21]. WESDR was the first large study to demonstrate an excess mortality risk of death in patients with diabetic retinopathy, independent of important CVD risk factors such as age, diabetes duration, glycemia, and gender [22]. Other studies confirmed this finding in several ethnic groups. Of note, this association, which was reported in type 2 diabetes, was less consistent in type 1 diabetes, mostly because of the role of age in CVD mortality. In a recent meta-analysis including over 19 000 patients from 20 studies, Kramer *et al.* [23] found that diabetic retinopathy was predictive for all-cause mortality both in type 1 and type 2 diabetes patients. The OR for the composite outcome in type 2 diabetic patients, when adjusted for CV risk factors, was 1.61 (95% CI 1.32–1.9) for any retinopathy, and 4.22 (95% CI 2.81–6.33) for advanced retinopathy. For type 1 diabetes, the corresponding OR for any retinopathy was 4.10 (95% CI 1.50–11.18), and 7.00 (95% CI 2.22–20.0) for advanced retinopathy. When limiting the analysis to the studies that reported all-cause mortality, the meta-analysis of the association between presence of retinopathy and all-cause mortality was approximately 2.5-fold for type 1 and type 2 diabetes.

Important lessons can also be learned from patients who survive diabetes for a long period of time. The Joslin 50 Year Medalist Study recently comprehensively described the prevalence of retinopathy in relation to other vascular complications and to important biochemical risk factors [24]. Of the patients studied, 42.6% remained free from advanced retinopathy, and 86.9% had no signs of kidney disease. Glycemic control in these patients was unrelated to complications, but elevated serum levels of the advanced glycation end products (AGE) carboxyethyllysine and pentosidine were strongly associated with complications. A subset of patients may also exist characterized by slow or absent progression over time. They remain free of further worsening of retinopathy. This characteristic can only be detected by continuous screening, as long as no other biomarkers are established to predict patient subgroups that are protected. The persistent absence of nephropathy is one possible protective marker.

From the DCCT study, it is known that the risk for retinopathy clusters in families [25]. Several candidate genes in type 1 and type 2 diabetes have been investigated, but, so far, only polymorphisms for aldose reductase, Vascular endothelial growth factor (VEGF) and erythropoietin have stood up convincingly [26–28]. In type 2 diabetes, studies found a few genetic variants associated with diabetic retinopathy, which could not be replicated in an independent cohort.

Pathogenesis of diabetic retinopathy

Given the evidence cited above that the implementation of improved control of blood glucose, blood pressure, and possibly also lipids leads to an overall decrease in the incidence of diabetic retinopathy, it can be concluded that these factors, together with the cumulative exposure to these factors by duration, have the greatest impact on the outcome of retinopathy in clinical studies. However, glycosylated hemoglobin (HbA1c) accounts for only 11% of the risk of retinopathy in type 1 diabetes, suggesting that many more components may have an impact on incidence and progression of retinopathy [29]. By evaluating these factors, it appears that the evolution and natural history of diabetic retinopathy is divided into two steps: one that is characterized by vasodegeneration, and one that is characterized by the response to this injury either with angiogenesis or with increased permeability.

In addition, two important novel aspects may be considered which can help with finding more efficient treatment modalities in future: (1) the impact of the neuroglia on the vasculature in the diabetic retina, and (2) the role that the kidney plays in retinopathy progression. While the neuroglia may be involved during the initial phase of retinopathy (i.e., incidence), the role of the kidney may be notably important during the progressive phase of retinopathy.

Elevated glucose levels are set in stone in the pathogenesis of diabetic retinopathy and nephropathy. Hyperglycemia leads to an increase in oxidative stress from different sources, including mitochondrial overproduction of reactive oxygen species (ROS), enzyme-mediated cytoplasmic ROS production, and receptor-mediated ROS production [30]. As the 50 or different cell types of the retina are *per se* variably equipped with glucose transporters responding to the ambient glucose levels, with receptors responding to reactive intermediates and advanced glycation products, and enzymes producing ROS in the cytoplasm, it is likely that not one single mechanism can entirely explain the clinical phenotype [31]. A second and third level of complexity may be introduced by the effect of high blood pressure and of individual tissue responses, including antioxidant, angiogenic, neurotrophic, and inflammatory mediators, which when permanently activated may damage rather than repair the affected organs [32, 33].

Oxidative stress from hyperglycemia induces the activation of major pathogenetic pathways affecting vascular and neuroglial cells in the retina: (1) increased formation of AGEs, (2) increased expression of the receptor for AGEs (RAGE), (3) activation of protein kinase C (PKC) isoforms, and (4) overactivation of the hexosamine pathway. These mechanisms are the result of a single upstream event, i.e., mitochondrial overproduction of ROS. A fifth pathway, the aldose reductase pathway, may be shorter than the others because the K_m of aldose reductase for glucose and the concentration of the aldehyde form of glucose, which is a better substrate for aldose reductase, are too low to have a major impact.

In general, AGEs form from glucose, glycolytic intermediates such as dicarbonyls, and intermediates of free fatty acid oxidation. Extracellular AGEs form from glucose and have slow formation characteristics. In contrast, intracellular AGEs form rapidly from glycolytic intermediates such as methylglyoxal, and can modify protein function, cellular function via altered receptor recognition, and by changes in matrix interactions. Binding of AGEs leaked into plasma or extracellular AGEs accumulating on the matrix to AGE receptors of various cells can activate the transcription factor NF-κB. In the diabetic retina, the receptor for AGE, RAGE, has been localized to the retinal glia (astrocytes and Müller cells) [34]. RAGE expression can be regulated by high glucose in cell cultures and in diabetic animals involving ROS-induced methylglyoxal, which increases NF-κB and AP-1 binding to the RAGE promoter [35]. AGEs can cooperate with the hexosamine pathway (see below) to modify transcriptional corepressors such as mSin3A, which then changes the transcriptional activation of growth factors such as angiopoietin-2 (Ang-2) [36]. Thus, AGEs can mimic hypoxia in complications of target tissues like the retina.

Several PKC isoforms have been implicated in altered cell functions of the diabetic retina, in particular pericyte loss (PKC δ), blood flow, and permeability (PKC β) [37]. Persistent PKC activation results from enhanced *de novo* synthesis of diacylglycerol from hyperglycemia-induced triose phosphate, which is available because mitochondrial ROS overproduction inhibits the glycolytic enzyme GAPDH (see below). PKC activation can also result from RAGE activation via AGEs. PKC δ activation leads to increased expression of SHP-1, a protein tyrosine phosphatase affecting platelet derived growth factor-β receptor downstream signaling and pericyte apoptosis. PKC activa-

tion may also affect VEGF transcription with effects on vascular permeability.

The fourth hyperglycemia-driven biochemical abnormality is the activation of the hexosamine pathway. Fructose-6-phosphate, diverted from glycolysis, is the substrate for fructose 6-phosphate amidotransferase (GFAT) and is converted into uridine diphosphate-N-acetylglucosamine (GlucNac). Specific transferases use GlucNac for modification of serine and threonine residues. As indicated earlier, AGE modification of the transcriptional repressor mSin3A increases the recruitment of such a transferase resulting in the modification of SP3, which causes a decrease in binding to the glucose-sensitive GC box in the Ang-2 promoter, inducing Ang-2 transcription and translation. Increased expression of Ang-2 precedes pericyte loss in the diabetic retina, and accelerated formation of acellular capillaries. Ang-2 has been implicated in pericyte migration as an alternate mechanism by which incipient pericyte loss in the diabetic retina can occur as well as from apoptosis [38]. The hexosamine pathway was also reported to be relevant for transforming growth factor-β1and plasminogen activator inhibitor-1 expression; its relevance in the diabetic retina is not entirely clear.

Given the inability to prevent complications by only targeting one of the above described abnormalities, a unifying mechanisms was introduced representing a common denominator of the biochemical abnormalities, and a mechanism by which hyperglycemic memory could be explained [39]. This mechanism is the overproduction of superoxide by the mitochondrial electron transport chain. It has been demonstrated that hyperglycemia induces an increased flux of electron donors into the mitochondrial electron transport chain. The resulting voltage gradient leaks superoxide because electron transfer is blocked at complex III of the electron chain. In endothelial cells exposed to high glucose in culture, superoxide and subsequent ROS production is increased. ROS overproduction through high glucose is prevented when either the gradient is collapsed by UCP-1 or when superoxide is degraded by superoxide dismutase. Cells without mitochondria do not increase ROS production when they lack mitochondria (rho zero cells). When the glycolysis and the TCA cycle have produced a sufficient voltage under high-glucose conditions, mitochondrial ROS production causes DNA damage which activates an enzyme system called poly-ADP ribose polymerase (PARP). PARP, which normally resides in the nucleus in its inactive form, translocates to the cytoplasm upon ROS activation causing polymers of ADP-ribose to form and inhibit GAPDH activity. Inhibition of GAPDH causes increases in the glycolytic intermediates that give rise to the biochemical pathway abnormalities described above.

The principle components of these alterations are found in the retina of diabetic rats [40]. There is ample evidence of hyperglycemia-induced ROS overproduction, PARP activation, increased availability of AGEs such as methylglyoxal, and activation of the PKC and the hexosamine pathways.

These abnormalities are more or less readily reversible upon glycemic re-entry with the exception of long-lasting modifications of matrix by AGEs. Several pieces of evidence from clinical and preclinical data, however, indicate that prolonged periods of glycemia—either normal or high—leave permanent changes in the diabetic vasculature. For example, diabetic dogs developed similar degrees of retinopathy when treatment from bad to good glycemic control was changed [41]. Clinically, patients with good glycemic control over 6.5 years in the Diabetes Control and Complication Trial continued to have much lower retinopathy progression during the subsequent 14 years of follow-up, although their glycemia had become identical to former control patients whose glycemia had been much worse during the initial

6.5 years only [42]. This glycemic memory effect has also been found in patients with type 2 diabetes, and only glucose, but not blood pressure control, produces such memory in target organ complication [43]. Part of the memory effect may be explained by epigenetic changes, caused by mitochondrial ROS overproduction. They can involve methyltransferases, which induce the sustained alteration of transcription factors as shown for NF-κB and subsequent proinflammatory genes as a paradigm. The changes, although only induced by relatively short hyperglycemic periods, persist for as long as 6 days in culture and for months in diabetic animals. They can be prevented by either blocking mitochondrial ROS overproduction or by activation of the methylglyoxal detoxifying enzyme glyoxalase I [44]. Accordingly, increased H4K2 methylation of SOD2 has been found to cause downregulation of the enzyme, and failure to correct this change upon euglycemic re-entry suggests a role in hyperglycemic memory.

The validity of this concept has been confirmed in preclinical animal models of experimental diabetic retinopathy. Both, catalytic antioxidants and metabolic signal blockers were effective in preventing retinal vasoregression [40, 45]. As outlined above, ROS lead to an inhibition of GAPDH activity, and an increased concentration of intermediates upstream of the enzyme block. The resultant increased flux through metabolic pathways calls upon a strategy that shifts glycolytic intermediates such as fructose-6-phosphate and glyceraldehyde-3-phosphate from the hexosamine and the AGE pathways to alternate less toxic pathways. Both metabolites are end products of the non-oxidative part of the pentose phosphate shuttle, of which transketolase is the rate-limiting enzyme. The cofactor of transketolase is thiamine, which can activate the enzyme by 25%. However, lipid-soluble benfotiamine activates the enzyme by 250% in endothelial cells. Long-term treatment using benfotiamine in models of retinopathy prevented acellular capillary formation.

Inhibition of PARP activation using chemically defined PARP inhibitors reduced transcriptional regulation of Ang-2, pericyte apoptosis, and the formation of acellular capillaries. Chronic application of the catalytic antioxidant α-lipoic acid has produced similar results in two independent experiments.

The most predominant factor involved in the pathogenesis of advanced stages of diabetic retinopathy is VEGF [46]. Properties of VEGF comply with angiogenesis and increased vascular permeability, both of which are mechanisms relevant to proliferative diabetic retinopathy and CSME [47]. The strongest signal for VEGF regulation is hypoxia, which most likely results from progressive vascular occlusion in the retina. However, VEGF is regulated in models which develop only scattered vascular occlusions and no neovascularizations, and, in diabetic animal models, VEGF is upregulated in the retina prior to significant capillary dropouts. Moreover, VEGF is not only regulated by hypoxia as the strongest stimulus, but can also be regulated by glycolytic intermediates, ROS and AGEs which may explain why VEGF regulation precedes, and does not follow, vasoregression.

Another hypoxia-driven vascular growth factor is Ang-2. It acts as the natural antagonist of angiopoietin-1, which stimulates the endothelial receptor tyrosine kinase Tie-2. This signal promotes vascular maturation, pericyte recruitment, and tightening of the endothelial barrier function. The antagonistic Ang-2 displaces Ang-1 from Tie-2 and cooperates with VEGF to induce angiogenesis. In the absence of VEGF, it leads to vasoregression. Its role in diabetic retinopathy can be summarized as follows: (1) Ang-2 is regulated by the combined action of enzymatic and non-enzymatic glycosylation; (2) Ang-2 is upregulated prior to peri-cyte dropout, (3) Ang-2 regulation appears to determine pericyte migration as alternative to pericyte apoptosis, (4) Ang-2 reduction reduces vasoregression in diabetic retinopathy [38, 48].

Inflammatory signaling has become a favorite subject of retinopathy research since leukocytes and monocytes have been found at increased numbers in the diabetic rat retina. Pattern recognition receptors such as RAGE mediate the response by regulation of inflammatory cytokines via NF-κB (see above). Since the absolute expression levels and the regulation in diabetes is lower than, for example, in sepsis, the term parainflammation may be more appropriate. Inhibition of genetic deletion of several mediators of parainflammation such as NF-κB, iNOS, COX, ICAM and interleukin (IL)-1β has been shown to improve early lesions in experimental retinopathy models. iNOS is predominantly expressed by macrophages and microglia in the diabetic retina, and microglia is activated in diabetic retinopathy, suggesting that this cell type mediates damage to the vasculature [33].

Interaction of AGEs with RAGE activates the endothelium by inducing the expression of adhesion molecules such as ICAM-1 and VCAM-1, which stimulate leukocyte adherence to the endothelium. This leukostasis is thought to contribute to microvascular damage by the release of toxic cytokines or by occluding capillaries [49]. Leukostasis is increased in the retina of diabetic animals in all three areas, i.e., arterioles, venoles, and capillaries. Leukostasis even occurs in the absence of overt hyperglycemia in obese rat strains, and the relationship between leukostasis and capillary regression is probably not causal because vasoregression can be prevented without correction of leukostasis [50, 51].

The concomitant presence of hypertension and diabetes multiplies the risk of nephropathy. The underlying mechanisms which define the cellular response phenotypes of this deadly couple are poorly understood. It is, however, suggested that hypertension, renal impairment, and increased shear stress impact on the pre-existing biochemical abnormalities induced by chronic hyperglycemia.

Lopes de Faria *et al.* [32] recently pointed out that hyperglycemia and hypertension cooperate in the generation of oxidative stress and inflammation causing an aggravation and acceleration of retinopathy and nephropathy. Hypertension *per se* induces oxidative stress through activation of the renin–angiotensin system, of PKC isoforms, and the overexpression of inflammatory cytokines, among others. Mechanical stress-induced upregulation of angiotensin II directly induces ROS production, VEGF upregulation independently of hypoxia and hyperglycemia, and vasoconstriction. Increased shear stress in hypertension may interact with hyperglycemic signaling also on the level of permanent NF-κB activation and subsequent inflammatory gene expression.

As pointed out by Calcutt *et al.* [31], metabolic and hemodynamic pathways can interact on various levels: both can determine formation of reactive intermediates, biochemical mediators, and ROS, and both can induce and modify intracellular signaling and expression of growth factors. As both can also modify shear stress-induced vasoreactivity and inflammation, the interaction may amplify injury and perpetuate microvascular disease progression. This may explain why various treatment modalities, such as metabolic signal blockers and catalytic antioxidants, have shown efficacy in experimental animal models, both for nephropathy and retinopathy. For example, benfotiamine and thiamine have been shown to reduce albuminuria together with a reduction of methylglyoxaltype AGEs and PKC activation in the diabetic kidney [52]. PARP inhibition reduced podocyte loss, mesangial expansion, and albuminuria, and α-lipoic acid reduced glomerular sclerosis indices and albuminuria [53].

As in the retina, VEGF was established as an important mediator of glomerular damage in the kidney. VEGF-A is constitutively expressed in glomerular podocytes which signal to VEGF-R bearing endothelial and mesangial cells [54]. Increased VEGF-A levels are associated with endothelial proliferation and neovascularization in the kidney. As in the retina, a constitutive level of VEGF-A is requisite for normal function, because both the absence and the overproduction of VEGF are associated with glomerular pathology and proteinuria. Neutralizing VEGF with an antibody was effective in normalizing albuminuria or proteinuria and glomerular sclerosis in diabetic animals [55].

Angiopoietins are also important for the regulation of the glomerular filtration barrier. Ang-1 is expressed in the normal podocyte, and Ang-2 is not detectable in the normal kidney. However, Ang-2 is deregulated when albuminuria develops in diabetic nephropathy and other glomerular diseases. Podocyte overexpression of Ang-2 causes albuminuria and glomerular endothelial cell apoptosis. Although these data suggest a role for Ang-2 in glomerular filtration, it needs to be clarified whether or not Ang-2 is a permeability factor. It has recently been shown that Ang-2 can act as a stimulus for Tie-2 under stress conditions [56].

Figure 12.2 summarizes the pathogenetic concept of diabetic microvascular damage.

Clinical treatment

Although many mechanism-based treatment options are currently validated in preclinical models and phase II–IV studies, our current concepts of prevention and intervention in diabetic retinopathy (and general vasculopathy) is being challenged by the re-evaluation of clinical trials. In a recent systematic review and meta-analysis of randomized clinical trials, the effect of targeting intensive glycemic control versus conventional control on retin-

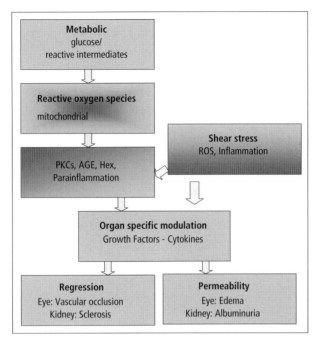

Proposed pathogenetic concept of diabetic microvascular complications. Hyperglycemia and reactive intermediates cause mitochondrial overproduction of reactive oxygen species. Biochemical pathways are overactivated and increased shear stress perpetuates and aggravates biochemical abnormalities and parainflammation. Tissue specific growth factors and cytokines determine the response to injury. AGE, advanced glycation end product; PKC, protein kinase C; ROS, reactive oxygen species.

opathy was 20%, but trial sequential analyses did not give sufficient evidence for a true effect [57]. These data suggest that the overall effect of glycemic control might have been overestimated, and that limitations of euglycemic treatment targets are considerable due to a 30% increase in the relative risk of severe hypoglycemia.

Blockade of RAS in normotensive type 1 diabetic patients slows the progression of established retinopathy independent of blood pressure [58]. Blood pressure control *per se* does not prevent the incidence of retinopathy in type 2 diabetes [59]. However, when blood pressure is elevated, a reduction is beneficial to prevent retinopathy progression [60].

Lipid control is yet another concept by which retinopathy may be treated, given the observation of lipid-rich hard exudates as one lesion. Results from the FIELD study suggest that fenofibrate treatment reduces the need for laser treatment in patients with type 2 diabetes and proliferative diabetic retinopathy and diabetic macular edema [61]. These effects were independent of the effect of fenofibrate on lipid concentrations. There was no effect on several other parameters such as retinopathy incidence, visual outcome, or hard exudates. Overall, the number of events was small, and the indication for laser treatment was not prespecified for all centers. In a substudy to ACCORD, the combination of fibrates with statins was assessed for the effect on retinopathy progression. A 40% reduction for the risk of a three-step retinopathy progression, laser treatment, or vitrectomy was reported [59].

Multifactorial treatment for glycemia, blood pressure, lipids, platelet aggregation, and lifestyle has been evaluated in microalbuminuric type 2 diabetic patients. There was a 55% risk reduction for the need of laser treatment, and a 43% risk reduction for retinopathy progression in this high-risk population [62].

The gold standard for treatment of proliferative diabetic retinopathy remains panretinal laser photocoagulation. This is 95% effective in the preventing loss of vision loss. In CSME, the effect of grid laser photocoagulation is only reduced by 50% over 3 years. Novel therapies addressing both the inflammatory epiphenomena of progressive vascular occlusion and ischemia in the diabetic eye, including steroids and anti-VEGF strategies, show benefits in subsets of patients with type 2 diabetes [63, 64]. For pseudophakic eyes, first-line treatment of diabetic macular edema is triamcinolone. For phakic eyes, anti-VEGF therapy with ranibizumab and deferred grid laser provide an additional visual benefit over triamcinolone over 2 years.

Overall, it appears that systemic therapy of diabetic microvascular complications needs to address shared pathophysiologic mechanisms of which the general targets have to be annotated. The more retinopathy and nephropathy progress and are overlayed by systemic factors such as prolonged metabolic and hemodynamic alterations, the more organ-specific proangiogenic (retina) and prosclerotic (kidney) epiphenomena take over. Identification of patients at risk for developing advanced organ damage is a perpetual challenge and addressed by ongoing studies. Until better markers are identified, renal involvement is an important risk indicator for both retinopathy progression and increased cardiovascular risk.

References

1. Friedman EA, L'Esperance FA Jr. *Diabetic renal-retinal syndrome. Therapy*. New York, NY: Grune & Stratton, 1986.

2. Antonetti DA, Klein R, Gardner TW. Diabetic retinopathy. *N Engl J Med* 2012; **366**:1227–39.

3. Frank RN. Diabetic retinopathy. *N Engl J Med* 2004;**350**:48–58.

4. Aguilar E, Friedlander M, Gariano RF. Endothelial proliferation in diabetic retinal microaneurysms. *Arch Ophthalmol* 2003;**121**:740–1.

5. Bresnick GH SP, Mattson D. Fluorescein angiographic and clinicopathologic findings. In: Little HL JR, Patz A, Forsham PH (eds) *Diabetic Retinopathy*. Stuttgart: Georg Thieme Verlag, 1983, pp. 37–71.

6. Browning DJ, Glassman AR, Aiello LP, *et al*. Relationship between optical coherence tomography-measured central retinal thickness and visual acuity in diabetic macular edema. *Ophthalmology* 2007;**114**:525–36.

7. Yau JW, Rogers SL, Kawasaki R, *et al*. Global prevalence and major risk factors of diabetic retinopathy. *Diabetes Care* 2012;**35**:556–64.

8. Klein R, Knudtson MD, Lee KE, *et al*. The Wisconsin Epidemiologic Study of Diabetic Retinopathy: XXII the twenty-five-year progression of retinopathy in persons with type 1 diabetes. *Ophthalmology* 2008;**115**:1859–68.

9. Hammes HP, Kerner W, Hofer S, *et al*. Diabetic retinopathy in type 1 diabetes-a contemporary analysis of 8,784 patients. *Diabetologia* 2011;**54**:1977–84.

10. Hovind P, Tarnow L, Rossing K, *et al*. Decreasing incidence of severe diabetic microangiopathy in type 1 diabetes. *Diabetes Care* 2003;**26**:1258–64.

11. Klein R, Klein BE. Are individuals with diabetes seeing better?: a long-term epidemiological perspective. *Diabetes* 2010;**59**:1853–60.

12. Klein R. Diabetic retinopathy and nephropathy. In: Cortes P, Mogensen CE

(eds) *The diabetic kidney*. Totowa, NJ: Humana Press, 2006, pp. 473–98.

13. Gilbert RE, Tsalamandris C, Allen TJ, *et al*. Early nephropathy predicts vision-threatening retinal disease in patients with type I diabetes mellitus. *J Am Soc Nephrol* 1998;**9**:85–9.

14. Jensen T, Deckert T. Diabetic retinopathy, nephropathy and neuropathy. Generalized vascular damage in insulin-dependent diabetic patients. *Horm Metab Res Suppl* 1992;**26**:68–70.

15. Kofoed-Enevoldsen A, Jensen T, Borch-Johnsen K, Deckert T. Incidence of retinopathy in type I (insulin-dependent) diabetes: association with clinical nephropathy. *J Diabet Complications* 1987; **1**:96–9.

16. Grunwald JE, Alexander J, Maguire M, *et al*. Prevalence of ocular fundus pathology in patients with chronic kidney disease. *Clin J Am Soc Nephrol* 2010;**5**:867–73.

17. Knudsen ST, Bek T, Poulsen PL, *et al*. Macular edema reflects generalized vascular hyperpermeability in type 2 diabetic patients with retinopathy. *Diabetes Care* 2002;**25**:2328–34.

18. Knudsen LL, Lervang HH, Lundbye-Christensen S, Gorst-Rasmussen A. The North Jutland County Diabetic Retinopathy Study (NCDRS) 2. Non-ophthalmic parameters and clinically significant macular oedema. *Br J Ophthalmol* 2007;**91**:1593–5.

19. Klein R, Klein BE, Moss SE, Cruickshanks KJ. The Wisconsin Epidemiologic Study of Diabetic Retinopathy: XVII. The 14-year incidence and progression of diabetic retinopathy and associated risk factors in type 1 diabetes. *Ophthalmology* 1998;**105**:1801–15.

20. Matsushita K, van der Velde M, Astor BC, *et al*. Association of estimated glomerular filtration rate and albuminuria with all-cause and cardiovascular mortality in general population cohorts: a collaborative meta-analysis. *Lancet* 2010;**375**:2073–81.

21. Liew G, Wang JJ, Mitchell P, Wong TY. Retinal vascular imaging: a new tool in microvascular disease research. *Circ Cardiovasc Imaging* 2008;**1**:156–61.

22. Klein R, Klein BE, Moss SE, Cruickshanks KJ. Association of ocular disease and mortality in a diabetic population. *Arch Ophthalmol* 1999;**117**:1487–95.

23. Kramer CK, Rodrigues TC, Canani LH, *et al*. Diabetic retinopathy predicts all-cause mortality and cardiovascular events in both type 1 and 2 diabetes: meta-analysis of observational studies. *Diabetes Care* 2011;**34**:1238–44.

24. Sun JK, Keenan HA, Cavallerano JD, *et al*. Protection from retinopathy and other complications in patients with type 1 diabetes of extreme duration: the Joslin 50-year medalist study. *Diabetes Care* 2011;**34**:968–74.

25. Clustering of long-term complications in families with diabetes in the diabetes control and complications trial. The Diabetes Control and Complications Trial Research Group. *Diabetes* 1997;**46**: 1829–39.

26. Tong Z, Yang Z, Patel S, *et al*. Promoter polymorphism of the erythropoietin gene in severe diabetic eye and kidney complications. *Proc Natl Acad Sci USA* 2008;**105**:6998–7003.

27. Abhary S, Burdon KP, Laurie KJ, *et al*. Aldose reductase gene polymorphisms and diabetic retinopathy susceptibility. *Diabetes Care* 2010;**33**:1834–6.

28. Al-Kateb H, Mirea L, Xie X, *et al*. Multiple variants in vascular endothelial growth factor (VEGFA) are risk factors for time to severe retinopathy in type 1 diabetes: the DCCT/EDIC genetics study. *Diabetes* 2007;**56**:2161–8.

29. Hirsch IB, Brownlee M. Beyond hemoglobin A1c–need for additional markers of risk for diabetic microvascular complications. *JAMA* 2010;**303**:2291–2.

30. Giacco F, Brownlee M. Oxidative stress and diabetic complications. *Circ Res* 2010;**107**:1058–70.

31. Calcutt NA, Cooper ME, Kern TS, Schmidt AM. Therapies for hyperglycaemia-induced diabetic complications: from animal models to clinical trials. *Nat Rev Drug Discov* 2009; **8**:417–29.

32. Lopes de Faria JB, Silva KC, Lopes de Faria JM. The contribution of hypertension to diabetic nephropathy and retinopathy: the role of inflammation and oxidative stress. *Hypertens Res* 2011;**34**:413–22.

33. Tang J, Kern TS. Inflammation in diabetic retinopathy. *Prog Retin Eye Res* 2011;**30**: 343–58.

34. Wang Y, Vom Hagen F, Pfister F, *et al*. Receptor for advanced glycation end product expression in experimental diabetic retinopathy. *Ann NY Acad Sci* 2008;**1126**:42–5.

35. Bierhaus A, Nawroth PP. Multiple levels of regulation determine the role of the receptor for AGE (RAGE) as common soil in inflammation, immune responses and diabetes mellitus and its complications. *Diabetologia* 2009;**52**:2251–63.

36. Yao D, Taguchi T, Matsumura T, *et al*. High glucose increases angiopoietin-2 transcription in microvascular endothelial cells through methylglyoxal modification of mSin3A. *J Biol Chem* 2007;**282**: 31038–45.

37. Geraldes P, King GL. Activation of protein kinase C isoforms and its impact on diabetic complications. *Circ Res* 2010; **106**:1319–31.

38. Pfister F, Feng Y, vom Hagen F, *et al*. Pericyte migration: a novel mechanism of pericyte loss in experimental diabetic retinopathy. *Diabetes* 2008;**57**: 2495–502.

39. Brownlee M. Biochemistry and molecular cell biology of diabetic complications. *Nature* 2001;**414**:813–20.

40. Hammes HP, Du X, Edelstein D, Ju Q, *et al*. Benfotiamine blocks three major pathways of hyperglycemic damage and prevents experimental diabetic retinopathy. *Nat Med* 2003;**9**:294–9.

41. Engerman RL, Kern TS. Progression of incipient diabetic retinopathy during good glycemic control. *Diabetes* 1987; **36**:808–12.

42. White NH, Sun W, Cleary PA, *et al*. Effect of prior intensive therapy in type 1 diabetes on 10-year progression of retinopathy in the DCCT/EDIC: comparison of adults and adolescents. *Diabetes* 2010;**59**:1244–53.

43. Holman RR, Paul SK, Bethel MA, *et al*. 10-year follow-up of intensive glucose control in type 2 diabetes. *N Engl J Med* 2008;**359**:1577–89.

44. El-Osta A, Brasacchio D, Yao D, *et al*. Transient high glucose causes persistent epigenetic changes and altered gene expression during subsequent normoglycemia. *J Exp Med* 2008;**205**: 2409–17.

45. Lin J, Bierhaus A, Bugert P, *et al*. Effect of R-(+)-alpha-lipoic acid on experimental diabetic retinopathy. *Diabetologia* 2006; **49**:1089–96.

46. Aiello LP, Avery RL, Arrigg PG, *et al*. Vascular endothelial growth factor in ocular fluid of patients with diabetic retinopathy and other retinal disorders. *The New England journal of medicine*. 1994;**331**:1480–7.

47. Duh E, Aiello LP. Vascular endothelial growth factor and diabetes: the agonist versus antagonist paradox. *Diabetes* 1999;**48**:1899–906.

48. Hammes HP, Lin J, Wagner P, *et al.* Angiopoietin-2 causes pericyte dropout in the normal retina: evidence for involvement in diabetic retinopathy. *Diabetes* 2004;**53**:1104–10.

49. Curtis TM, Gardiner TA, Stitt AW. Microvascular lesions of diabetic retinopathy: clues towards understanding pathogenesis? *Eye (Lond)* 2009;**23**: 1496–508.

50. Li G, Tang J, Du Y, Lee CA, Kern TS. Beneficial effects of a novel RAGE inhibitor on early diabetic retinopathy and tactile allodynia. *Mol Vis* 2011;**17**:3156–65.

51. Wang Q, Gorbey S, Pfister F, *et al.* Long-term treatment with suberythropoietic Epo is vaso- and neuroprotective in experimental diabetic retinopathy. *Cell Physiol Biochem* 2011; **27**:769–82.

52. Babaei-Jadidi R, Karachalias N, Ahmed N, *et al.* Prevention of incipient diabetic nephropathy by high-dose thiamine and benfotiamine. *Diabetes* 2003;**52**:2110–20.

53. Szabo C, Biser A, Benko R, *et al.* Poly(ADP-ribose) polymerase inhibitors ameliorate nephropathy of type 2 diabetic Leprdb/db mice. *Diabetes* 2006;**55**:3004–12.

54. Karalliedde J, Gnudi L. Endothelial factors and diabetic nephropathy. *Diabetes Care* 2011;**34**(Suppl 2):S291–6.

55. Flyvbjerg A, Dagnaes-Hansen F, De Vriese AS, *et al.* Amelioration of long-term renal changes in obese type 2 diabetic mice by a neutralizing vascular endothelial growth factor antibody. *Diabetes* 2002;**51**:3090–4.

56. Woolf AS, Gnudi L, Long DA. Roles of angiopoietins in kidney development and disease. *J Am Soc Nephrol* 2009;**20**:239–44.

57. Hemmingsen B, Lund SS, Gluud C, *et al.* Intensive glycaemic control for patients with type 2 diabetes: systematic review with meta-analysis and trial sequential analysis of randomised clinical trials. *BMJ* 2011;**343**:d6898.

58. Mauer M, Zinman B, Gardiner R, *et al.* Renal and retinal effects of enalapril and losartan in type 1 diabetes. *N Engl J Med* 2009;**361**:40–51.

59. Chew EY, Ambrosius WT, Davis MD, *et al.* Effects of medical therapies on retinopathy progression in type 2 diabetes. *N Engl J Med* 2010;**363**:233–44.

60. Tight blood pressure control and risk of macrovascular and microvascular complications in type 2 diabetes: UKPDS 38. UK Prospective Diabetes Study Group. *BMJ* 1998;**317**:703–13.

61. Keech AC, Mitchell P, Summanen PA, *et al.* Effect of fenofibrate on the need for laser treatment for diabetic retinopathy (FIELD study): a randomised controlled trial. *Lancet* 2007;**370**:1687–97.

62. Gaede P, Lund-Andersen H, Parving HH, Pedersen O. Effect of a multifactorial intervention on mortality in type 2 diabetes. *N Engl J Med* 2008;**358**: 580–91.

63. Rajendram R, Fraser-Bell S, Kaines A, *et al.* A 2-Year prospective randomized controlled trial of intravitreal bevacizumab or laser therapy (BOLT) in the management of diabetic macular edema: 24-month data: report 3. *Arch Ophthalmol* 2012 (in press).

64. Dewan V, Lambert D, Edler J, *et al.* Cost-effectiveness analysis of ranibizumab plus prompt or deferred laser or triamcinolone plus prompt laser for diabetic macular edema. *Ophthalmology* 2012;**119**:1679–84.

Part III

Prevention and Therapy

Reducing progression of diabetic nephropathy by antihyperglycemic treatment

Christoph Hasslacher

Diabetesinstitut Heidelberg, Heidelberg, Germany

Key points

- The quality of metabolic control is an essential component of the multifactorial strategy that is currently recommended for primary and secondary prevention of diabetic nephropathy.
- Implementation of an optimized metabolic control improves not only the course of the nephropathy, but also the prognosis of patients.
- The target of glycemic control, i.e., glycosylated hemoglobin (HbA1c) values, depends on various clinical findings such as age, concomitant diseases, and risk of hypoglycemia.
- With declining renal function, attention must be paid to the altered pharmacokinetics of the administered agents in order to prevent hypoglycemia.

- Monitoring of metabolic control in renally impaired diabetic patients is extremely important in view of the high risk of hypoglycemia because of the altered therapeutic conditions.
- Reliable methods are available both for blood glucose self-monitoring and the monitoring of long-term glycemic control. With renal insufficiency, however, confounding factors may come into play which must be considered when interpreting measurements.

The progression of diabetic nephropathy from the initial appearance of persistent microalbuminuria to terminal renal insufficiency is slow. If diagnosed early, there is ample time available for therapeutic intervention. Numerous factors are known to modulate the course of nephropathy, including diabetes and hypertension, dyslipidemia, cigarette smoking, anemia status, obesity, and protein consumption. These are all treatable factors that are of varying degrees for different patients, and which are differentially susceptible to influence for changing the

---

Diabetes and Kidney Disease, First Edition. Edited by Gunter Wolf.
© 2013 John Wiley & Sons, Ltd. Published 2013 by John Wiley & Sons, Ltd.

clinical course of a nephropathy. The "multifactorial" presence of treatable influence factors has led to the current recommendation to always align therapeutic intervention for diabetic nephropathy in an multifactorial manner, i.e., to treat all possible factors at the same time wherever possible. This strategy has led to more intensive antihypertensive and lipid therapy, which has improved the prognosis of diabetic nephropathy when considering the relative reduction in risk [1]. The target of improved diabetes control has not been approached in clinical studies, however, so that intensification of this component of multifactorial treatment is certainly called for [2].

Diabetes control and development of nephropathy (primary prevention)

The prime importance of diabetes management for primary prevention of diabetic nephropathy is now well documented. In *patients with type 1 diabetes* this relationship had already been demonstrated in the 1980s in small intervention studies with a short monitoring period [3].

The Diabetes Control and Complications Trial (DCCT) study was able to confirm and expand these findings [4, 5]. A total of 1441 patients were treated with either intensive or conventional insulin therapy for an average of 9 years. The improved metabolic control with intensified therapy [mean glycosylated hemoglobin (HbA1c) 7.0%] resulted in a lower incidence of microalbuminuria than that which was observed under standard treatment (mean HbA1c 8.9%): as such, the cumulative incidence in the "primary prevention group" (patients with short duration of diabetes without retinopathy) was 16% under intensified therapy and 27% under standard therapy. In the "secondary prevention group" (patients with longer duration of diabetes and pre-existing retinopathy), the corresponding inci-

dences were 26% and 42%. Also, the occurrence of advanced stage microalbuminuria (albumin excretion >70 µg/min) or the occurrence of macroalbuminuria (albumin excretion >200 µg/min) was significantly reduced under intensified metabolic control. The calculated risk reductions are presented in Figure 13.1 [4, 5].

Most patients in the DCCT study (n = 1375) participated in further monitoring (DCCT/EDIC; [6]). The treatment was now no longer performed by trial centers, but rather by general practitioners. In the intensified treatment group there was a slight deterioration of metabolic control (HbA1c 7.9%) whereas in the conventionally treated group there was an improvement (HbA1c 8.2%). Despite the change in mode of the metabolic control, the beneficial effect of intensive insulin therapy on nephropathy development persisted: after 4 years of follow-up the reduction in risk for the occurrence of microalbuminuria was 53% while that for macroalbuminuria was 86%.

Results on the course of renal function have recently been reported after a total of 22 years of monitoring [7]. Here, too, the positive impact of prior intensive diabetes therapy could be shown: impaired renal function, i.e., a glomerular filtration rate (GFR) <60 mL/min/1.73 m^2, appeared in 24 patients of the intensively and 46 patients of the conventionally treated group. The development of terminal renal insufficiency was also only half as high in the initially intensively treated group (8 versus 16 patients). The lower the HbA1c in the intensive group, the lower was the risk of an impaired GFR.

In patients with type 2 diabetes it could also be shown in four large intervention studies (UKPDS, ACCORD, ADVANCE, and VADT) that there was a beneficial influence of improved metabolic control on the primary prevention of diabetic nephropathy. The main characteristics of these studies are illustrated in Table 13.1, whereas the results for the occurrence of micro- or macroalbuminuria are given in Table 13.2.

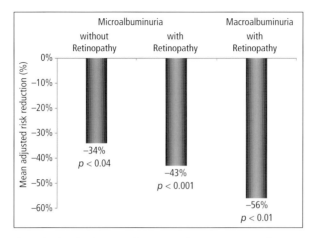

Mean adjusted risk reduction regarding onset of micro- or macroalbuminuria in type 1 diabetic patients of the intensified treated group. According to The effect of intensive treatment of diabetes on the development and progression of long-term complications in insulin-dependent diabetes mellitus. The Diabetes Control and Complications Trial Research Group. *N Engl J Med* 1993 Sep 30;**329**(14):977–86. and Effect of intensive therapy on the development and progression of diabetic nephropathy in the Diabetes Control and Complications Trial. The Diabetes Control and Complications (DCCT) Research Group. *Kidney Int* 1995 Juni;**47**(6):1703–20.

Main characteristics of patients at start of study

	UKPDS	ACCORD	ADVANCE	VADT
Patients (*n*)	3867	10251	11140	1791
Age (years)	54	62	66	60
Known diabetes (years)	0	10	8	11,5
HbA1c (%)	7,1	8,1	7,2	9,5
Known cardiovascular complications (%)	0	35	32	40

Risk reduction (RR) regarding onset of renal endpoints due to intensified glucose control in four intervention studies with type 2 diabetic patients

	UKPDS	ACCORD	ADVANCE	VADT
HbA1c (%) intensive group	7.0	6.4	6.4	6.9
HbA1c (%) standard group	7.9	7.5	7.0	8.4
Treatment period (years)	12	3.5	5.0	6.25
RR microalbuminuria	−33%	−21%	−9%	n.s.
RR macroalbuminuria	−34%	−31%	−30%	n.s.
RR doubling S-creatinine	−74%	n.d.	n.s.	n.d.

n.s., not significant; n.d., not done.

In the UKPDS study [8], newly identified patients with type 2 diabetes were monitored under a conventional or intensive treatment with oral antidiabetic drugs and/or insulin for 15 years. The HbA1c in the intensified treatment group was reduced by about 0.9% throughout the entire study. This led to a significant decrease in nephropathy risk, as shown in Table 13.2 for various end point measures. There was no difference regarding the chosen form of therapy, i.e., whether oral hypoglycemic agents or insulin were used. These findings could be confirmed in a UKPDS follow-up study over 10 years [9].

In the ACCORD study [10], antidiabetic therapy was characterized by the multiple use of oral hypoglycemic agents and insulin. In the intensively treated group almost all patients received metformin (95%), glitazone (92%), and sulfonylureas (87%), whereas insulin therapy was given to 77% of the patients. In the control group with "standard therapy" the prevalences were lower (metformin 87%, glitazone 58%, sulfonylureas 74%, and insulin 55%). Under improved metabolic control in the intensified treatment group, a highly significant reduction in risk for the occurrence of micro- or macroalbuminuria was evident after 3.5 years of monitoring (Table 13.2).

After the study was terminated due to increased mortality among the patients undergoing intensified therapy, the patients were then assigned to the "standard treatment" group and treatment continued in that way. In antidiabetic therapy in the subsequent period, less insulin (52%) and rosiglitazone (25%) was administered. After a total of 5 years of follow-up, HbA1c in the originally intensively treated group at 7.2% was still significantly lower than it was in the standard therapy group (7.6%). Just as with the UKPDS, the risk reductions regarding the occurrence of micro- or macroalbuminuria remained (−15% and −28%, respectively).

In the ADVANCE study [11] the proportions of patients treated in the intensive arm were 94% for sulfonylurea (gliclazide), 74% for metformin, and 17% for glitazone. Forty-one percent of the patients received insulin. In the standard therapy arm the prevalences were correspondingly lower: sulfonylureas 62%, metformin 67%, glitazone 11%, and insulin 24%. The group with intensified metabolic therapy achieved a mean HbA1c of 6.49%, which was maintained over 5 years. Compared with the conventionally treated group with an HbA1c of 7.2% there was a significant reduction in the risk for the occurrence of micro- and macroalbuminuria (Table 13.2). There was no effect on the end point "doubling of serum creatinine". This was probably related to the short period over which the patients were monitored.

In the VADT study [12], which included almost exclusively male patients, no significant influence on the primary prevention of diabetic nephropathy was detected. The diabetes treatment was characterized by a high prevalence of insulin (90% in the intensive and 74% in the standard group). The prevalences for metformin, sulfonylurea, or glitazone dosing were similar (60%, 55%, 72%).

Practical consequences

The presented studies show that in patients with type 1 and type 2 diabetes there is a close relationship between the quality of metabolic control (HbA1c) and the development of diabetic nephropathy (micro/macroalbuminuria).

For primarily preventing diabetic nephropathy in patients with type 1 diabetes and type 2 diabetes at a younger age and without concomitant cardiovascular complications, near-normal glycemic control aiming for HbA1c levels of <6.5% is suggested.

In type 2 diabetes afflicting older patients or in the presence of cardiovascular complications, HbA1c levels in the range 6.5–7.5% should be targeted.

The choice of antidiabetic drug has no impact on the development of nephropathy.

The progression of nephropathy in its early stages (micro/macroalbuminuria with normal renal function) can be prevented or at least slowed down by tight glycemic control. For type 1 diabetes this was shown by a combined analysis of the STENO studies I and II, in which 51 patients with microalbuminuria were analyzed for progression to macroalbuminuria after 5 or 8 years of treatment with intensified or conventional insulin therapy [13]. As Figure 13.2 shows, the progression rate was significantly lower with better metabolic control. Similar results were also revealed by the EDIC study [6]: from type 1 diabetics who revealed a microalbuminuria at the end of the DCCT study, only 8% of the intensively treated, but 31% of the conventionally treated diabetics, developed macroalbuminuria (Figure 13.2). The recently published study following 22

years of monitoring confirmed these findings and also showed that a high percentage (40%) of patients can undergo a normalization of the albuminuria under intensive therapy [14].

Intervention studies concerning type 1 diabetic patients with impaired renal function have not been published. Monitoring studies on smaller cohorts also revealed a positive effect of good metabolic control in combination with good blood pressure control for nephropathy progression [15, 16]. One Italian study [16] showed that after multifactorial treatment, i.e., near-normal glycemic control (mean HbA1c 6.5%), intensive blood pressure therapy with an angiotensin-converting enzyme (ACE) inhibitor (mean blood pressure 120/75 mmHg) and normalization of protein intake (0.8–1.0 g/kg body weight/day), progression of renal impairment could be arrested or even reversed (Figure 13.3).

For patients with type 2 diabetes and microalbuminuria it could also be demonstrated that good metabolic control can reduce the progression of nephropathy [1, 17, 18]. In the STENO-II study, type 2 diabetics with microalbuminuria were randomly assigned to receive either an intensive or a conventional treatment regimen [1]. In addition to the goal

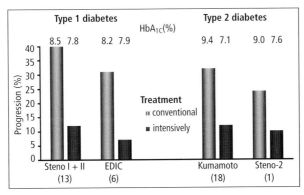

Metabolic control and progression of nephropathy from microalbuminuria to macroalbuminuria in studies with type 1 and type 2 diabetic patients.

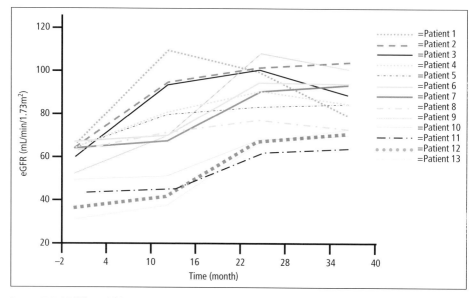

Figure 13.3 Multifactorial intervention and course of nephropathy in type 1 diabetic patients with advanced stages of nephropathy. Reproduced from Manto A, Cotroneo P, Marra G, Magnani P, Tilli P, Greco AV, et al. Effect of intensive treatment on diabetic nephropathy in patients with type I diabetes. *Kidney Int* 1995; **47**(1):231–5.

of achieving near-normal metabolic control (HbA1c <6.5%), the intensive therapy regimen also included routine administration of an ACE inhibitor and aspirin as well as intensified lipid therapy. Under these measures the progression of nephropathy to macroalbuminuria was considerably lower at 10% versus 24% (Figure 13.2).

These findings were recently confirmed by the VADT study and a study from China [19, 20]. Owing to intensified metabolic and anti-hypertension treatment, a significant reduction in the progression of albumin excretion and GFR decline could be achieved in patients with an elevated albumin/creatinine ratio at the study onset.

The benefits of a multifactorial intervention with advanced nephropathy were shown recently in the SURE study [21]. This study investigated the influence of a "structured" versus a "conventional" treatment in 205 type 2 diabetic patients with elevated serum creatinine (1.7–3.0 mg/dL) where the end point measure was terminal renal insufficiency. The patients assigned to the structured treatment group received multifactorial therapy with the following therapeutic targets: blood pressure <130/80 mmHg, HbA1c <7.0%, low-density lipoprotein cholesterol <100 mg/dL, triglycerides <175 mg/dL, and treatment with ACE inhibitors/AT1-blockers. The patients were advised at regular intervals by diabetology professionals, whereas for the control group the therapeutic goals and medication were left to the patient's family doctor. In the structured treatment group, the metabolic control was better than controls, but for blood pressure and lipid levels no differences were found. The structured therapy resulted in a marked slowing of progression to

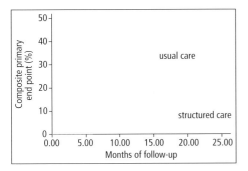

Effects of structured versus usual care on renal endpoint in type 2 diabetic patients with advanced stages of nephropathy. Reproduced from Chan JC, So W-Y, Yeung C-Y, Ko GT, Lau I-T, Tsang M-W, *et al*. Effects of structured versus usual care on renal endpoint in type 2 diabetes: the SURE study: a randomized multicenter translational study. *Diabetes Care* 2009;**32**(6):977–82.

the primary end point, terminal renal insufficiency, with the relative risk being reduced by 60% (Figure 13.4).

To delay the progression of a manifest diabetic nephropathy, good metabolic control is an essential component of any multifactorial therapeutic strategy.

In type 1 diabetes and younger type 2 diabetics without cardiovascular complications, the HbA1c value should lie below 7.0% in order to reduce the progression.

In type 2 diabetes afflicting older patients or in the presence of cardiovascular complications, HbA1c levels over a range 7.0–7.5% should be targeted.

In the presence of a hypoglycemia detection disorder or frequently occurring hypoglycemias, the HbA1c target can be revised upwards, at least temporarily.

With declining renal function attention must be paid to the altered pharmacokinetics of the administered agents in order to prevent hypoglycemia.

The life expectancy of dialysis patients with diabetes is significantly worse than that of non-diabetics. Although one major reason for this is the high cardiovascular morbidity of diabetic patients at the onset of dialysis, other complications such as infection, shunt problems, or electrolyte imbalances can also occur more frequently. Whether good diabetes management has an influence on the outcome of these patients, no intervention studies have yet been reported to address this. In the 1990s, observational studies on mostly smaller cohorts showed that good metabolic control was associated with improved survival prognosis [22, 23].

Two retrospective studies on data from major suppliers of dialysis equipment in the USA (Fresenius Medical Care and DaVita) confirmed the initial findings. Kalantar-Zadeh *et al*. [24] examined mortality in 23 000 dialysis patients with diabetes over a 3-year monitoring period (2001–2004) as a function of metabolic control. As Figure 13.5 shows, there was a clear association between increasing HbA1c levels and an increase in mortality (including cardiovascular mortality). Furthermore, it was also apparent in this study that a further reduction in HbA1c to below 5.0% was associated with an increased mortality. The results from Williams *et al*. [25] in a similar cohort confirmed these results: high mortality with low (<6.0%) and high HbA1c values (>11.0%). After biometric adjustment for numerous confounders, increased mortality with poor metabolic control persisted. In patients with type 1 diabetes who were examined in a substudy, however, a close association between HbA1c and life prognosis was demonstrated. It could not be deduced from the data whether the increase in mortality at low HbA1c values was a sign of malnutrition or increased morbidity,

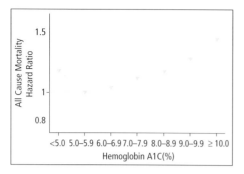

Figure 13.5 Relation between metabolic control and all cause mortality (hazard ratio) in diabetic patients under dialysis therapy and normal hemoglobin level. Reproduced from Kalantar-Zadeh K, Kopple JD, Regidor DL, Jing J, Shinaberger CS, Aronovitz J, et al. A1C and survival in maintenance hemodialysis patients. Diabetes Care 2007;**30**(5):1049–55.

or whether it pointed towards an increased risk of hypoglycemia with consecutively increased cardiovascular complications.

In the prospective 4D study the association between metabolic control and survival could be shown very clearly. Drechsler et al. [26] in 1255 hemodialysis patients with type 2 diabetes revealed a highly significant correlation between HbA1c and sudden cardiac death: for HbA1c >8.0% the risk for a sudden death was twice as high as it was with HbA1c <6.0 % (Figure 13.6); for every percentage point that HbA1c was raised, the risk for sudden death was increased by 18%, whereas that for overall mortality was raised by 8%. An association with metabolic was not recognized with the other chosen cardiovascular end points, i.e., stroke and heart attack.

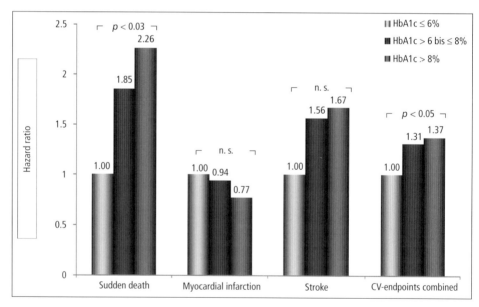

Figure 13.6 Relation between metabolic control and hazard ratio of sudden death, myocardial infarction, and stroke in diabetic patients under dialysis therapy. Reproduced from Drechsler C, Krane V, Ritz E, März W, Wanner C. Glycemic control and cardiovascular events in diabetic hemodialysis patients. Circulation 2009; **120**(24):2421–8.

The present studies show that with terminal renal insufficiency and under dialysis therapy, better metabolic control is associated with an improved prognosis.

The specification of HbA1c target values with terminal renal insufficiency and under renal replacement therapy is difficult not only because of the lack of any relevant studies, but also because the HbA1c value may not accurately reflect the metabolic situation. According to available observations, an HbA1c value within the range 6.5–8.0% would appear to be useful.

The metabolic control of a renally impaired diabetic patient is extremely important in view of the high risk of hypoglycemia due to altered therapeutic conditions. Reliable methods are available both for blood glucose self-monitoring and the monitoring of long-term glycemic control. With renal insufficiency, however, confounding factors may come into play which must be considered when interpreting measurements.

Blood glucose self-monitoring is an integral part of any diabetes therapy, especially for insulin-dependent patients. The implementation can, however, be impaired in patients with renal insufficiency due to various factors.

Interfering substances

Several deaths have been described in recent years that were due to incorrect blood glucose measurements leading to incorrectly calculated insulin injections [27]. The faulty readings arose because of the inclusion of maltose when using the test strips contained in the glucose dehydrogenase pyrroloquinoline quinone (GDH-PQQ) system. Increased maltose levels can arise for example with peritoneal dialysis

using an icodextrin-containing dialysate, or when administering maltose-containing immunoglobulins. As a result, most manufacturers using the GDH-PQQ system have now withdrawn the test strips from the market, or plan to do so in the foreseeable future.

However, even when using glucose oxidase test strips, possible interferences from reducing substances needs to be considered. These include substrates occurring naturally in the blood, such as uric acid, bilirubin, or drugs such as acetaminophen, ascorbic acid, and acetylsalicylic acid, etc. The newer generations of test strips appear to be freer from interference because the confounding factors mentioned only start to take effect at very high concentrations. The instructions for using the test strips must always be strictly followed if any interference errors are to be avoided.

Changes in hematocrit

In patients with diabetic nephropathy a reduction in hemoglobin occurs earlier than is the case for non-diabetic patients with kidney failure. Changes in the hematocrit (HCT), i.e., the ratio of the liquid and corpuscular components of the blood to one another, are generally accompanied by changes in glucose concentration: an HCT drop leads to an increase in glucose concentration, an HCT rise to a decrease in glucose concentration. In addition, however, changes in hematocrit per se lead to interference of hand-held blood glucose monitoring devices. According to the manufacturer's instructions, newer instruments can detect hematocrit changes and correct for them, so that the measured blood glucose levels in the HCT range can be 30–60% regardless of HCT status. Research from various working groups has recently revealed, however, that even newer blood glucose monitoring devices are significantly susceptible to interference from hematocrit changes within the low and high ranges [28].

A newer instrument for glucose monitoring, the continuous glucose monitoring system (CGMS) has until now been used rarely in dialysis patients. Marshall *et al.* [29] described findings from eight patients with diabetes undergoing continuous ambulatory peritoneal dialysis treatment for the first time in 2003. They found a very good agreement between the venous and the CGMS measured blood glucose levels.

Riveline *et al.* [30] recently investigated 19 hemodialysis and 39 non-dialysis-requiring type 2 diabetic patients with the Medtronic CGMS. The agreement between the blood glucose levels upon capillary self-control and the simultaneously measured sensor values was also highly significant, regardless of any dialysis requirement. In a comparison of the profiles during the first 3 hours under dialysis treatment and during a corresponding period on the following day revealed significant differences: on dialysis days the glucose profile was markedly lower. Milder cases of hypoglycemia were not rare, and were found in 35% of patients during the day and 47% at night. All the reported episodes, however, were only short term and non-symptomatic forms of hypoglycemia. In another study [31], about a quarter of the 17 studied hemodialysis patients with diabetes suffered reductions in blood glucose below 50/dL that lasted 30 minutes. Another study group who investigated only eight patients reported results intermediary between these two other studies [32].

The investigations showed that continuous monitoring of glucose concentrations in the interstitium operates reliably under dialysis conditions, i.e., with strong fluctuations in electrolyte and fluid content. It is also able to detect mild hypoglycemia episodes, which occur in a significant proportion of diabetics upon dialysis. By applying appropriate corrective therapy or timely initiation of control measures these could, however, be avoided.

Three clinical parameters are currently available for long-term blood sugar monitoring: glycosylated hemoglobin (HbA1c), fructosamine, and glycosylated albumin (GA).

HbA1c

The diagnostic reliability of HbA1c as a "classic" instrument for monitoring the quality of long-term diabetes control can be impaired by various factors in terminal renal insufficiency or under dialysis therapy. It has long been known that increasing urea levels can lead to carbamylation of the hemoglobin molecule, which with some HbA1c assay methods (e.g., older ion exchange methods) can also be recorded. These HbA1c values are erroneously reported as higher than they should be. By selecting a suitable HbA1c assay method [immunological tests, modern high-performance liquid chromatography method (HPLC)] this problem can be circumvented.

Upon deterioration of renal function, patients with diabetes show an early anemia that is frequently due to iron deficiency [33]. Iron deficiency can lead to a change in glycosylation. In one population study, a shift in HbA1c towards higher values was detected in the presence of iron deficiency, although the magnitude of this change was not very large [34]. In non-diabetic expectant mothers, a negative association was observed between parameters of iron deficiency (ferritin, transferrin saturation) and HbA1c values, thus confirming this relationship [35].

Conversely, iron therapy in the presence of iron deficiency or administration of erythropoietin (EPO) in the presence of renal anemia in non-diabetic patients led to a significant decrease in HbA1c levels unrelated to blood glucose concentrations [36, 37]. In patients with diabetes and impaired renal function (eGFR 20–44 mL/min) and anemia, Ng *et al.* [38] found a decrease in HbA1c by 0.4% after iron administration and by 0.7% under EPO administration. Simultaneously implemented seven-point glucose measurements revealed no changes in metabolic control during the monitoring period.

Such blood sugar independent HbA1c alterations are due to a displacement of the erythrocyte population towards younger forms in which the rate of glycosylation is decelerated. Because of the shortened lifespan of erythrocytes in renal insufficiency, the exposure time in the diabetic milieu is reduced, which can also lead to lower HbA1c values. Among the modern methods used in dialysis therapy, reduced erythrocyte survival has been cast into doubt. Studies by Joy *et al.* [39] were able to show only a weak association between red cell survival time and HbA1c levels.

The aforementioned CGMS study of Riveline *et al.* [30] was still able to show a significant correlation in dialysis patients between the blood glucose profiles and HbA1c values. However, the slope of the relationship line was different for diabetic and non-diabetic patients (Figure 13.7). When interpreting HbA1c levels in dialysis-dependent diabetics, the above-cited confounding factors also need to be taken into account, since this laboratory parameter can be included without reservations for assessing the metabolic state. Uzu *et al.* [40] proposed conversion factors for HbA1c values which take into account hematocrit and EPO dose as confounding factors.

Fructosamine

Fructosamine is a general measure for glycosylated proteins in the body and represents an integral parameter reflecting metabolic control for the previous 2–3 weeks. Although it is not influenced by the factors that confound HbA1c measurements, it does have its own battery of potential confounders.

High uric acid concentrations, for example, can lead to erroneous measurements. Sch-

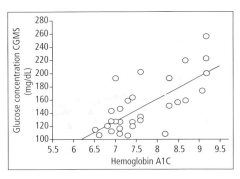

Correlation between mean glucose obtained through the continuous glucose monitoring system (CGMS) and glycosylated hemoglobin (HbA1c) in type 2 diabetic patients on dialysis therapy and type 2 diabetic patients without dialysis therapy. Correlation in dialyzed patients—triangles (*r* = 0.47; *p* = 0.042). Correlation in non-dialyzed patients—circles (*r* = 0.71; *p* ≤ 0.001 [30]). Reproduced from Riveline J-P, Teynie J, Belmouaz S, Franc S, Dardari D, Bauwens M, *et al.* Glycaemic control in type 2 diabetic patients on chronic haemodialysis: use of a continuous glucose monitoring system. *Nephrol Dial Transplant* 2009;**24**(9): 2866–71.

leicher *et al.* [41] showed that only about 50% of the reducing activity is determined by specific non-enzymatic glycosylation of proteins. A further disadvantage of this parameter lies in the fact that it illustrates the glycosylation levels of numerous proteins with differing turnovers. Erroneously low values can be reported in disorders of protein metabolism, e.g., with nephrotic syndrome or liver cirrhosis. Regarding the incidence of diabetes-typical complications, fructosamine has not been adequately assessed in a clinical setting. In a recent study on dialysis-dependent diabetics, in which fructosamine was corrected to the albumin concentration, an association with an increased susceptibility to infection and hospitalization was found [42].

Glycosylated albumin

An alternative to HbA1c determination that has been introduced in recent years is glycosylated albumin, which today can be measured easily by HPLC and an enzymatic assay [43, 44]. Owing to the shorter half-life of albumin than glycosylated hemoglobin, albumin reflects a shorter period of diabetes control and is unaffected by hemoglobin metabolism disorders. In comparative studies on HbA1c and glycosylated albumin, almost all studies concluded that an uncorrected HbA1c underestimates the metabolic situation, and that the percentage of glycosylated albumin therefore reflects it better. Compared with HbA1c, however, glycosylated albumin has not been properly validated in long-term monitoring. Initial investigations have shown that a high level of glycosylated albumin is associated with increased vascular stiffness, increased cardiovascular morbidity, and shortened survival in dialysis patients [45–47]. It is also unclear which glycosylated albumin value should be targeted. Ultimately, confounding factors also need to be considered with this parameter. As such, diseases that are associated with changes in albumin metabolism, including proteinuria, liver disease, thyroid dysfunction, or chronic inflammation, can also affect this marker.

References

1. Gaede P, Vedel P, Parving HH, Pedersen O. Intensified multifactorial intervention in patients with type 2 diabetes mellitus and microalbuminuria: the Steno type 2 randomised study. *Lancet* 1999;**353**: 617–22.
2. Rossing P, de Zeeuw D. Need for better diabetes treatment for improved renal outcome. *Kidney Int* 2011;**79**(Suppl 120): S28–32.
3. Wang PH, Lau J, Chalmers TC. Meta-analysis of effects of intensive blood-glucose control on late complications of type I diabetes. *Lancet* 1993;**341**:1306–9.
4. The Diabetes Control and Complications Trial Research Group. The effect of intensive treatment of diabetes on the development and progression of long-term complications in insulin-dependent diabetes mellitus. *N Engl J Med* 1993;**329**: 977–86.
5. The Diabetes Control and Complications (DCCT) Research Group. Effect of intensive therapy on the development and progression of diabetic nephropathy in the Diabetes Control and Complications Trial. *Kidney Int* 1995; **47**:1703–20.
6. The Diabetes Control and Complications Trial/Epidemiology of Diabetes Interventions and Complications Research Group. Retinopathy and nephropathy in patients with type 1 diabetes four years after a trial of Intensive therapy. *N Engl J Med* 2000; **342**:381–9.
7. de Boer IH, Sun W, Cleary PA, Lachin JM, Molitch ME, Steffes MW, *et al.* Intensive diabetes therapy and glomerular filtration rate in type 1 diabetes. *N Engl J Med* 2011;**365**:2366–76.
8. UK Prospective Diabetes Study (UKPDS) Group. Intensive blood-glucose control with sulphonylureas or insulin compared with conventional treatment and risk of complications in patients with type 2 diabetes (UKPDS 33). *Lancet* 1998; **352**:837–53.
9. Holman RR, Paul SK, Bethel MA, *et al.* 10-year follow-up of intensive glucose control in type 2 diabetes. *N Engl J Med* 2008;**359**:1577–89.
10. Ismail-Beigi F, Craven T, Banerji MA, *et al* Effect of intensive treatment of hyperglycaemia on microvascular outcomes in type 2 diabetes: an analysis of the ACCORD randomised trial. *Lancet* 2010;**376**:419–30.
11. Patel A, MacMahon S, Chalmers J, *et al.* Intensive blood glucose control and vascular outcomes in patients with

type 2 diabetes. *N Engl J Med* 2008;
358:2560–72.

12. Duckworth W, Abraira C, Moritz T, *et al.*
Glucose Control and Vascular
Complications in Veterans with Type
2 Diabetes. *N Engl J Med* 2009;**360**:
129–39.

13. Feldt-Rasmussen B, Mathiesen ER, Jensen
T, *et al.* Effect of improved metabolic
control on loss of kidney function in
type 1 (insulin-dependent) diabetic
patients: an update of the Steno studies.
Diabetologia 1991;**34**:164–70.

14. de Boer IH, Rue TC, Cleary PA, *et al*
Long-term renal outcomes of patients
with type 1 diabetes mellitus and
microalbuminuria: an analysis of the
Diabetes Control and Complications
Trial/Epidemiology of Diabetes
Interventions and Complications cohort.
Arch Intern Med 2011;**171**:412–20.

15. Nyberg G, Blohmé G, Nordén G. Impact
of metabolic control in progression of
clinical diabetic nephropathy.
Diabetologia 1987;**30**:82–6.

16. Manto A, Cotroneo P, Marra G, *et al.*
Effect of intensive treatment on diabetic
nephropathy in patients with type I
diabetes. *Kidney Int* 1995;**47**:231–5.

17. Ohkubo Y, Kishikawa H, Araki E, *et al.*
Intensive insulin therapy prevents the
progression of diabetic microvascular
complications in Japanese patients with
non-insulin-dependent diabetes mellitus:
a randomized prospective 6-year study.
Diabetes Res Clin Pract 1995;**28**:103–17.

18. Shichiri M, Kishikawa H, Ohkubo Y,
Wake N. Long-term results of the
Kumamoto Study on optimal diabetes
control in type 2 diabetic patients.
Diabetes Care 2000;**23**(Suppl 2):B21–29.

19. Agrawal L, Azad N, Emanuele NV, *et al.*
Observation on renal outcomes in the
Veterans Affairs Diabetes Trial. *Diabetes
Care* 2011;**34**:2090–4.

20. Hsieh M-C, Hsieh Y-T, Cho T-J, *et al.*
Remission of diabetic nephropathy in
type 2 diabetic Asian population: role of
tight glucose and blood pressure control.
Eur J Clin Invest 2011;**41**:870–878.

21. Chan JC, So W-Y, Yeung C-Y, *et al.* Effects
of structured versus usual care on renal
endpoint in type 2 diabetes: the SURE
study: a randomized multicenter
translational study. *Diabetes Care* 2009;
32:977–82.

22. Wu MS, Yu CC, Yang CW, *et al.* Poor
pre-dialysis glycaemic control is a
predictor of mortality in type II diabetic
patients on maintenance haemodialysis.
Nephrol Dial Transplant 1997;**12**:
2105–10.

23. Morioka T, Emoto M, Tabata T, *et al.*
Glycemic control is a predictor of survival
for diabetic patients on hemodialysis.
Diabetes Care 2001;**24**:909–13.

24. Kalantar-Zadeh K, Kopple JD, Regidor DL,
et al. A1C and survival in maintenance
hemodialysis patients. *Diabetes Care* 2007;
30:1049–55.

25. Williams ME, Lacson E Jr, Wang W, *et al.*
Glycemic control and extended
hemodialysis survival in patients with
diabetes mellitus: comparative results of
traditional and time-dependent Cox
model analyses. *Clin J Am Soc Nephrol*
2010;**5**:1595–601.

26. Drechsler C, Krane V, Ritz E, *et al.*
Glycemic control and cardiovascular
events in diabetic hemodialysis patients.
Circulation 2009;**120**:2421–8.

27. Frias JP, Lim CG, Ellison JM, Montandon
CM. Review of adverse events associated
with false glucose readings measured by
GDH-PQQ-based glucose test strips in the
presence of interfering sugars. *Diabetes
Care* 2010;**33**:728–9.

28. Kristensen GBB, Monsen G, Skeie S,
Sandberg S. Standardized evaluation of
nine instruments for self-monitoring of

blood glucose. *Diabetes Technol Ther* 2008; **10**:467–77.

29. Marshall J, Jennings P, Scott A, *et al.* Glycemic control in diabetic CAPD patients assessed by continuous glucose monitoring system (CGMS). *Kidney Int* 2003;**64**:1480–6.

30. Riveline J-P, Teynie J, Belmouaz S, *et al.* Glycaemic control in type 2 diabetic patients on chronic haemodialysis: use of a continuous glucose monitoring system. *Nephrol Dial Transplant* 2009;**24**:2866–71.

31. Kazempour-Ardebili S, Lecamwasam VL, Dassanyake T, *et al.* Assessing glycemic control in maintenance hemodialysis patients with type 2 diabetes. *Diabetes Care* 2009;**32**:1137–42.

32. Jung HS, Kim HI, Kim MJ, *et al.* Analysis of hemodialysis-associated hypoglycemia in patients with type 2 diabetes using a continuous glucose monitoring system. *Diabetes Technol Ther* 2010;**12**:801–7.

33. Hsu C-Y, McCulloch CE, Curhan GC. Iron status and hemoglobin level in chronic renal insufficiency. *J Am Soc Nephrol* 2002;**13**:2783–6.

34. Kim C, Bullard KM, Herman WH, Beckles GL. Association between iron deficiency and A1C Levels among adults without diabetes in the National Health and Nutrition Examination Survey, 1999–2006. *Diabetes Care* 2010;**33**:780–5.

35. Hashimoto K, Noguchi S, Morimoto Y, *et al.* A1C but not serum glycated albumin is elevated in late pregnancy owing to iron deficiency. *Diabetes Care* 2008;**31**:1945–8.

36. Gram-Hansen P, Eriksen J, Mourits-Andersen T, Olesen L. Glycosylated haemoglobin (HbA1c) in iron- and vitamin B12 deficiency. *J Intern Med* 1990;**227**:133–6.

37. Nakao T, Matsumoto H, Okada T, *et al.* Influence of erythropoietin treatment on hemoglobin A1c levels in patients with chronic renal failure on hemodialysis. *Intern Med* 1998;**37**:826–30.

38. Ng JM, Cooke M, Bhandari S, *et al.* The effect of iron and erythropoietin treatment on the A1C of patients with diabetes and chronic kidney disease. *Diabetes Care* 2010;**33**:2310–3.

39. Joy MS, Cefalu WT, Hogan SL, Nachman PH. Long-term glycemic control measurements in diabetic patients receiving hemodialysis. *Am J Kidney Dis* 2002;**39**:297–307.

40. Uzu T, Hatta T, Deji N, *et al.* Target for glycemic control in type 2 diabetic patients on hemodialysis: effects of anemia and erythropoietin injection on hemoglobin A(1c). *Ther Apher Dial* 2009;**13**:89–94.

41. Schleicher ED, Mayer R, Wagner EM, Gerbitz KD. Is serum fructosamine assay specific for determination of glycated serum protein? *Clin Chem* 1988;**34**: 320–3.

42. Mittman N, Desiraju B, Fazil I, *et al.* Serum fructosamine versus glycosylated hemoglobin as an index of glycemic control, hospitalization, and infection in diabetic hemodialysis patients. *Kidney Int Suppl* 2010;**117**:S41–45.

43. Inaba M, Okuno S, Kumeda Y, *et al.* Glycated albumin is a better glycemic indicator than glycated hemoglobin values in hemodialysis patients with diabetes: effect of anemia and erythropoietin injection. *J Am Soc Nephrol* 2007;**18**:896–903.

44. Peacock TP, Shihabi ZK, Bleyer AJ, *et al.* Comparison of glycated albumin and hemoglobin A(1c) levels in diabetic subjects on hemodialysis. *Kidney Int* 2008;**73**:1062–8.

45. Kumeda Y, Inaba M, Shoji S, *et al.* Significant correlation of glycated albumin, but not glycated haemoglobin, with arterial stiffening in haemodialysis patients with type 2 diabetes. *Clin Endocrinol* 2008;**69**:556–61.

46. Okada T, Nakao T, Matsumoto H, *et al.* Association between markers of glycemic control, cardiovascular complications and survival in type 2 diabetic patients with end-stage renal disease. *Intern Med* 2007;**46**:807–14.

47. Fukuoka K, Nakao K, Morimoto H, *et al.* Glycated albumin levels predict long-term survival in diabetic patients undergoing haemodialysis. *Nephrology* 2008;**13**:278–83.

Chapter 14

Dosage of antihyperglycemic drugs in patients with renal insufficiency

Alexander Sämann and Ulrich A. Müller

Jena University Hospital, Jena, Germany

Key points

- Metformin lowers diabetic late complications and death rate in obese people with diabetes.
- There is no general agreement at which glomerular filtration rate metformin should be stopped, usually at chronic kidney disease stage 3.
- Glibenclamide prevents microsvascular complications.
- Glibenclamide may cause hypoglycemia, especially in people with near-normal glycosylated hemoglobin (HbA1c) short diabetes duration and renal insufficiency.
- Glibenclamide should be stopped at chronic kidney disease (CKD) stage 4.

- Gliquidon and glinides have no limitations in CKD; however the evidence for lesser hypoglycemia is weak.
- Sitagliptin and linagliptin have no limitations in CKD, but long-term benefit or harm is unknown
- Insulin has no limitations in any stages of CKD including dialysis.
- Adjustment of insulin dose is necessary in advanced stages of CKD.
- Structured diabetes education prevents hypoglycemia and diabetic foot syndrome.

Introduction

The prevalence of type 2 diabetes, as well as micro- and macrovascular complications due to type 1 and 2 diabetes is high [1–4]. The cardiovascular risk in type 2 diabetes is similar to non-diabetic individuals who have already had a cardiovascular event [5].

Declining renal function has contrary effects on blood glucose metabolism. Peripheral insulin resistance increases while renal gluconeogenesis and hypoglycemic counter-regulation decreases [6, 7]. The clearance of insulin and other antihyperglycemic agents declines, which results in pharmacokinetic and pharmacodynamic changes with increased risk of

Diabetes and Kidney Disease, First Edition. Edited by Gunter Wolf.
© 2013 John Wiley & Sons, Ltd. Published 2013 by John Wiley & Sons, Ltd.

hypoglycemia [8]. The failure to notice asymptomatically declining renal function can hinder necessary dosage adjustments.

While insulin therapy is the only therapeutic option in type 1 diabetes, the treatment algorithms in type 2 diabetes are more complex. The basic intervention should be non-pharmacological by weight reduction, dietary adjustments, and lifestyle intervention. If glycemic goals are not achieved, oral antihyperglycemic mono- and combination therapy can be added. Insulin therapy should be the last step [9, 10].

There are eight groups of antihyperglycemic medicines involving biguanides, sulfonylureas, meglitinides, glitazones, glucosidase inhibitors, gliptins, glucagon-like peptide (GLP)-1 analogues, and insulin. All agents are well evaluated regarding the effects on surrogate parameters such as blood glucose and HbA1c. But only for insulin, metformin, and glibenclamide has an improvement in diabetes-related complications been shown [11, 12]. Head-to-head studies on long-term outcomes and side effects of antihyperglycemic mono- and combination therapy in patients with and without diabetes-related complications are still lacking. National drug permissions differ. This chapter adopts the regulations of the European Medicines Agency (EMA) on dose adjustments or contraindications in renal insufficiency.

Near-normal glycemia can reduce micro- and might reduce macrovascular complications in type 1 and type 2 diabetes [11–15]. Overly aggressive blood glucose lowering in aged, multimorbid patients with type 2 diabetes and polypharmacy can increase severe hypoglycemia and mortality [16]. Therefore, individual glycemic goals should be set while taking account of life expectancy, comorbidities, ability to undertake diabetes therapy, and to control side effects, as well as personal health wishes and values [17–20]. An HbA1c between 6.5% and 7.5% (47–58 mmol/mol) should be aimed for, to avoid microvascular complications [9, 10]. Less tight glucose control is necessary to stop hyperglycemic symptoms and acute complications (HbA1c 8–10%; 66–86 mmol/mol).

History

The antihyperglycemic properties of demethyl-biguanid and its derivatives were first described in the 1920s [21, 22]. It took 30 years until the biguanids metformin, phenformin, and buformin entered clinical practice. The University Group Diabetes Project (UGDP study) and recurrent reports on fatal lactic acidosis due to phenformin and buformin ended the clinical use of these agents in 1977/78 [23]. Metformin remained in use for a much lower incidence of lactic acidosis. As a result of the United Kingdom Prospective Diabetes Study (UKPDS), metformin experienced a renaissance in 1998 for its then proven, favorable effects on micro- and macrovascular complications in type 2 diabetes [11].

Mechanism of action

Metformin lowers pre- and postprandial blood glucose without the risk of hypoglycemia. Metformin delays intestinal glucose uptake, suppresses hepatic gluconeogenesis and glycogenolysis, and might improve peripheral insulin sensitivity by activation of AMP-activated protein kinase [24–26]. Metformin improves serum lipid profiles by increasing lipid oxidation, and may have beneficial renal pleiotropic effects by influencing insulin resistance, oxidative stress, and chronic inflammation [27–29].

Indications and contraindications

Metformin is indicated in adults with type 2 diabetes, particularly in obese patients who fail glycemic goals even though non-pharmacological interventions are adequate. Metformin is indicated in mono- and combination therapy with other antihyperglycemic agents including insulin.

Metformin is contraindicated in diabetic ketoacidosis, coma, cardiac, or respiratory failure, recent myocardial infarction, hepatic insufficiency, acute alcohol intoxication, alcoholism, and lactation. Furthermore, acute diseases with the potential to impair renal function, including dehydration, severe infection, shock, and intravascular administration of iodinated contrast agents, are contraindications.

Chronic kidney disease

Metformin can be given in chronic kidney disease (CKD) stage 1–2 without dosage adjustment. In elderly people, metformin administration has to be re-evaluated regularly because of possible changes in kidney function. However, there is controversy on when to stop metformin in CKD, i.e., German Diabetes Association, glomerular filtration rate (GFR) $\leq 60\,mL/min$; EMA, serum creatinine $\geq 110\,\mu mol/L$ (females) and $\geq 135\,\mu mol/L$ (males); other authors, $\leq 35\,mL/min$ or serum creatinine $\geq 150\,\mu mol/L$ [30–32].

Comedication which can deteriorate renal function, e.g., diuretics, angiotensin-converting enzyme inhibitors, non-steroidal antirheumatic drugs, requires careful monitoring. In planned surgery with general anesthesia and administration of iodinated contrast agents, metformin should be discontinued 48 hours before and after. Kidney function should be monitored before readministration of metformin therapy.

Side effects

In about 10% of patients, metformin causes gastrointestinal symptoms, including nausea,

vomiting, abdominal pain, and loss of appetite. These symptoms can resolve spontaneously. Starting low and increasing dosage slowly can prevent gastrointestinal discomfort.

Medical conditions with possible metformin accumulation can cause lactic acidosis. Lactic acidosis is infrequent but potentially fatal (mortality rate 25–50%), with estimates of three to four cases per 100 000 patient-years in routine care [24, 33, 34]. Most patients with metformin-associated lactic acidosis had severely impaired renal function. However, a Cochrane review, with pooled data from 347 prospective trials, revealed no cases of fatal or non-fatal lactic acidosis in 70 490 well-documented patient-years of metformin use [35].

Lactic acidosis presents with metabolic acidosis, hyperventilation, abdominal pain, and disturbed vigilance followed by coma. Laboratory findings include metabolic acidosis, increased anion gap, and plasma lactate level. Lactic acidosis is a medical emergency which requires intensive care monitoring and supportive treatment. Hemodialysis is the most effective method to remove lactate and metformin, and to correct electrolyte and acid–base disturbances [34, 36]. There is only anecdotal evidence of the controversy about when to initiate hemodialysis in patients without terminal kidney failure [37, 38].

Evaluation

Metformin lowers HbA1c by about 1%. The UKPDS was a landmark study in type 2 diabetes therapy. It compared intensive and conventional antihyperglycemic therapy using metformin, chlorpropamide, glibenclamide, glipizide, or insulin. Metformin monotherapy was superior in the reduction of any diabetes-related complication, myocardial infarction, diabetes-related mortality, and overall mortality (Table 14.1) [11, 12]. According to a Cochrane review, metformin is the first antihyperglycemic

United Kingdom Prospective Diabetes Study: outcomes of antihyperglycemic therapy in type 2 diabetes

Therapy group	Any diabetes-related end point[a]	Myocardial Infarction[a]	Diabetes-related mortality[a]	Overall mortality[a]
Metformin monotherapy (HbA1c 7.4%)[b]	30	11	8	14
Sulfonylurea/insulin (HbA1c 7.4%)[b]	40	14	10	19
Diet (HbA1c 8%)[b]	43	18	13	21

[a]Events/1000 patient-years. [b]Mean HbA1c over 10 years of follow-up [11].
Reproduced from Effect of intensive blood-glucose control with metformin on complications in overweight patients with type 2 diabetes (UKPDS 34). UK Prospective Diabetes Study (UKPDS) Group. *Lancet* 1998; **352**(9131):854–65. Epub 1998/09/22.

choice in obese patients with type 2 diabetes because of its benefits on vascular complications, glycemic control, body weight, serum lipids, insulinemia, and diastolic blood pressure [39].

The metformin controversy in moderate to severe chronic kidney disease

Metformin has evaluated advantages on macrovascular complications in type 2 diabetes [11]. The extremely low risk of lactic acidosis in CKD limits use. But there are arguments against this paradigm. Since metformin is frequently used, it might be an "innocent bystander" in severely ill patients with lactic acidosis and sepsis, hypovolemia, or myocardial infarction [40]. There is evidence that might support the safe use of appropriate doses of metformin in patients with chronic but otherwise stable renal impairment [41]. Alternative antihyperglycemic agents could carry a greater risk of serious side effects, notably hypoglycemia [42]. Other traditional contraindications to metformin use such as heart failure are also being re-evaluated, as the benefits of metformin in these patients are increasingly recognized [43].

History

During the typhoid fever epidemic in Montpellier in 1942, Marcel Janbon and colleagues described severe hypoglycemic side effects of the antimicrobial agent sulfonamidothiodiazol [44]. In 1956, systematic research work yielded the first oral antidiabetic sulfonylurea (SU), cerbutamid, which still had antimicrobial effects. By changing an amino- to a methyl group the next agents were tolbutamide and chlorpropramide, which lost its antimicrobial properties. The development of more effective antihyperglycemic SUs resulted in the classification of first- (lead substance: tolbutamide), second- (glibenclamide) and third-generation SUs (glimepiride) by Ernst-Friedrich Pfeiffer in 1971 [45].

Mechanism of action

Sulfonylureas (SUs) trigger insulin secretion by closing ATP-sensitive potassium channels at the β-cell. There are isoforms of SU receptors (SURs) in different tissues, i.e., SUR-1 in pancreatic β-cells, SUR-2A in cardiac cells and SUR-2B in smooth muscle cells. SUs become metabolized by hepatic cytochrome P450 CYP2C9 [46, 47]. Moreover SUs can improve insulin sensitivity by stimulation of transmembranous glucose transporters in muscle and fat cells, and lowering of hepatic inactivation.

Indications and contraindications

SUs are mainly indicated in non-obese patients with type 2 diabetes, when non-pharmacological interventions fail to achieve glycemic goals. SUs can be given as mono- and combination therapy including insulin.

SUs should not be used in insulin-dependent diabetes, diabetic coma, ketoacidosis, lactation, pregnancy, and/or severe renal or hepatic failure.

Chronic kidney disease

SUs can be applied in CKD stages 1–3. Dosage adjustment may become necessary in CKD stage 3. Gliquidon is fecal eliminated and, therefore, has a theoretically lower risk of hypoglycemia in CKD.

Side effects

SUs can increase body weight, i.e., 1.7 kg more than placebo within 10 years, which limits their use in obese patients [12, 48]. Severe hypoglycemia is the most serious and potentially life-threatening complication of SUs. The individual risk of severe hypoglycemia depends on multiple factors, including diabetes duration, therapy goals, diabetes education, isoforms of CYP2C9, short duration of therapy with SU, near-normal glycaemia, history of severe hypoglycemia and hypoglycemia unawareness, comorbidities, and socioeconomic status [49–52]. Meals cannot be skipped or taken at irregular intervals. Other factors which favor hypoglycemia include alterations of diet, increased physical activity, alcohol consumption, acute renal or hepatic failure, or overdosage. Prolonged or recurrent hypoglyc-

emia should be considered, especially in third-generation SUs.

Evaluation

SUs lower HbA1c by about 1%. The UKPDS has shown a 3.9% absolute (34% relative) risk reduction regarding microvascular end points for 5467 person-years with SUs compared with placebo. This favorable result was sustained 10 years after the end of the main trial [11, 53].

The controversy about myocardial infarction

In 1970, the UGDP study gave rise to concerns of tolbutamide-associated cardiovascular mortality [54]. SUs are suspected of reducing ischemic preconditioning in patients with stable coronary heart disease [55]. This might lower myocardial ischemic tolerance in acute coronary syndrome. The importance of this mechanism is unclear. The 10-year observational follow-up of the UKPDS did not show increased cardiovascular complications compared with insulin or metformin [11, 12, 53]. But since patients with known coronary heart disease were excluded, the UKPDS data cannot prove the cardiovascular safety of SUs. Epidemiological studies indicate differences in the cardiovascular risk of various SUs [56, 57].

Meglitinides

History

The German pharmaceutical company Dr. Karl Thomae investigated meglitinides from 1983. Thomae was later acquired by Boehringer-Ingelheim, which licensed the agent to Novo Nordisk. Novo Nordisk developed repaglinide and gained the marketing authorization for Prandin and Novonorm in 1997. The patent ended in 2009, and generic medicines appeared.

The marketing of nateglinide and mitiglinide started in 2000 and 2004.

Mechanism of action

Repaglinide and mitiglinide are benzoic acid derivatives, and nateglinide, a D-phenylalanine derivative, exhibits insulinotropic effects by stimulating pancreatic SURs. Compared with SU, meglitinides receptor activation is more rapid and shorter. Repaglinide is hepatic-metabolized and fecal-eliminated, while nateglinide is hepatic-metabolized and renal-excreted by about 80%.

Indications and contraindications

Meglitinides are indicated in type 2 diabetes when glycemic goals are not achieved through adequate non-pharmacological interventions. Repaglinide can be given in mono- or combination therapy with metformin. Nateglinide can only be given in combination with metformin.

Contraindications involve ketoacidosis, severe liver failure, and comedication with gemfibrozil.

Chronic kidney disease

Repaglinide may be given in all stages of renal failure. Dosage adjustments should be considered at CKD stage 4–5. Nateglinide should be combined with metformin, which means a contraindication at CKD stage 3–5.

Side effects

Meglitinides can cause hypoglycemia similar to SUs (please also compare the concerns of cardiovascular risk of severe hypoglycemia).

Evaluation

Repaglinide and nateglinide/metformin lower HbA1c by about 1%. The effect on patient-relevant long-term outcomes has not been investigated. The safety data of repaglinide in progressed renal failure is limited. Only one study with 3 months of follow-up compared repaglinide in 108 patients with mild to moderate renal failure, and 22 patients with severe to preterminal renal failure [58]. There was a non-significant trend to greater and more severe side effects in decreasing renal function.

Thiazolidinediones

History

Troglitazone was the first thiazolidinedione (TZD), which was authorized in early 1997. Marketing ended in 1997 and 2000 because of serious liver complications [59, 60]. Supposedly some 100 patients died from acute liver failure or received liver transplants [61]. The "troglitazone story" underlines the importance of robust pharmacovigilance systems and independent, critical, appraisal of new medicines by regulatory authorities and the medical community. Rosiglitazone, the next TZD was substantially less liver toxic but was withdrawn in 2010 because of serious cardiovascular and osteoskeletal complications, as well as congestive heart failure [62, 63].

Mechanism of action

TZDs activate the nuclear PPAR γ-type receptor (peroxisome proliferator activated γ-receptor), which acts as a transcription factor for various genes. TZDs increase insulin sensitivity of muscle, adipose, and hepatic tissues without influencing insulin secretion. Hepatic CYP2C8 and other cytochromes metabolize TZDs. Polymorphism of hepatic cytochromes can impact on the action and side effects of TZDs [64].

Indications and contraindications

Pioglitazone is the only TZD left on the market. Pioglitazone is indicated in combination therapy in type 2 diabetes when non-pharmacological interventions fail to achieve glycemic goals. Pioglitazone can be used as monotherapy if metformin cannot be given. Pioglitazone is contraindicated in congestive heart failure [New York Heart Association (NYHA) I–IV], reduced liver function, pregnancy, lactation, and bladder cancer.

Chronic kidney disease

Pioglitazone can be administered until the GFR declines to 4 mL/min, but not if renal replacement therapy has been initiated. The coincidence of CKD and congestive heart failure is frequent, pioglitazone should be carefully considered and monitored accordingly [65].

Side effects

Pioglitazone causes fluid retention and exacerbates congestive heart failure [66]. Pioglitazone increases fracture risk in women [67].The EMA performed a thorough review of the clinical data of more than 12 000 patients on pioglitazone in 2011 and reported an increased risk of bladder cancer (prevalence 0.15% versus 0.07%). The use of pioglitazone has been suspended in France, and reimbursement was stopped in Germany in 2011.

Evaluation

Pioglitazone lowers HbA1c by about 1%. The benefit–risk ratio remains unclear. A Cochrane review found no evidence that pioglitazone improves patient-oriented outcomes, including mortality, morbidity, adverse effects, costs, and health-related quality of life [68].

Glucosidase inhibitors

History

In the late 1960s, the pharmaceutical company Bayer investigated agents inhibiting enteric car-

bohydrate digestion. Since 1970, Bodo Junge and collaborators at Bayer isolated and developed the agent acarbose, a pseudo-tetrasaccharide which was derived from the bacterium *Actinoplanes* [69]. In 1990, Bayer started the marketing of the first glucosidase inhibitor, acarbose. Sanofi licensed Miglitol from Bayer, and brought it to the market in 1998. Voglibose, the third glucosidase inhibitor, is marketed in India and Japan.

Mechanism of action

Glycosidases such as glucoamylase, lactase, isomaltase, and saccharase are located in the brush border of the small intestine mucosa, and break up enteral polysaccharides [70]. Acarbose, miglitol, and voglibose inhibit enteric glucosidases competitively and reversibly. This mechanism reduces pre- and postprandial blood glucose peaks. The agent acts locally but has multiple side effects on gastrointestinal hormones [71, 72].

Indications and contraindications

Glucosidase inhibitors are indicated in type 2 diabetes when glycemic goals are not achieved through adequate weight reduction, dietary adjustments and life style interventions. Combination therapy with SUs is possible.

Contraindications are bowel inflammation, stenosis, ulceration and passage disturbances, hernias, and impaired enteral uptake. Glucosidase inhibitors are contraindicated during pregnancy and lactation.

Chronic kidney disease

Acarbose, miglitol, and voglibose can be given in CKD stage 1–3 without dosage adjustments.

Side effects

The gastrointestinal side effects including abdominal discomfort, diarrhea, and flatulence, are caused by the mechanism of action. The symptoms can decline over time and with dietary adjustments.

Evaluation

Glucosidase inhibitors lower HbA1c by 0.5–0.8%. The association of postprandial glycemic peaks in diabetes and cardiovascular complications is well documented in various epidemiological, but not in interventional, studies [73]. The effect of glucosidase inhibitors on mortality, morbidity, and quality of life in patients with type 2 diabetes remains unclear [74].

History

In the mid-1960s, experiments on the difference of insulin release after oral and intravenous administered glucose postulated unknown glucoregulatory intestinal hormones, so-called incretins. Further research elucidated two incretins, glucose-dependent insulinotropic peptide (GIP) in 1970 and, 15 years later, the glucagon-like peptide (GLP-1). Since both hormones are rapidly inactivated by the enzyme dipeptidylpeptidase-4 (DPP-4), pharmaceutical research focused on the development of long-acting GLP-1 and agents which stabilize endogenous GLP-1. The first long-acting GLP-1 analogue exenatid (Byetta) was originally found in the saliva of the Gila monster in 1992 by John Eng, and received marketing permission in 2005. The first DPP-4 inhibitor, sitagliptin, was authorized in 2006.

Mechanism of action

DPP-4 is expressed in many tissues, including intestine, kidneys, liver, lung, T-cells, B-cells and natural killer cells [75]. Incretins inhibit glucagon secretion and stimulate insulin release in a blood glucose-dependent manner

[76]. Incretins trigger almost 70% of postprandial insulin secretion and lower pre- and postprandial glycemia. DPP-4 inhibitors bind selectively to DPP-4 and prevent the rapid hydrolysis of incretin. DPP-4 inhibitors cannot trigger hypoglycemia. DPP-4 inhibitors become inactivated by hepatic metabolism or hydrolysis.

The injectable GLP-1 agonist exenatide has only limited homology with GLP-1 [77]. This increases its resistance to DPP-4 and prolongs its half-life time. Liraglutide is a long-acting true GLP-1 analogue, which received approval in 2009. Oral variants are under investigation. GLP-1 analogues reduce body weight and body fat mass through reducing hunger and energy intake.

Indications and contraindications

DPP-4 inhibitors and GLP-1 agents are indicated in patients with type 2 diabetes when glycemia is inadequately controlled by weight reduction, dietary adjustments and lifestyle interventions. The indication for mono- and combination therapies with other oral antihyperglycemic agents and insulin varies (please compare with Table 14.4 below).

Contraindications involve mild to severe hepatic impairment, pregnancy, and lactation. Vildagliptin is not recommended in congestive heart failure NYHA class III–IV. Thyroid adverse events, including increased blood calcitonin, goiter, and thyroid neoplasm, have been reported in clinical trials in particular in patients with pre-existing thyroid disease [78].

Side effects

DPP-4 inhibitors prolong the action of neuropeptides, growth hormone-releasing hormone, chemokines (stromal cell derived factor 1, macrophage-derived chemokine), regulate the specific and non-specific cellular immune system, the migration of CD34+ progenitor cells, and hematopoietic stem cells [79]. The long-term safety has still to be investigated. DPP-4 inhibitors and GLP-1 analogues can increase the risk of hemorrhagic and necrotizing pancreatitis (linagliptin 2 events in 2566 patients versus zero in 1183 patients receiving placebo) [80]. Patients should be informed of the risk and symptoms of pancreatitis.

Renal insufficiency

The limitations in renal impairment differ and may change in future (Tables 14.2–14.4).

Evaluation

GLP-1 analogues and DPP-4 inhibitors lower HbA1c by about 0.5–1% without triggering hypoglycemia [80, 81]. GLP-1 analogues can lower body weight by 3 kg [82]. The effects of incretin-based therapy on mortality, morbidity, and quality of life and long-term safety is unclear. A cancer registry has been established to monitor a possible increased cancer risk over the next 15 years.

Insulin

History

The discovery of insulin has saved millions of lives to date. It is a brilliant piece of modern scientific medical history involving the outstanding personalities of Paul Langerhans, Oscar Minkowski, Sir Frederick Grant Banting, Charles Herbert Best, James Bertram Collip, Hans Christian Hagedorn, and others. The next milestones of antidiabetic insulin therapy were the development of blood glucose self-monitoring stripes in the 1960s, followed by the introduction of structured patient education programs for diabetes self-management in the 1970s by Michael Berger and colleagues. In 1993, the landmark study Diabetes Control and Complications Trial proved the concept of near-normoglycemic intensive, flexible insulin therapy.

Mechanism of action

Human insulin and insulin analogues act as physiological substitutes on insulin receptors and correct a relative or absolute insulin deficiency. Although endogenous insulin becomes inactivated within minutes, the pharmacodynamic properties of short-, intermediate- and long-acting insulin and insulin analogues are modified, and result in the intrinsic risk of hypoglycemia. Insulin becomes inactivated by endocytosis of the insulin–receptor complex, and hepatic and renal clearance [83].

Indications and contraindications

Insulin and insulin analogues are indicated in the treatment of diabetes mellitus in adults and children. It can be combined with all oral antihyperglycemic medicines except certain DPP-4 inhibitors (Table 14.4).

Side effects

Hypoglycemia is the most relevant side effect of insulin therapy. In elderly patients, during acute illness, in glycemia-modifying comedication, intensive physical activity, renal or hepatic impairment, and other conditions with high risk of hypo- and hyperglycemia, glucose monitoring and insulin dose adjustment should be intensified on an individual basis.

Renal insufficiency

Insulin and insulin analogues can be used in all stages of CKD. In CKD, insulin action can change individually in an unpredictable manner; therefore, general advice on dose adjustments cannot be given. Glucose monitoring and insulin dose adjustment should be

Pharmacokinetic properties of antihyperglycemic agents

	Mean $t_{1/2}$ plasma (h)	Metabolism	Active metabolites	Urinary excretion (%)	Accumulation in CKD	Caveat in CKD
Metformin	6.5	None	No	90	Yes	Stop at GFR <60 mL/min
Glibenclamide	1.5–2	Hepatic	Yes	50	Yes	Reduce dose at GFR <60 mL/min
Gliquidon*	3	Hepatic	No	5	Yes	and stop at GFR <30 mL/min
Glipizide	2–4	Hepatic	Yes	65	Yes	*no dose adjustment in gliquidon.
Glimepiride	5–8	Hepatic	Yes	50	Yes	
Glibornuride	8	Hepatic/renal	No	33	Yes	
Gliclazide	20	Hepatic	No	85	Yes	
Repaglinide	1	Hepatic	No	<10	No	Reduce dose at GFR <30 mL/min
Nateglinide	1–2	Hepatic	Yes	83	No	
Mitiglinide	1.2	Hepatic	No	54–74	Yes	
Pioglitazone	3–7	Hepatic	No	15–30	No	Stop in dialysis and NYHA I–IV
Acarbose	9–13	Intestinal	No	<2	No	Stop at GFR <25 mL/min
Miglitol	2–3	Renal	No	95	Yes	
Voglibose	No uptake	No	No	No	No	
Linagliptin	12	Hepatic/renal	No	5	Yes	Compare with Table 14.4 for
Sitagliptin	12	Hepatic/renal	No	87	Yes	adjustment of dosage
Saxagliptin	3–4	Renal	Yes	75	Yes	
Vildagliptin	3	Renal	No	85%	Yes	
Exenatide	2.4	Renal	No	Not known	Yes	Stop at GFR <30 mL/min
Liraglutide	13	Not known	No	Not known	Not known	Stop at GFR <60 mL/min

GFR, glomerular filtration rate; CKD, chronic kidney disease.

Table 14.3 Indications of antihyperglycemic medicines depending on stage of chronic kidney disease (CKD), GFR-glomerular filtration rate

CKD stage	1	2	3	4	5
Metformin	Indicated in GFR >60 mL/min				
Nateglinide/metformin	Indicated in GFR >60 mL/min				
Liraglutide	Indicated in GFR >60 mL/min				
Exenatide	Indicated in GFR >30 mL/min, adjust dose if GFR <50		mL/min		
Glibenclamide	Indicated in GFR >30 mL/min, adjust dose if GFR <60		mL/min		
Gliclazide	Indicated in GFR >30 mL/min, adjust dose if GFR <60		mL/min		
Glimepiride	Indicated in GFR >30 mL/min, adjust dose if GFR <60		mL/min		
Gliquidon	Indicated in GFR >30 mL/min, adjust dose if GFR <60		mL/min		
Acarbose	Indicated in GFR >25 mL/min, no dose adjustment				
Miglitol	Indicated in GFR >25 mL/min, no dose adjustment				
Pioglitazone	Indicated in GFR >4 mL/min, no dose adjustment, contraindicated in dialysis				
Repaglinide	No limitation, consider dose adjustment				
Linagliptin	No limitation, consider dose adjustment				
Sitagliptin	No limitation, consider dose adjustment				
Normal insulin	No limitation, consider dose adjustment				
Insulin lispro	No limitation, consider dose adjustment				
NPH insulin	No limitation, consider dose adjustment				
Insulin glargine	No limitation, consider dose adjustment				

Table 14.4 Indications and renal limitations of DPP-4 inhibitors, stage of chronic kidney disease (CKD) displayed

	Exenatide	Liraglutide	Linagliptin	Saxagliptin	Sitagliptin	Vildagliptin
Monotherapy			CKD 1–5		CKD 1–5	
Combined with Metformin	CKD 1–2	CKD 1–2	CKD 1–2	CKD 1–2	CKD 1–2	CKD 1–2
Combined with sulfonylurea	CKD 1–3	CKD 1–2		CKD 1–3	CKD 1–3	CKD 1–2
Combined with pioglitazone	CKD 1–3			CKD 1–5*	CKD 1–5	CKD 1–2
Combined with metformin and sulfonylurea	CKD 1–2	CKD 1–2	CKD 1–2		CKD 1–2	
Combined with metformin and pioglitazone	CKD 1–2	CKD 1–2			CKD 1–2	
Combined with insulin				CKD 1–5*	CKD 1–5	

*Not in dialysis.

intensified on an individual basis. Patient education is an effective method of decreasing the risk of severe hypoglycemia while improving glycemic control.

Evaluation

Insulin therapy reduces microvascular diabetes-related complications in type 1 and type 2 diabetes [12, 15]. The effect of insulin therapy on macrovascular morbidity and overall mortality is less well investigated [12, 14]. The risk of severe hypoglycemia can be reduced by structured diabetes self-management programs [84].

1. Levey AS, Atkins R, Coresh J, *et al*. Chronic kidney disease as a global public health problem: approaches and initiatives—a position statement from Kidney Disease Improving Global Outcomes. *Kidney Int* 2007;**72**:247–59.
2. Stamler J, Vaccaro O, Neaton JD, Wentworth D. Diabetes, other risk factors, and 12-yr cardiovascular mortality for men screened in the Multiple Risk Factor Intervention Trial. *Diabetes Care* 1993;**16**:434–44.
3. Manson JE, Colditz GA, Stampfer MJ, *et al*. A prospective study of maturity-onset diabetes mellitus and risk of coronary heart disease and stroke in women. *Arch Intern Med* 1991;**151**:1141–7.
4. Hagen B, Altenhofen L, Blaschy S, *et al*. Annual quality assurance report on the Disease-Management-Programs in Nordrhein in 2009. 2010 (http://www.kvno.de/downloads/quali/qualbe_dmp09.pdf) (In German).
5. Haffner SM, Lehto S, Ronnemaa T, *et al*. Mortality from coronary heart disease in subjects with type 2 diabetes and in nondiabetic subjects with and without prior myocardial infarction. *N Engl J Med* 1998;**339**:229–34.
6. Svensson M, Yu ZW, Eriksson JW. A small reduction in glomerular filtration is accompanied by insulin resistance in type I diabetes patients with diabetic nephropathy. *Eur J Clin Invest* 2002;**32**:100–9.
7. Stumvoll M. Glucose production by the human kidney–its importance has been underestimated. *Nephrol Dial Transplant* 1998;**13**:2996–9.
8. Rave K, Heise T, Pfutzner A, *et al*. Impact of diabetic nephropathy on pharmacodynamic and pharmacokinetic properties of insulin in type 1 diabetic patients. *Diabetes Care* 2001;**24**:886–90.
9. Nathan DM, Buse JB, Davidson MB, *et al*. Medical management of hyperglycaemia in type 2 diabetes mellitus: a consensus algorithm for the initiation and adjustment of therapy: a consensus statement from the American Diabetes Association and the European Association for the Study of Diabetes. *Diabetologia* 2009;**52**:17–30.
10. Scottish Intercollegiate Guidelines Network. *Management of diabetes. A national clinical guideline*. Edinburgh: SIGN, 2010.
11. UK Prospective Diabetes Study (UKPDS) Group. Effect of intensive blood-glucose control with metformin on complications in overweight patients with type 2 diabetes (UKPDS 34). *Lancet* 1998;**352**:854–65.
12. UK Prospective Diabetes Study (UKPDS) Group. Intensive blood-glucose control with sulphonylureas or insulin compared with conventional treatment and risk of complications in patients with type 2 diabetes (UKPDS 33). *Lancet* 1998;**352**:837–53.
13. Hemmingsen B, Lund SS, Gluud C, *et al*. Targeting intensive glycaemic control

versus targeting conventional glycaemic control for type 2 diabetes mellitus. *Cochrane Database Syst Rev* 2011(6): CD008143.

14. Nathan DM, Cleary PA, Backlund JY, *et al.* Intensive diabetes treatment and cardiovascular disease in patients with type 1 diabetes. *N Engl J Med* 2005;**353**: 2643–53.

15. The Diabetes Control and Complications Trial Research Group. The effect of intensive treatment of diabetes on the development and progression of long-term complications in insulin-dependent diabetes mellitus. *N Engl J Med* 1993; **329**:977–86.

16. Action to Control Cardiovascular Risk in Diabetes Study G, Gerstein HC, Miller ME, Byington RP, *et al.* Effects of intensive glucose lowering in type 2 diabetes. *N Engl J Med* 2008;**358**:2545–59.

17. Winocour PH. Effective diabetes care: a need for realistic targets. *BMJ* 2002;**324**: 1577–80.

18. Buse JB. Type 2 diabetes mellitus in 2010: individualizing treatment targets in diabetes care. *Nat Rev Endocrinol* 2011;**7**: 67–8.

19. Stewart J, Kendrick D, Nottingham Diabetes Blood Pressure Study G. Setting and negotiating targets in people with Type 2 diabetes in primary care: a cross sectional survey. *Diabet Med* 2005;**22**: 683–7.

20. Olson DE, Norris SL. Diabetes in older adults. Overview of AGS guidelines for the treatment of diabetes mellitus in geriatric populations. *Geriatrics* 2004; **59**:18–24; quiz 5.

21. Hesse E, Taubmann G. Die Wirkung des Biguanids und seiner Derivate auf den Zuckerstoffwechsel. [The effect of biguanid and its derivates on glucose metabolism]. *Arch Exptl Patho Pharmakol* 1929;**142**:290–308.

22. Werner E, Bell J. The preparation of methylguanidine, and of β-dimethylguanidine by the interaction of dicyanodiamide, and methylammonium and dimethylammonium chlorides respectively. *J Chem Soc Trans* 1921; **121**:1790–5.

23. University Group Diabetes Program. A study on the effects of hypoglycemic agents on vascular complications on patients with adult-onset diabetes: V. Evaluation of phenformin therapy. *Diabetes* 1975;**24**(Suppl 1):65–184.

24. Bailey CJ, Turner RC. Metformin. *N Engl J Med* 1996;**334**:574–9.

25. Musi N, Hirshman MF, Nygren J, *et al.* Metformin increases AMP-activated protein kinase activity in skeletal muscle of subjects with type 2 diabetes. *Diabetes* 2002;**51**:2074–81.

26. Kim YD, Park KG, Lee YS, *et al.* Metformin inhibits hepatic gluconeogenesis through AMP-activated protein kinase-dependent regulation of the orphan nuclear receptor SHP. *Diabetes* 2008;**57**:306–14.

27. Tonelli M, Sacks F, Pfeffer M, *et al.* Biomarkers of inflammation and progression of chronic kidney disease. *Kidney Int* 2005;**68**:237–45.

28. Morales AI, Detaille D, Prieto M, *et al.* Metformin prevents experimental gentamicin-induced nephropathy by a mitochondria-dependent pathway. *Kidney Int* 2010;**77**:861–9.

29. Collier CA, Bruce CR, Smith AC, *et al.* Metformin counters the insulin-induced suppression of fatty acid oxidation and stimulation of triacylglycerol storage in rodent skeletal muscle. *Am J Physiol Endocrinol Metab* 2006;**291**:E182–9.

30. Marshall SM, Flyvbjerg A. Diabetic Nephropathy. In: Holt RIG (ed.) *Textbook of diabetes*, 4th edn. Oxford: Wiley-Blackwell, 2010.

31. Matthaei S, Bierwirth R, Fritsche A, *et al*. In German: Pharmacological Antihyperglycemic Therapy of Type 2 Diabetes mellitus. Update of the Evidence-Based Guidelines of The German Diabetes Association. *Diabetologie* 2009;**4**:32–64.

32. Jones GC, Macklin JP, Alexander WD. Contraindications to the use of metformin. *BMJ* 2003;**326**:4–5.

33. Misbin RI. The phantom of lactic acidosis due to metformin in patients with diabetes. *Diabetes Care* 2004;**27**: 1791–3.

34. Peters N, Jay N, Barraud D, *et al*. Metformin-associated lactic acidosis in an intensive care unit. *Crit Care* 2008;**12**: R149.

35. Salpeter SR, Greyber E, Pasternak GA, *et al*. Risk of fatal and nonfatal lactic acidosis with metformin use in type 2 diabetes mellitus. *Cochrane Database Syst Rev* 2010(2):CD002967.

36. Nguyen HL, Concepcion L. Metformin intoxication requiring dialysis. *Hemodialy Int* 2011;**15**(Suppl 1):S68–71.

37. Guo PY, Storsley LJ, Finkle SN. Severe lactic acidosis treated with prolonged hemodialysis: recovery after massive overdoses of metformin. *Sem Dial* 2006; **19**:80–3.

38. Panzer U, Kluge S, Kreymann G, Wolf G. Combination of intermittent haemodialysis and high-volume continuous haemofiltration for the treatment of severe metformin-induced lactic acidosis. *Nephrol Dial Transplant* 2004;**19**:2157–8.

39. Saenz A, Fernandez-Esteban I, Mataix A, *et al*. Metformin monotherapy for type 2 diabetes mellitus. *Cochrane Database Syst Rev* 2005(3):CD002966.

40. Lalau JD, Race JM. Lactic acidosis in metformin therapy: searching for a link with metformin in reports of

"metformin-associated lactic acidosis". *Diabetes Obes Metab* 2001;**3**:195–201.

41. Nye HJ, Herrington WG. Metformin: the safest hypoglycaemic agent in chronic kidney disease? *Nephron Clin Pract* 2011; **118**:c380–3.

42. Bodmer M, Meier C, Krahenbuhl S, *et al*. Metformin, sulfonylureas, or other antidiabetes drugs and the risk of lactic acidosis or hypoglycemia: a nested case-control analysis. *Diabetes Care* 2008;**31**:2086–91.

43. Eurich DT, McAlister FA, Blackburn DF, *et al*. Benefits and harms of antidiabetic agents in patients with diabetes and heart failure: systematic review. *BMJ* 2007;**335**:497.

44. Loubatieres A. The hypoglycemic sulfonamides: history and development of the problem from 1942 to 1955. *Ann NY Acad Sci* 1957;**71**:4–11.

45. Joost HG, Hasselblatt A. Insulin release by tolbutamide and glibenclamide. A comparative study on the perfused rat pancreas. *Naunyn-Schmiedeberg's Arch Pharmacol* 1979;**306**:185–8.

46. Niemi M, Cascorbi I, Timm R, Kroemer HK, Neuvonen PJ, Kivisto KT. Glyburide and glimepiride pharmacokinetics in subjects with different CYP2C9 genotypes. *Clin Pharmacol Ther* 2002; **72**:326–32.

47. Becker ML, Visser LE, Trienekens PH, *et al*. Cytochrome P450 2C9 *2 and *3 polymorphisms and the dose and effect of sulfonylurea in type II diabetes mellitus. *Clin Pharmacol Ther* 2008; **83**:288–92.

48. United Kingdom Prospective Diabetes Study Group. United Kingdom Prospective Diabetes Study 24: a 6-year, randomized, controlled trial comparing sulfonylurea, insulin, and metformin therapy in patients with newly diagnosed type 2 diabetes that could not be

controlled with diet therapy. *Ann Intern Med* 1998;**128**:165–75.

49. Group UKHS. Risk of hypoglycaemia in types 1 and 2 diabetes: effects of treatment modalities and their duration. *Diabetologia* 2007;**50**:1140–7.

50. Amiel SA. Hypoglycemia: from the laboratory to the clinic. *Diabetes Care* 2009;**32**:1364–71.

51. Holstein A, Plaschke A, Egberts EH. Clinical characterisation of severe hypoglycaemia—a prospective population-based study. *Exp Clin Endocrinol Diabetes* 2003;**111**:364–9.

52. Asplund K, Wiholm BE, Lithner F. Glibenclamide-associated hypoglycaemia: a report on 57 cases. *Diabetologia* 1983; **24**:412–7.

53. Holman RR, Paul SK, Bethel MA, *et al.* 10-year follow-up of intensive glucose control in type 2 diabetes. *N Engl J Med* 2008;**359**:1577–89.

54. Meinert CL, Knatterud GL, Prout TE, Klimt CR. A study of the effects of hypoglycemic agents on vascular complications in patients with adult-onset diabetes. II. Mortality results. *Diabetes* 1970;**19**(Suppl):789–830.

55. Meier JJ, Gallwitz B, Schmidt WE, *et al.* Is impairment of ischaemic preconditioning by sulfonylurea drugs clinically important? *Heart* 2004;**90**: 9–12.

56. Pantalone KM, Kattan MW, Yu C, *et al.* The risk of overall mortality in patients with type 2 diabetes receiving glipizide, glyburide, or glimepiride monotherapy: a retrospective analysis. *Diabetes Care* 2010;**33**:1224–9.

57. Schramm TK, Gislason GH, Vaag A, *et al.* Mortality and cardiovascular risk associated with different insulin secretagogues compared with metformin in type 2 diabetes, with or without a previous myocardial infarction: a nationwide study. *Eur Heart J* 2011;**32**: 1900–8.

58. IQWiG (Institute for Quality and Efficiency in Health Care). Glinids as a therapy in type 2 diabetes mellitus (German). report no. 48. Final report A05–05C. 2009.

59. Gale EA. Lessons from the glitazones: a story of drug development. *Lancet* 2001; **357**:1870–5.

60. Gale EA. Troglitazone: the lesson that nobody learned? *Diabetologia* 2006; **49**:1–6.

61. Graham D, Green L. *Memorandum. Final report: Liver failure risk with troglitazone (Rezulin) NDA: 20-720*. Bethesda, MD: USDHHS, FDA, Center for Drug Evaluation and Research, 2000.

62. Nissen SE, Wolski K. Effect of rosiglitazone on the risk of myocardial infarction and death from cardiovascular causes. *N Engl J Med* 2007;**356**:2457–71.

63. Habib ZA, Havstad SL, Wells K, *et al.* Thiazolidinedione use and the longitudinal risk of fractures in patients with type 2 diabetes mellitus. *J Clin Endocrinol Metab* 2010;**95**:592–600.

64. Kirchheiner J, Thomas S, Bauer S, *et al.* Pharmacokinetics and pharmacodynamics of rosiglitazone in relation to CYP2C8 genotype. *Clin Pharmacol Ther* 2006;**80**:657–67.

65. Patel UD, Hernandez AF, Liang L, *et al.* Quality of care and outcomes among patients with heart failure and chronic kidney disease: A Get With the Guidelines – Heart Failure Program study. *American Heart J* 2008;**156**:674–81.

66. Dormandy JA, Charbonnel B, Eckland DJ, *et al.* Secondary prevention of macrovascular events in patients with type 2 diabetes in the PROactive Study (PROspective pioglitAzone Clinical Trial In macroVascular Events): a randomised controlled trial. *Lancet* 2005;**366**:1279–89.

67. Loke YK, Singh S, Furberg CD. Long-term use of thiazolidinediones and fractures in type 2 diabetes: a meta-analysis. *Can Med Assoc J* 2009;**180**:32–9.

68. Richter B, Bandeira-Echtler E, Bergerhoff K, *et al.* Pioglitazone for type 2 diabetes mellitus. *Cochrane Database Syst Rev* 2006; (4):CD006060.

69. Benz G, Hahn R, Reinhardt C. 100 Jahre chemisch-wissenschaftliches Laboratorium der Bayer AG in Wuppertal-Elbersfeld 1898–1996. *Leverkusen* 1996:88–90.

70. Scott LJ, Spencer CM. Miglitol: a review of its therapeutic potential in type 2 diabetes mellitus. *Drugs* 2000;**59**:521–49.

71. Holstein A, Beil W. Oral antidiabetic drug metabolism: pharmacogenomics and drug interactions. *Expert Opin Drug Metab Toxicol* 2009;**5**:225–41.

72. *Precose Prescribing Information*. Leverkusen: Bayer Pharmaceuticals Corporation. 3/2011.

73. Holman RR, Cull CA, Turner RC. A randomized double-blind trial of acarbose in type 2 diabetes shows improved glycemic control over 3 years (U.K. Prospective Diabetes Study 44). *Diabetes Care* 1999;**22**:960–4.

74. Van de Laar FA, Lucassen PL, Akkermans RP, *et al.* Alpha-glucosidase inhibitors for type 2 diabetes mellitus. *Cochrane Database Syst Rev* 2005;(2):CD003639.

75. Thornberry NA, Weber AE. Discovery of JANUVIA (Sitagliptin), a selective dipeptidyl peptidase IV inhibitor for the treatment of type 2 diabetes. *Curr Topics Med Chem* 2007;**7**:557–68.

76. Joy SV, Rodgers PT, Scates AC. Incretin mimetics as emerging treatments for type 2 diabetes. *Ann Pharmacother* 2005; **39**:110–8.

77. Cvetkovic RS, Plosker GL. Exenatide: a review of its use in patients with type 2 diabetes mellitus (as an adjunct to metformin and/or a sulfonylurea). *Drugs* 2007;**67**:935–54.

78. EMA. Assessment report. Victoza. Procedure No: EMEA/H/C/001026/ II/0005/G. 2011.

79. Green BD, Flatt PR, Bailey CJ. Dipeptidyl peptidase IV (DPP IV) inhibitors: A newly emerging drug class for the treatment of type 2 diabetes. *Diabetes Vascular Dis Res* 2006;**3**:159–65.

80. European Medicines Agency. Trajenta: EPAR—Summary for the public. 06/10/2011.

81. Richter B, Bandeira-Echtler E, Bergerhoff K, Lerch CL. Dipeptidyl peptidase-4 (DPP-4) inhibitors for type 2 diabetes mellitus. *Cochrane Database Syst Rev* 2008;(2):CD006739.

82. Vilsboll T, Christensen M, Junker AE, *et al.* Effects of glucagon-like peptide-1 receptor agonists on weight loss: systematic review and meta-analyses of randomised controlled trials. *BMJ* 2012;**344**:d7771.

83. Duckworth WC, Bennett RG, Hamel FG. Insulin degradation: progress and potential. *Endocr Rev* 1998;**19**:608–24.

84. Samann A, Muhlhauser I, Bender R, *et al.* Glycaemic control and severe hypoglycaemia following training in flexible, intensive insulin therapy to enable dietary freedom in people with type 1 diabetes: a prospective implementation study. *Diabetologia* 2005;**48**:1965–70.

Chapter 15

Reducing progression of diabetic nephropathy by antihypertensive treatment

Anita Hansen, Ivo Quack and Lars Christian Rump

Heinrich-Heine University Düsseldorf, Düsseldorf, Germany

Key points

- Achieving low blood pressure levels is the most important goal to prevent diabetic nephropathy in patients with type 2 diabetes. The higher the initial blood pressure the greater is the treatment effect.
- Blockers of the renin–angiotensin system should be preferred as first-line treatment in hypertensive type 1 and type 2 diabetics with proteinuria/albuminuria and/or advanced nephropathy.
- A pronounced antiproteinuric response to antihypertensive treatment indicates a better prognosis of diabetic nephropathy.
- Renin–angiotensin system blockers are antiproteinuric independent of their blood pressure-lowering effect in diabetic nephropathy and this effect seems to be dose dependent.

- Combinations of different blockers of the renin–angiotensin system should be avoided in patients with type 2 diabetes and/or with chronic kidney disease defined as a glomerular filtration rate <60 mL/min/1.73 m^2. Combination therapy with a renin inhibitor and angiotensin-converting enzyme inhibitors or AT1-blockers is contraindicated according to an announcement by the European Medical Association in February 2012.
- In type 2 diabetics individualized blood pressure targets lower than 140/90 mmHg should be achieved in the range of 130–139/80–85 mmHg or even lower if tolerable, adjusted to age and concomitant diseases.

Introduction

Diabetic nephropathy is the leading cause of end-stage renal disease [1]. Microalbuminuria defined as urinary albumin excretion rate of 30 mg/g creatinine or greater is the first detectable sign of diabetic nephropathy. Antihypertensive treatment does not only reduce blood pressure but also albuminuria and is expected to slow the decline of glomerular filtration rate (GFR). Another beneficial side effect is the reduction of cardiovascular risk. This review

Diabetes and Kidney Disease, First Edition. Edited by Gunter Wolf.
© 2013 John Wiley & Sons, Ltd. Published 2013 by John Wiley & Sons, Ltd.

focuses on prevention and slowing of progression of diabetic nephropathy by antihypertensive treatment.

In diabetics, glomerular hyperfiltration and microinflammation are thought to be early and important mechanisms of kidney injury. Lowering blood pressure by renin–angiotensin system (RAS) blockers may therefore be a possible approach to prevent diabetic nephropathy. This hypothesis was tested in two main trials in type 2 diabetes [2, 3] and in two trials with type 1 diabetes [4, 5].

BENEDICT and ROADMAP

The Bergamo Nephrologic Diabetes Complications Trial (BENEDICT) investigated whether angiotensin-converting enzyme (ACE) inhibitors and non-dihydropyridine calcium channel blockers alone or in combination prevent microalbuminuria in type 2 diabetics [2]. In this double-blind randomized trial 1204 normoalbuminuric patients were enrolled. Blood pressure levels at baseline were higher than 130/85 mmHg, creatinine <1.5 mg/dL and diabetes duration less than 25 years. Patients were randomized to four groups receiving trandolapril in combination with verapamil (2/180 mg), trandolapril alone (2 mg), verapamil alone (240 mg) and placebo with baseline blood pressures between 150.1 ± 13.1/87.5 ± 7.2 mmHg and 151.9 ± 15.4/87.7 ± 7.6 mmHg. Target blood pressure level was 120/80 mmHg and additional antihypertensive drugs were allowed. The primary end point was the development of persistent micoalbuminuria. After a median of 3.6 years, 5.7% of patients treated with the combination therapy of trandolapril with verapamil developed microalbuminuria compared with 10% in subjects receiving placebo, 6% in

patients with trandolapril alone and 11.9% in patients with verapamil alone. Thus, treatment with trandolapril in combination with verapamil or alone significantly delayed the onset of microalbuminuria by a factor of 2.6 and 2.1 compared with placebo or verapamil alone.

The achieved mean blood pressure levels were slightly lower in the trandolapril groups with 139 ± 10/80 ± 6 mmHg (combination therapy), 139 ± 12/81 ± 6 mmHg (trandolapril) compared with 141 ± 12/83 ± 6 mmHg (verapamil) and 142 ± 12/83 ± 6 mmHg (placebo). Nevertheless, the beneficial effect of trandolapril persisted after adjustment for systolic and diastolic blood pressure. In all treatment groups, the creatinine (0.9 ± 0.2 mg/dL) was similar and did not change during follow-up. A *post hoc* analysis revealed that the benefit mainly occurred in patients with a systolic blood pressure higher than 139 mmHg during follow-up [6]. Thus, the BENEDICT trial demonstrated that type 2 diabetics with hypertension, normoalbuminuria, and normal renal function benefit from treatment with an ACE inhibitor by a decrease in the rate of microalbuminuria of about 53%. Whether similar benefits occur with an angiotensin receptor blocker (ARB) in lower blood pressure ranges (<130/80 mmHg) was investigated by the Randomized Olmesartan and Diabetes Microalbuminuria Prevention (ROADMAP) Trial in a much larger cohort of patients [3]. This randomized placebo-controlled, double-blind trial assessed whether 40 mg of olmesartan would delay or prevent the occurrence of microalbuminuria in type 2 diabetes and normoalbuminuria over a study period of 3.2 years. A total of 4447 patients were enrolled, with a mean blood pressure level of 136 ± 15/81 ± 10 mmHg at baseline. Additional antihypertensive drugs except ACE inhibitors or ARBs were allowed so that the target blood pressure of less than 130/80 mmHg could be reached. Baseline characteristics were not significantly different in both groups and serum creatinine was

77.5 ± 16.2 µmol/L (0.88 ± 0.18 mg/dL) according to a mean GFR of 84.9 ± 17.2 mL/min/1.73 m². The primary end point was defined as the first onset of microalbuminuria; the second end points were renal and cardiovascular events. The target blood pressure level was achieved in nearly 80% of the patients taking olmesartan and 71% taking placebo. Mean blood pressure levels during follow-up were 125/74.3 mmHg (olmesartan) versus 128.7/76.2 mmHg (placebo). Microalbuminuria developed in 8.2% of patients with olmesartan and 9.8% with placebo. Olmesartan was associated with an increased time to onset of microalbuminuria by 23%. The beneficial effect of olmesartan remained after adjustment for differences in blood pressure levels, which were lower in the olmesartan group than in the placebo group by approximately 3.1/1.9 mmHg. The estimated GFR declined in both groups (from 85.0 ± 17.0 to 80.1 ± 18.5 mL/min/1.73 m² in the olmesartan group and from 84.7 ± 17.3 to 83.7 ± 18.3 mL/min/1.73 m² in the placebo group ($p < 0.001$ for the between-group comparison of the change from baseline). Patients with a GFR below (<83.8 mL/min/1.73 m²) or an urinary albumin-to-creatinine ratio above the median (>4) showed a tendency to have a greater benefit. The same was true for patients with systolic blood pressure ≥135 mmHg at baseline.

Thus, BENEDICT showed that hypertensive type 2 diabetics with normoalbuminuria benefit from treatment with an ACE inhibitor, and in addition ROADMAP showed a benefit of an ARB even in normotensive type 2 diabetic patients. The most likely explanation for the greater effect in BENEDICT than in ROADMAP could be associated with the higher blood pressure levels in BENEDICT at baseline and during follow-up. One could speculate that higher blood pressure levels may reflect greater RAS activity resulting in greater treatment effects in prevention of diabetic neph-

ropathy. Both studies suggest that RAS blockers are capable to delay the onset of diabetic nephropathy beyond their blood pressure-lowering effects. A similar question had been previously addressed in a smaller cohort of patients by the ABCD trial (Appropriate Blood Pressure Control in Diabetes) [7].

ABCD trial

In the ABCD trial (normotensive arm) 480 type 2 diabetics were randomized to moderate (diastolic 80–89 mmHg) versus intensive (diastolic decrease of 10 mmHg, intensive group) blood pressure goals. Baseline blood pressure levels were 135.6 ± 0.8/84.4 ± 0.2 versus and 137.2 ± 0.9/84.4 ± 0.2. Patients in the moderate group received placebo and patients in the intensive group were treated with the calcium channel blocker nisoldipine (10 mg/day titrated up to a maximum of 60 mg/day) or the ACE inhibitor enalapril (5 mg/day titrated up to 40 mg/day). In the intensive group, 9.3% of patients had overt albuminuria versus 12% in the moderate group. Microalbuminuria was found in 21% versus 25%. Over a period of 5.3 years, the mean blood pressure level in the intensive group was 128 ± 0.8/75 ± 0.3 mmHg versus 137 ± 0.7/81 ± 0.3 mmHg in the moderate group. The estimated GFR was stable in both groups, but there was a lower percentage of patients in the intensive group who developed microalbuminuria or progressed from microalbuminuria to overt albuminuria. This effect was independent of the antihypertensive agent. This suggests that intensive blood pressure control in type 2 diabetics is more important than the antihypertensive used to prevent microalbuminuria. However, the cohort of normoalbuminuric patients was only a subgroup and considerably smaller than those in ROADMAP and BENEDICT. However, there have been other studies with a lack of a beneficial effect by RAS blockers on microalbuminuria in type 2 diabetes.

DIRECT

The DIRECT-Renal analysis was a subgroup analysis of three related trials in the DIRECT program to study the incidence of microalbuminuria in normoalbuminuric diabetics who were normotensive or had a blood pressure (≤160/90 mmHg) [4]. The DIRECT program was designed to investigate whether candesartan (32 mg) could prevent diabetic retinopathy in type 1 or type 2 diabetes over a median of 4.7 years. The incidence of microalbuminuria was a prespecified end point. The program comprised three studies: DIRECT-Prevent 1 with 1421 normotensive and normoalbuminuric type 1 diabetics without retinopathy, DIRECT-Protect 1 with 1905 normotensive and normalbuminuric type 1 diabetics with mild to moderate retinopathy, and DIRECT-Protect 2 with 1905 normoalbuminuric type 2 diabetics with mild to moderate retinopathy who were normotensive or had "controlled" hypertension (≤160/90 mmHg). Patients with a GFR <90 mL/min/1.73 m^2 were excluded. The type 2 diabetes study population had a mean blood pressure level of 123 ± 8.7/75 ± 6.4 mmHg in the candesartan group versus 123 ± 9/76 ± 6.5 mmHg in the placebo group, and 139 ± 12.7/79 ± 6.9 mmHg versus 139 ± 12.0/80 ± 7.1 mmHg in the patients with controlled hypertension. Candesartan did not have a significant effect on the incidence of microalbuminuria. However, DIRECT was not powered for renal end points.

In line with this, the DIRECT-Renal analysis showed no preventive effect of candesartan on the incidence of microalbuminuria in the 3326 type 1 diabetics over a study period of 4.7 years. Another trial which investigated the effects of an early blockade of the renin–angiotensin system in type 1 diabetes is the Renin–Angiotensin System Study (RASS) by Mauer et al. [5]. This 5-year randomized, double-blind trial compared the effects of the ACE inhibitor enalapril (10–20 mg) and the ARB losartan (50–100 mg) with placebo on structural changes from diabetic nephropathy in 285 normoalbuminuric patients (GFR >90 mL/min) with type 1 diabetes. The primary end point was a change in the fraction of the glomerular volume occupied by mesangium; secondary renal end points included changes in other glomerular, vascular, tubular, and interstitial variables, and changes in the albumin excretion rate and GFR. Blood pressure levels at baseline were 120 ± 13/71 ± 8 mmHg (enalapril group), 120 ± 11/70 ± 8 mmHg (losartan group), and 119 ± 11/70 ± 8 mmHg (placebo group), and were significantly lower during the study in the enalapril (113 ± 9/66 ± 6 mmHg) and losartan (115 ± 8/66 ± 6 mmHg) group than in the placebo (117 ± 8/68 ± 5 mmHg) group. There were no significant effects on progression of structural changes, albuminuria, or GFR. Unexpectedly, the incidence of microalbuminuria was higher in the losartan group.

The most likely explanations for these negative results could be young age of study patients (29–31 years), and low blood pressure levels of 117/73 mmHg and ~120/70 mmHg. The baseline urinary albumin excretion rate (UAER) of 5 µg/min in DIRECT-Renal was low, and the effect of candesartan on the rate of change in albumin excretion was very small. Thus, the rate of change in UAER from baseline may be too slow to detect an effect of treatment over 4.7 years. Moreover, many of these patients may never develop nephropathy. The cumulative incidence in type 1 diabetes is only 40% after 40 years. Thus, a much longer duration of follow-up would be necessary [4]. Therefore, the role of a RAS blockade in normotensive normoalbuminuric type 1 diabetics is unclear. In type 2 diabetics the differing effects of RAS blockade to prevent diabetic nephropathy may be due to (1) lack of power for renal end points in DIRECT-Renal, and (2) different blood pressure levels in RASS and DIRECT-Renal (low) than in BENEDICT and ROADMAP (higher).

Slowing progression of established diabetic nephropathy by antihypertensives

There have been several studies which focused on slowing progression in diabetic nephropathy and the role of antihypertensive treatment.

Type 1 diabetics

In 1993 Lewis *et al.* demonstrated beneficial effects of the ACE inhibitor captopril on progression of diabetic nephropathy in insulin-dependent diabetic patients [8]. In this 3-year randomized placebo-controlled, double-blind trial of 409 patients with insulin-dependent diabetes mellitus for at least 7 years with onset before the age of 30, all patients had diabetic nephropathy at baseline with an albuminuria of more than 500 mg/day and a serum creatinine ≤2.5 mg/dL. The treatment group received 3 × 25 mg captopril per day. Blood pressure lower than 140/90 mmHg was the goal. Captopril retarded the rate of loss of renal function in these patients. The risk reduction of the primary end point doubling serum creatinine was 48% and 50% of the combined end point (dialysis, death and transplantation). The beneficial effect of captopril was not explained by the differences in blood pressure between the two groups: 135/86 mmHg at baseline (captopril group) versus 138/86 mmHg (placebo) and during follow-up 128–134/77–82 mmHg versus 129–136/80–84 mmHg. Similar results were demonstrated by a smaller study in normotensive patients with insulin-dependent diabetes and persistent microalbuminuria. Captopril

therapy significantly prevented the increase in the urinary albumin excretion rate and the progression to clinical proteinuria [9].

Type 2 diabetics with advanced diabetic nephropathy

Two landmark studies with advanced diabetic nephropathy and hypertension were presented in 2001, the Irbesartan Diabetic Nephropathy Trial (IDNT), with 1715 patients [10], and the Reduction of End Points in NIDDM with the Angiotensin II-Antagonist Losartan Study (RENAAL), with 1513 patients [11]. Both randomized controlled trials evaluated the beneficial use of an ARB (irbesartan 300 mg and losartan 100 mg daily) in protecting against the progression of diabetic nephropathy over a treatment period of 2.6 and 3.4 years, respectively. The primary end point was the composite end point of doubling of serum creatinine, end-stage renal disease, or death. In IDNT the effect of losartan was tested and compared with 10 mg of amlodipine and placebo; RENAAL was placebo controlled. All patients were hypertensive with baseline blood pressure levels of about 160/87 mmHg and 152/82 mmHg and overt albuminuria (~1.9 g/day and ~1.2 g/day). Target blood pressure levels were lower than 140/90 mmHg; at the end of the studies the mean blood pressure level was 140/77–74 mmHg. The primary end point was reduced in both trials. There was a significant risk reduction of 33% for doubling serum creatinine and of 23% for end-stage renal disease in IDNT. Treatment with losartan reduced the risk reduction of the composite end point by 16%, doubling of serum creatinine by 25% and end-stage renal disease by 28%. In RENAAL, losartan reduced proteinuria by 35% in contrast to patients treated with placebo, who tended to show an increase in proteinuria. Thus, IDNT and RENAAL revealed a significant benefit of two different ARBs beyond blood pressure in advanced diabetic nephropathy.

Albuminuria and antihypertensive treatment

Is albuminuria a target for diabetic nephropathy? A retrospective analysis of the RENAAL trial evaluated risk factors for doubling serum creatinine or the development of end-stage renal disease [12]. Proteinuria, serum creatinine, serum albumin, and hemoglobin levels were demonstrated to be four independent risk factors; however, proteinuria was the single most powerful predictor of adverse renal outcomes in association with progression of nephropathy in patients with type 2 diabetes and diabetic nephropathy. Further analysis of the RENAAL patient cohort examined the importance of albuminuria on renal outcome [13]. Patients with a high baseline albuminuria of 3 g/day or higher had a 5.2-fold increased risk for reaching the composite renal end point of doubling serum creatinine and end-stage renal disease and a 8.1-fold increased risk for progressing to end-stage renal disease compared with the group with low albuminuria <1.5 g/day. Every 50% reduction in albuminuria in the first 6 months of therapy was associated with a risk reduction of 36% for a renal end point and 45% for end-stage renal disease during later follow-up. Residual albuminuria after 6 months of treatment showed a linear relationship with renal outcome. Losartan reduced albuminuria by 28% while placebo increased albuminuria by 4%. Thus, the higher albuminuria, the greater is the renal risk. Reduction of albuminuria was associated with a proportional effect on renal protection. Therefore, type 2 diabetics with nephropathy benefit from using an ARB through better blood pressure control, slowing of GFR decline, and reduction of albuminuria. Furthermore, the dose of the ARB seems to be important.

IRMA-2, MARVAL and DETAIL

Parving *et al.* [14] showed in the IRMA-2 (IRbesartan in MicroAlbuminuria, Type 2 Diabetic Nephropathy) trial that irbesartan in two different doses (150 mg and 300 mg) reduces albuminuria in 590 patients with type 2 diabetes. Despite similar blood pressure control, irbesartan 300 mg was significantly more effective (38% albuminuria reduction) than irbesartan 150 mg (24% albuminuria reduction). IRMA-2 underlines that proteinuria as a target in diabetic nephropathy requires higher doses of ARB for renoprotection. Side effects like hyperkalemia or deterioration of renal function may be problems in daily practice and need careful monitoring. However, these adverse events were not significantly prevalent in the above-mentioned well-controlled studies. If there is an increase in serum creatinine after starting RAS blocker therapy, renal artery stenosis should be excluded. However, stopping this medication early may not be advisable. *Post hoc* analyses of IDNT and RENAAL have shown that those patients with a stronger initial decline of GFR in the first months may still benefit from treatment with RAS blockers in the long run [15, 16]. Beneficial effects of ARBs were confirmed by the MicroAlbuminuria Reduction With Valsartan (MARVAL) study, which evaluated the blood pressure-independent effect of valsartan on the UAER in type 2 diabetics with microalbuminuria [17]. 332 patients were included with or without hypertension. They were randomly assigned to 80 mg valsartan or 5 mg amlodipine, which was doubled if the target blood pressure of 135/85 mmHg was not achieved. The primary end point was change in UAER from baseline to 24 weeks. Baseline blood pressure levels were about 147/85 mmHg in both groups. There was a significant decrease in albuminuria by 44% in the valsartan group, but of only 8% in the amlodipine group, despite similar blood pressure levels. With valsartan more patients regressed to normoalbuminuria. This effect of valsartan was independent of the hypertensive status. Thus, reduction of blood pressure is essential to slow progression of diabetic nephropathy, and the use of ARBs in type 2 diabetics shows additional protection. Results from the DETAIL study (Diabetic Exposed to Telmisartan and Enalapril) underline that an ARB (telmisartan) is not inferior to an ACE inhibitor (enalapril) in preventing the progressive decline of GFR in type 2 diabetics with early nephropathy [18]. A total 250 hypertensive type 2 diabetics having early diabetic nephropathy with a GFR higher than $70\,mL/min/1.73\,m^2$ were randomly assigned to receive either 80 mg telmisartan or 20 mg enalapril over 5 years. The GFR was measured by plasma clearance of iohexol. Mean change was $-18.7\,mL/min/1.73\,m^2$ in the telmisartan and $-15.8\,mL/min/1.73\,m^2$ in the enalapril group, resulting in a non-inferiority of telmisartan relative to enalapril.

ADVANCE

A completely different approach was followed in the ADVANCE study. They asked whether routine administration of an ACE inhibitor/diuretic (perindopril/indapamide) combination has advantages in type 2 diabetics irrespective of the initial blood pressure levels or current medication. Use of ACE inhibitors was excluded, but ARBs were allowed [19]. A total of 11 140 patients with increased cardiovascular risk were randomized. The mean age was 66 years, 4% had macroalbuminuria and 26% microalbuminuria. Renal function was near normal, with creatinine of 87 µmol/L. There was a relative risk reduction of new-onset or progressive proteinuria of 18%. Active treatment was associated with a significant reduction of 21% in all renal events with a borderline reduction in new or worsening nephropathy (18%), and a significant reduction in the development of microalbuminuria (21%). The positive results regarding the renoprotective effect by add-on combination therapy of perindopril/indapamide is most likely due to the lower blood pressure levels in the treatment group. However, a specific drug effect cannot be

excluded. At baseline, blood pressure levels were ~145/81 mmHg and were reduced over a mean follow up of 4.3 years by an average of 5.6 mmHg systolic and 2.2 mmHg diastolic in patients with active treatment. The benefit of blood pressure-lowering independent of the drug used had been shown in the UKPDS trial with 1148 hypertensive type 2 diabetics with higher target blood pressures [20]. Tight blood pressure control lower than 150/85 mmHg over 8.4 years achieved a clinically important reduction in the risk of deaths and other complications related to diabetes independent of the drug used (atenolol versus captopril).

Renin-inhibition and RAS blocker combinations

It was assumed that double blockade of RAS in diabetic nephropathy may be renoprotective and that additional direct renin inhibition by aliskiren would intensify this effect.

ONTARGET

As part of the prespecified analyses of the Ongoing Telmisartan Alone and in combination with Ramipril Global Endpoint Trial (ONTARGET) Mann et al. [21] examined the effects of telmisartan (80 mg), ramipril (10 mg), and their combination on renal outcomes in a large population of 25 620 patients at age 55 years or older. All patients were at high cardiovascular risk with established atherosclerotic vascular disease or with diabetes with end-organ damage over 56 months. About 37% of patients in this cohort were diabetics. The primary renal outcome was a composite end point of dialysis, doubling of serum creatinine, and death. This was similar for telmisartan and ramipril, but significantly more frequent with combination therapy than with ramipril alone. Similar results were seen for the secondary renal outcome, defined as dialysis or doubling of serum creatinine, which was increased in the combination therapy. With regard to the highest renal risk group—patients with overt diabetic nephropathy, patients with hypertension and diabetes, and patients with a GFR below 60 mL/min/1.73 m^2—combination therapy had no clear benefit. Only 13.1% of all participants presented with microalbuminuria: 29.7% of those with diabetes, macroalbuminuria was seen in 4% of all participants and in 12.2% of diabetics. The urinary albumin excretion rate increased in the whole patient cohort over study period; however, the increase was lower in patients treated with telmisartan or combination therapy and the risk of developing micro- or macroalbuminuria was lower in the group with combination therapy. Thus, in patients at high cardiovascular risk, the effect of telmisartan on major renal outcomes was similar to ramipril. However, combination therapy of an ACE inhibitor and an ARB was associated with more renal events, although there were contrasting beneficial effects on reduction of proteinuria. To investigate whether low renal function and/or albuminuria is associated with an increased ability to benefit from a dual RAS blockade in patients at high cardiovascular risk, a *post hoc* analysis of ONTARGET was performed [22]. A cohort of 23 422 patients including 37.5% patients with diabetes from the ONTARGET population were analyzed. A total 1287 patients had macroalbuminuria, and 5623 patients had a GFR <60 mL/min/1.73 m^2. A total of 608 patients of those with low GFR were macroalbuminuric. Overall, dual therapy was associated with more primary renal events than monotherapy. No subgroup showed renal benefit with dual RAS blockade, even those with low GFR and macroalbuminuria, and there was a trend for dual therapy to increase chronic dialysis or doubling of serum creatinine in this highest risk group. Dual therapy led to more acute dialysis-dependent renal failure and more hyperkalemia than monotherapy. Discontinuation because of hypotension was more frequent with dual

therapy. So, both analyses do not support dual RAS blocker therapy over monotherapy in high cardiovascular risk patients with low GFR or albuminuria. Similar results were postulated in the Olmesartan reducing Incidence of End-stage Renal Disease in Diabetic Nephropathy Trial (ORIENT) [23]. Combination therapy of an ACE inhibitor and ARB over 3.2 years did not show an additional benefit on the composite end point of doubling serum creatinine, end-stage renal disease, and death in 577 type 2 diabetics with advanced diabetic nephropathy. Blood pressure and proteinuria were reduced by combination therapy compared with placebo. It has to be mentioned that cardiovascular death was more frequent in the olmesartan group, although the study was not powered for cardiovascular outcome.

AVOID and ALTITUDE

In AVOID, 599 hypertensive type 2 diabetics with an estimated GFR of >30 mL/min/1.73 m^2 were treated with 100 mg of losartan for 3 months [24]. Then they were assigned to receive 150 mg of aliskiren for 3 months followed by 300 mg for 3 months versus placebo on top of the ARB. Baseline blood pressure levels were around 135/78 mmHg, and urinary albumin excretion about 500 mg/g creatinine in all groups. There was no significant difference in blood pressure levels at the end of the study between groups. A reduction in albuminuria of 50% or more was seen in 24.7% of patients who received aliskiren, compared with 12.5% of patients who received placebo. The mean rate decline of GFR was not significantly different between both groups. Thus, addition of a direct renin inhibitor has a beneficial effect on proteinuria independent of blood pressure effects and seemed to be safe in type 2 diabetics. However, the ALTITUDE (Aliskiren Trial in Type 2 Diabetes Using Cardiovascular and Renal Disease Endpoints), which tested a combination of aliskiren with an ACE inhibitor or

ARB in a large cohort of diabetics [25], has been stopped due to an increased risk of stroke and renal events. Thus, combination therapy of aliskiren and other RAS blockers is now contraindicated in type 2 diabetics and patients with a GFR <60 mL/min according to an EMA (European Medical Association) announcement from February 2012.

Target blood pressure levels in patients with diabetic nephropathy

Guidelines have suggested a target blood pressure level of less than 130/80 mmHg in patients with diabetes regardless of renal function. However, recently these low blood pressure levels have been questioned.

Previous recommendations were mainly based on findings of the Hypertension Optimal Treatment (HOT) study [26]. This study suggested a significant risk reduction for cardiovascular events in patients achieving a diastolic blood pressure lower than 80 mmHg compared with higher blood pressure levels over a study period of 36 months. A total of 18 790 patients with hypertension and a mean diastolic blood pressure of 105 mmHg were randomly assigned to a target diastolic blood pressure ≤90 mmHg versus ≤85 mmHg versus ≤80 mmHg. The mean age was 61.5 years, and about 8% of patients were diabetics. During follow-up, mean diastolic blood pressure levels were described as 85.2 mmHg versus 83.2 mmHg versus 81.2 mmHg. The lowest incidence of major cardiovascular events, defined as fatal and non-fatal myocardial infarctions, fatal and non-fatal strokes, and all other cardiovascular death, occurred at a mean achieved diastolic blood pressure of 82.6 mmHg and lowest risk of cardiovascular mortality at a diastolic blood pressure level of 86.5 mmHg. The authors described that further reductions below these levels were safe. With regard to the subgroup of diabetics, the risk of major cardiovascular events was halved in the lowest target group (≤80 mmHg) compared with the group with diastolic blood pressure ≤90 mmHg; the risk reduction for stroke was about 30% and cardiovascular mortality was also significantly lower.

Insights from other studies suggested that blood pressure levels less than 130/80 mmHg in diabetic patients may be associated with more adverse events. Therefore, the discussion about the optimal blood pressure target was resumed and the Action to Control Cardiovascular Risk in Diabetes (ACCORD) trial was designed to evaluate the effect of a target blood pressure below 120 mmHg systolic as compared to below 140 mmHg on major cardiovascular events defined as non-fatal myocardial infarction, non-fatal stroke, or death from cardiovascular disease among 4733 high-risk patients with type 2 diabetes [27]. Patients were randomly (non-blinded) assigned to intensive therapy with systolic blood pressure targets of less than 120 mmHg and to standard therapy (<140 mmHg) over a mean study period of 4.7 years. The mean age of patients was 62.2 years and baseline characteristics were similar in both groups. Baseline blood pressure levels were about 139.2/76 mmHg, renal function was near normal with an estimated GFR of 91.6 mL/min/1.73 m^2, and the median urinary albumin excretion rate was 14.3 mg/g creatinine; 33.7% of the patients had cardiovascular disease. Treatment strategies that were currently available were used to lower blood pressure. Despite the fact that the achieved blood pressure levels in the intensive treatment group were definitely lower than the standard treatment group (119.3/64.4 mmHg versus 133.5/70.5 mmHg), the two groups did not differ significantly between the primary composite end point (1.87% versus 2.09% per year) and most of the secondary end points, except that the rate of total stroke and non-fatal stroke was significantly lower in the intensive treatment group. However, the intensive treatment group had a significantly higher rate of adverse events attributed to antihypertensive treatment. The mean estimated GFR was lower, and they had higher rates of hypokalemia and elevations in serum creatinine. The results from ACCORD provide no evidence of a benefit from intensive blood pressure control lower than 120 mmHg systolic in patients at high cardiovascular risk with type 2 diabetes. There is no reduction in major cardiovascular events, and adverse events may be increased with lower blood pressure due to medications.

Also, in ROADMAP it was noted that the small number of cardiovascular deaths occurred in the olmesartan group, possibly related to too low blood pressure levels, especially in patients with coronary artery disease and systolic blood pressure levels lower than 120 mmHg. Comparable results had been noted in *post hoc* analyses of the ONTARGET and INVEST trial [28, 29].

Thus, the actual recommendations for target blood pressure levels were challenged, and retrospective analysis of the HOT trial revealed that diabetic patients in particular had never achieved the assigned low blood pressure levels in the HOT trial. Patients assigned to the group <80 mmHg had achieved only a mean blood pressure of 139.7/81 mmHg. In the UKPDS trial the mean achieved blood pressure was 144/82 mmHg, which showed a reduction in micro- and macrovascular events. These trials demonstrated that there is a beneficial effect for patients with lower blood pressure levels, but the achieved levels were about 130–139/80–85 mmHg, and there was no evidence for a benefit of blood pressure lowering less than 130/80 mmHg.

With regards to the above-mentioned new insights, most guidelines were updated recently; the update of the seventh report of the Joint National Committee on Prevention, Evaluation and Treatment of High Blood Pressure (JNC-7) is expected. Currently, the committee recommends that blood pressure in diabetics should be controlled to levels of 130/80 mmHg or lower and treatment with an ACE inhibitor or ARB should be preferred [30]. The National Institute for Health and Clinical Excellence (NICE) presented their last update for treatment recommendations in diabetic patients in 2009 and approved a blood pressure level of <140/80 mmHg [31]. If there is kidney, eye, or cerebrovascular damage, blood pressure should be lower than 130/80 mmHg. The reappraisal of the guidelines of the European Society of Hypertension was published in 2009 [32]. They advise that blood pressure in patients with diabetes should be lower than 140/90 mmHg (~130–139/80–85 mmHg), particularly in patients with microalbuminuria; however, they no longer support the previously recommended blood pressure goal of <130/80 mmHg in diabetic patients because of the lack of evidence from large controlled trials. German guidelines from the DHL (Deutsche Hochdruckliga) were updated in 2011, and they also recommend a blood pressure goal of 130–140/80–85 mmHg in patients with diabetes. In addition to this, they suggest a blood pressure goal of <130/80 mmHg in diabetic patients with chronic kidney disease, which should be lowered to ≤125/75 mmHg if proteinuria of 1 g/day or more is present [33]. All the above-mentioned guidelines recommend a preferential antihypertensive treatment with an ACE inhibitor or ARB, especially in patients with microalbuminuria. The guideline for hypertension in chronic kidney disease of the committee of KDIGO (Kidney Disease: improving Global Outcomes) is under development; however, actual blood pressure targets were presented to the meeting of the American Society of Nephrology 2012. They recommend that patients with diabetes and chronic kidney disease with a urine albumin excretion (UAE) lower than 30 mg/24 hours (or equivalent) and office blood pressure levels >140 mmHg systolic or >90 mmHg diastolic should be treated with antihypertensives to maintain a blood

Table 15.1 Current guideline recommendations for blood pressure targets in diabetic patients

	JNC-7 (2003)	NICE (2009)	ESH (2009)	DHL (2011)	KDIGO (2012)
Target blood pressure level in diabetic patients (mmHg)	≤130/80	<140/80	<140/90	≤140/90	≤140/90
with microalbuminuria/ CKD	n.d.	<130/80	n.d.	≤130/80	≤130/80
with macroalbuminuria or proteinuria >1 g	n.d.	n.d.	n.d.	≤125/75	≤130/80
ACE inhibitor or ARB as first line therapy	+	+	+	+	+

JNC-7, Seventh Report of the Joint National Committee on Prevention, Evaluation and Treatment of High Blood Pressure; NICE, National Institute for Health and Clinical Excellence; ESH, European society of hypertension; DHL, Deutsche Hochdruckliga; KDIGO, Kidney Disease: improving Global Outcomes; CKD: chronic kidney disease; ACE inhibitor, angiotensin-converting enzyme inhibitor; ARB, angiotensin-receptor blocker; n.d.: not defined.

pressure consistently ≤140 mmHg systolic and ≤90 mmHg diastolic. Diabetic patients with a UAE >30 mg/day and office blood pressure levels >130/80 mmHg should be treated with blood pressure-lowering drugs to maintain a blood pressure consistently ≤130 mmHg systolic and ≤80 mmHg diastolic. They recommend an ARB or ACE inhibitor as first-line therapy in those patients with a UAE of 30–300 mg/day irrespective of blood pressure and in those patients with a UAE of >300 mg in whom treatment with antihypertensives is indicated. A summary of the current guideline recommendations for blood pressure targets in diabetic patients is also shown in Table 15.1.

References

1. U S Renal Data System (2011) USRDS 2011 Annual data report: atlas of chronic kidney disease and end-stage renal disease in the United States. Bethesda, MD: National Institutes of Health.
2. Ruggenenti P, Fassi A, Ilieva A, et al. Preventing microalbuminuria in type 2 diabetes. N Engl J Med 2004;351: 1941–51.
3. Haller H, Ito S, Izzo J Jr, et al. Olmesartan for the Delay or prevention of microalbuminuria in type 2 diabetes. N Engl J Med 2011; 364:907–17
4. Bilous R, Chaturvedi N, Sjølie A, et al. Effect of candesartan on microalbuminuria and albumin excretion rate in diabetes. Ann Intern Med 2009; 151:11–20
5. Mauer M, Zinman B, Gardiner R, et al. Renal and retinal effects of enalapril and losartan in type 1 diabetes. N Engl J Med 2009;361:40–51.
6. Ruggenenti P, Perna A, Ganeva M, et al. for the BENEDICT Study Group. impact of blood pressure control and angiotensin-converting enzyme inhibitor therapy on new-onset microalbuminuria in type 2 diabetes: a post hoc analysis of the BENEDICT trial. J Am Soc Nephrol 2006;17:3472–81.
7. Schrier RW, Estacio RO, Esler A, et al. Effects of aggressive blood pressure control in normotensive type 2 diabetic patients on albuminuria, retinopathy and strokes. Kidney Int 2002;61: 1086–97.

8. Lewis E, Hunsicker L, Bain R, *et al*. The effect of angiotensin-converting-enzyme inhibition on diabetic nephropathy. *N Engl J Med* 1993;**329**:1456–62.

9. Viberti G, Mogensen CE, Groop LC, *et al*. Effect of captopril on progression to clinical proteinuria in patients with insulin-dependent diabetes mellitus and microalbuminuria. European Microalbuminuria Captopril Study Group. *JAMA* 1994;**271**:275–79.

10. Lewis E, Hunsicker L, Clarke W, *et al*. Renoprotective effect of the angiotensin-receptor antagonist irbesartan in patients with nephropathy due to type 2 diabetes *N Engl J Med* 2001;**345**:851–60.

11. Brenner B, Cooper M, de Zeeuw D. Effects of losartan on renal and cardiovascular outcomes in patients with type 2 diabetes and nephropathy. *N Engl J Med* 2001;**345**:861–9.

12. Keane WF, Brenner BM, de Zeeuw D, *et al*. The risk of developing end-stage renal disease in patients with type 2 diabetes and nephropathy: the RENAAL study. *Kidney Int* 2003;**63**:1499–1507.

13. de Zeeuw D, Remuzzi G, Parving H-H, *et al*. Proteinuria, a target for renoprotection in patients with type 2 diabetic nephropathy: lessons from RENAAL. *Kidney Int* 2004;**65**:2309–20.

14. Parving H, Lehnert H., *et al*. The effect of irbesartan on the development of diabetic nephropathy in patients with type 2 diabetes. *N Engl J Med* 2001;**345**:870–8.

15. Evans M, Bain S, Hogan S, *et al*. Irbesartan delays progression of nephropathy as measured by estimated glomerular filtration rate: post hoc analysis of the Irbesartan Diabetic Nephropathy Trial. *Nephrol Dial Transplant* **201**;0:1–9.

16. Holtkamp F, de Zeeuw D, Thomas M *et al*. An acute fall in estimated glomerular filtration rate during treatment with losartan predicts a slower decrease in long-term renal function. *Kidney Int* 2011;**80**:282–87.

17. Viberti G, Wheeldon NM for the MicroAlbuminuria Reduction With VALsartan (MARVAL) Study Investigators. Microalbuminuria reduction with valsartan in patients with type 2 diabetes mellitus: a blood pressure-independent effect. *Circulation* 2002;**106**:672–78.

18. Barnett A, Bain S, Bouter P, *et al*. Angiotensin-receptor blockade versus converting–enzyme inhibition in type 2 diabetes and nephropathy. *N Engl J Med* 2004;**351**:1952–61.

19. Patel A for the ADVANCE Collaborative Group. Effects of a fixed combination of perindopril and indapamide on macrovascular and microvascular outcomes in patients with type 2 diabetes mellitus (the ADVANCE trial): a randomised controlled trial. *Lancet* 2007; **370**:829–40.

20. UK Prospective Diabetes Study Group. Tight blood pressure control and risk of macrovascular and microvascular complications in type 2 diabetes: UKPDS 38. *BMJ* 1998;**317**:703–13.

21. Mann JFE, Schmieder RE, McQueen M, *et al*. Renal outcomes with telmisartan, ramipril, or both, in people at high vascular risk (the ONTARGET study): a multicentre, randomised, double-blind, controlled trial. *Lancet* 2008;**372**: 547–53.

22. Tobe SW, Clase CM, Gao P, *et al*. Cardiovascular and renal outcomes with telmisartan, ramipril, or both in people at high renal risk: results from the ONTARGET and TRANSCEND studies. *Circulation* 2011;**123**:1098–107.

23. Imai E, Chan JCN, Ito s, *et al*. Effects of olmesartan on renal and cardiovascular outcomes in type 2 diabetes with overt nephropathy: a multicenter, randomized,

placebo-controlled study. *Diabetologia* 2011;**54**:2978–86.

24. Parving H-H, Persson F, Lewis JB, *et al.* for the AVOID Study Investigators. Aliskiren combined with losartan in type 2 diabetes and nephropathy. *N Engl J Med* 2008;**358**:2433–46.

25. Parving H-H, Brenner BM, McMurray JJ, *et al.* Baseline characteristics in the Aliskiren Trial in Type 2 Diabetes Using Cardio-Renal Endpoints (ALTITUDE). *J Renin Angiotensin Aldosterone Syst* 2012 (http://jra.sagepub.com/content/early/ 2012/02/14/1470320311434818).

26. Hansson L, Zanchetti A, Carruthers S, *et al.* Effects of intensive blood-pressure lowering and low-dose aspirin in patients with hypertension: principal results of the Hypertension Optimal Treatment (HOT) randomised trial. *Lancet* 1998;**351**:1755–62

27. Cushman WC, Evans GW, Byington RP, *et al.* Effects of Intensive Blood-Pressure Control in Type 2 Diabetes Mellitus. *N Engl J Med* 2010;**362**:1575–85.

28. Redon J, Mancia G, Sleight P, *et al.* Safety and efficacy of low blood pressures among patients with diabetes: subgroup analyses from the ONTARGET (ONgoing Telmisartan Alone and in combination with Ramipril Global Endpoint Trial). *J Am Coll Cardiol* 2012;**59**:74–83.

29. Cooper-DeHoff R, Gong Y. Tight Blood Pressure Control and Cardiovascular Outcomes Among Hypertensive Patients With Diabetes and Coronary Artery Disease. *JAMA* 2010,**304**:61–68.

30. Chobanian AV, Bakris GL, Black HR, *et al.* Seventh report of the Joint National Committee on Prevention, Detection, Evaluation, and Treatment of High Blood Pressure. *Hypertension* 2003;**42**:1206–52.

31. NICE. CG87 Type 2 diabetes—newer agents (a partial update of CG66): NICE guideline. (http://guidance.nice.org.uk/ CG87/NICEGuidance/pdf/English).

32. Mancia G, Laurent S, Agabiti-Rosei E, *et al.* Reappraisal of European guidelines on hypertension management: a European Society of Hypertension Task Force document. *J Hypertens* 2009;**27**: 2121–58.

33. Aktuelle Leitlinien zur Behandlung der arteriellen Hypertonie. (http:// www.hochdruckliga.de/bluthochdruck- behandlung-leitlinien.html).

Treatment of the patient with end-stage diabetic nephropathy

Muriel Ghosn and Fuad N. Ziyadeh

American University of Beirut, Beirut, Lebanon

Key points

- The multiple comorbidities associated with end-stage diabetic nephropathy (ESDN) (including anemia, bone disorders, hyperglycemia, dyslipidemia, hypertension and cardiovascular disease) require a detailed understanding of the pathophysiologic mechanisms of each condition and a systematic treatment approach that takes into account the prevailing diabetic state, the presence of kidney failure, and the renal replacement modality.
- One of the most important steps in the management of ESDN is the recognition that cardiovascular disease is the leading cause of morbidity and mortality and that major attention should be directed to preventing and treating coronary artery disease (CAD) in this high-risk population.
- The choice of the optimal renal replacement modality for the patient with ESDN includes considerations of the advantages and disadvantages of peritoneal dialysis and hemodialysis as well as whether kidney transplantation is feasible or is the preferred alternative.

The National Kidney Foundation (NKF) defines anemia in chronic kidney disease (CKD) as a hemoglobin level $<13.5\,g/dL$ in men and $<12.0\,g/dL$ in women. The incidence of anemia increases as the glomerular filtration rate (GFR) declines, and is estimated at 40% in CKD stage 3, and progressively increases to reach more than 70% in stage 5. Recent data clearly indicate that in the subset of diabetic patients, anemia is more frequent, occurs at earlier stages of CKD, and is often more severe [1]. The reasons for this increased frequency and severity of anemia in diabetes are not obvious.

Diabetes and Kidney Disease, First Edition. Edited by Gunter Wolf.
© 2013 John Wiley & Sons, Ltd. Published 2013 by John Wiley & Sons, Ltd.

Anemia in diabetic patients with CKD shares the same pathogenesis as in non-diabetic patients. Some of the important contributory factors are discussed below.

Erythropoietin deficiency and hyporesponsiveness

In CKD, erythropoietin (EPO) production by the renal cortical interstitial cells is reduced. Moreover, virtually all patients with end-stage renal disease (ESRD) suffer from hyporesponsiveness to EPO, attributed mostly to the state of systemic inflammation induced by the uremic environment, and is defined by the requirement of high doses of erythropoiesis-stimulating agents (ESAs) to achieve the target level of hemoglobin in the absence of iron deficiency.

Iron deficiency

Iron deficiency is a common problem in patients with CKD, whether they are on hemodialyis or not, and if not corrected is a major cause of hyporesponsiveness to ESAs. Absolute iron deficiency in CKD patients is defined by serum ferritin level <100 ng/mL or a transferrin saturation of <20%. Usual causes are reduced dietary iron intake, impaired intestinal iron absorption, and gastrointestinal bleeding as a consequence of stress-induced ulcerations of the gastric or small intestinal mucosa.

Anemia of chronic disease

Acute and chronic inflammatory conditions can lead to anemia of chronic disease, which is defined by a ferritin level >100 ng/mL along with reduced iron saturation. High levels of inflammatory cytokines such as interleukin-6 stimulate the production of hepcidin by the liver. Hepcidin, in turn, inhibits intestinal iron absorption and impairs its transport from the reticuloendothelial system to bone marrow, leading to iron sequestration and relative iron deficiency.

Decreased survival of red blood cells

This mechanism is largely specific to diabetic patients and is thought to be due to increased osmotic stress as a result of accumulation of sorbitol. Another proposed hypothesis is the abnormal composition of the red blood cell membrane, which increases the risk of trapping and sequestration of these cells in the microcirculation of the reticuloendothelial system.

Miscellaneous factors contributing to anemia

Several conditions in the diabetic patient with CKD may contribute to anemia, including (1) severe hyperparathyroidism with consequent bone marrow fibrosis; (2) sporadic aluminum toxicity; (3) folate and vitamin B12 deficiency; and (4) drugs that intercept the renin–angiotensin system. Angiotensin-converting enzyme (ACE) inhibitors and angiotensin receptor blockers cause a reversible decrease in hemoglobin concentration attributed to a direct blockade of the proerythropoietic effects of angiotensin II on red blood cell precursors, among other mechanisms. Attention directed at these miscellaneous factors will be important in treating or reversing anemia.

In diabetic patients with CKD, anemia has been associated with cognitive and sexual dysfunction as well as with a decline in exercise capacity. There is some evidence that anemia may also contribute to the progression of kidney disease. Most importantly, it is established as a major cardiovascular risk factor in patients with various stages of CKD, especially those suffering from diabetes and including those on maintenance dialysis [2–4]. Consequently, treatment of anemia with ESAs was proposed to reduce excessive cardiovascular morbidity and mortality. Early trials showed that anemia treatment decreased mortality and hospitalization rates [5] along with an improvement in quality of life and a reduction in transfusion rates [6]. However, such data, largely derived from observational studies and small interventional trials, were challenged by large randomized controlled trials (RCTs) that tested the impact of anemia correction on mortality and cardiovascular and renal outcomes. These trials (Table 16.1) also showed a significant improvement in the quality of life and a reduction in the transfusion rates with complete correction of anemia. However, a trend toward worse cardiac and cerebrovascular outcomes was observed. In an attempt to explain these findings, it has been hypothesized that it is the exposure to high doses of ESAs rather than the higher hemoglobin (Hb) or hematocrit (Hct) levels achieved that could be the direct cause of worse outcomes [7]. Currently, there are no specific recommendations for the management of anemia in patients with ESDN on maintenance dialysis, and such patients are treated in clinical practice according to the general guidelines issued on the overall ESRD patient population.

Recommendations for anemia treatment

Target Hb level

Considerable controversy has surrounded the target Hb level, and it was initially suggested that the higher the level the better the outcomes. However, after the Normal Hematocrit study conducted in 1998 showed worse outcomes with higher hematocrit levels, the 2001 version of the NKF-K/DOQI anemia guidelines

recommended a target Hb of 11–12 g/dL in ESA-treated anemic patients with CKD. The 2006 update of the same guidelines changed the target levels to 11–13 g/dL. In 2007, based on the results of the CHOIR and CREATE trials, the FDA changed the package insert for epoetin and darbepoetin to state that the physician should "individualize dosing to achieve and maintain hemoglobin levels within the range of 10 to 12 g/dL" in all patients with CKD, and the NKF-K/DOQI anemia workgroup recommended that the Hb target should be 11.0–12.0 g/dL (moderately strong evidence) and that the Hb target should not exceed 13 g/dL in all CKD patients [8].

Iron therapy

The 2006 NKF-K/DOQI anemia guidelines state that (1) iron status tests should be performed every month during initial ESA treatment and then every 3 months during stable ESA treatment; (2) serum ferritin levels should be kept >200 ng/mL for hemodialysis patients and >100 ng/mL for non-hemodialysis patients receiving ESAs; (3) serum transferrin saturation with iron should be kept >20 % in patients receiving ESAs with or without hemodialysis; (4) the preferred route of administration of iron is intravenously in patients with CKD on hemodialysis (strong recommendation); and (5) the route of iron administration can be either oral or intravenously in CKD patients not on hemodialysis.

Adverse effects of anemia therapy

Some of the side effects of ESAs include hypertension, local pain or tissue reaction to subcutaneous injections, flu-like symptoms within hours or days of the administration of an ESA, and arterial and venous thromboembolic events. ESAs have also been associated with a rare but serious from of pure red cell aplasia. In the TREAT trial, in the subgroup of patients with malignant conditions, darbepoetin-alfa

Table 16.1 Randomized controlled trials of anemia treatment with erythropoiesis-stimulating agents (ESAs) in patients with chronic kidney disease including diabetic patients

	N	Diabetes (%)	Study design	CKD stage	Hb target	Follow-up (months)	Primary outcome	Results	Secondary outcome	Results
NHS (1998)	1233 All CAD	54–58	Open label	Hemodialysis	30 vs 42 (Hct)	29	Death or non-fatal myocardial infarct	Worse in high Hct arm		
CHOIR (2006)	1432	47–51	Open label	3–4	11.3 vs 13.5	16	Death and cardiovascular events	Worse in high Hb arm	Need for renal replacement therapy	No difference
CREATE (2006)	603	77–80	Open label	3–4	10.5–11.5 vs 13–15	36	Death and cardiovascular events	No difference	1. Progression of CKD 2. Change in left ventricular mass index	No difference
ACORD (2007)	176	100	Open label	1–3	13–15 vs 10.5–11.5	18	Left ventricular hypertrophy	No difference	Renal function	No difference
TREAT (2009)	4038	100	RCT	3–4	9 vs 13	29	1. Death and cardiovascular events 2. Death and ESRD	No difference		

was associated with a higher incidence of cancer-related deaths. Oral iron use can give rise to adverse gastrointestinal side effects. Serious but very rare anaphylactic reactions occur with the intravenous preparations especially iron dextran.

Diabetic patients are at a higher risk of developing metabolic bone disease than non-diabetic subjects [9] and this is further enhanced by the coexistence of CKD, which is also typically associated with bone and mineral metabolism disorders (BMDs) [10].

Pathogenesis of BMD in diabetes and CKD

Renal osteodystrophy has been historically attributed to secondary hyperparathyroidism. However, it appears that in diabetic patients on maintenance hemodialysis, low-turnover bone disorders including adynamic bone disease (and rarely aluminum toxicity) predominate while osteitis fibrosa cystica is distinctly uncommon. It has been hypothesized that insulin is a cofactor for parathyroid hormone (PTH) secretion and bone turnover; consequently, low-turnover bone diseases may reflect either insulin lack and/or resistance within the parathyroid glands and bone [11]. Thiazolidinediones use, in particular, can contribute to bone loss in diabetic patients with or without CKD [12].

25-Hydroxyvitamin D deficiency has recently emerged as an important contributor to BMD in patients with CKD. The prevalence of vitamin D deficiency is significantly higher in CKD patients than the general population, particularly in the subgroup of non-dialysis-dependent patients with diabetic nephropathy [13]. However, and as relates to vascular calci-

fication, no significant relationship could be demonstrated between vitamin D levels on one hand and coronary artery calcification on the other hand [13]. Nonetheless, the frequent 25-hydroxoyvitamin D deficiency in patients with CKD is multifactorial and can be attributed to the following [14]: (1) reduced exposure to sunlight; (2) reduced endogenous synthesis of vitamin D3 in the skin following adequate exposure to sunlight; (3) reduced ingestion of foods that are natural sources of vitamin D; and (4) urinary losses of 25-hydroxyvitamin D and vitamin D-binding protein in CKD patients with nephrotic-range proteinuria.

Of considerable interest, a vitamin D receptor activator, paricalcitol, has recently been shown to reduce the magnitude of albuminuria in the CKD population in general [15] and in diabetic patients in particular [16], suggesting a potential renoprotective benefit of vitamin D supplementation in patients with CKD which is beyond the indications for BMD management.

Treatment of BMD in diabetic patients with CKD

To date, specific guidelines for the management of BMD in ESDN are lacking and such patients continue to be treated according to the general recommendations issued for all CKD patients including ESRD. However, particular care should be taken to avoid excessive PTH suppression and the consequent risk of low-turnover bone diseases. Adynamic bone disease in stage 5 CKD should be treated by allowing plasma levels of PTH to rise in order to increase bone turnover (opinion) and this can be accomplished by decreasing doses of calcium-based phosphate binders and vitamin D or eliminating such therapy (opinion) [14]. The general recommendations [14] state that hyperphosphatemia should be corrected and the target serum phosphorus level should be

<4.6 mg/dL in patients with CKD stage 3 and 4 (opinion) and <5.5 mg/dL in patients with CKD stage 5 and in those on dialysis (evidence). The serum calcium–phosphorus product should be maintained at <55 mg^2/dL^2 (evidence). Calcium-based phosphate binders should not be used in cases of hypercalcemia (corrected calcium >10.2 mg/dL), or when PTH <150 pg/mL (evidence). Non-calcium-containing phosphate binders are preferred in dialysis patients with severe vascular and/or other soft-tissue calcifications (opinion). In cases of vitamin D deficiency, current recommendations are to supplement with vitamin D if the serum level of 25-hydroxyvitamin D is <30 ng/mL in patients with CKD stage 3 and 4 (opinion). In patients with CKD stage 5 and those on dialysis, and irrespective of whether there is vitamin D deficiency, active vitamin D (calcitriol or analogues) should be provided if PTH level >300 pg/mL (opinion). Serum levels of total CO_2 should be maintained at >22 mEq/L (evidence) since acidosis is a major contributor to bone loss.

Glycemic control in diabetic patients with ESRD

It is well established that the treatment of diabetes in the general population and in patients with early stages of CKD not only delays the development of diabetic nephropathy or slows its progression but is also associated with a reduction in mortality and cardiovascular events. Unfortunately, data are scarce on how diabetes should best be treated in patients with ESDN and whether such treatment is beneficial.

Glycemia in the diabetic end-stage renal disease patient

In dialysis patients the serum glucose levels fluctuate widely with a tendency to both hyper- and hypoglycemia. Also, ESRD signifi-

cantly affects the excretion of many hypoglycemic agents and the level of glycosylated hemoglobin (HbA1c), making the management of diabetic dialysis patients particularly challenging. Impaired glucose tolerance is due to many factors in the ESDN patient [17], including (1) insulin resistance, which can be attributed to many disorders such as the accumulation of unidentified uremic toxins, anemia, malnutrition, and metabolic acidosis; (2) impaired insulin secretion due to 1,25-dihydroxyvitamin D deficiency and/or hyperparathyroidism; and (3) glucose loading from dialysis solution, particularly in patients on peritoneal dialysis. On the other hand, hypoglycemic events are common in diabetic patients with ESRD and carry a poor prognostic implication; they are due to the combination of malnutrition, impaired insulin clearance, defective renal gluconeogenesis, counter-regulatory hormone deficiency, and concomitant administration of hypoglycemic agents.

Diagnostic tools of glycemic control in ESRD

Shortened red blood cell life span and the common use of ESAs in ESRD patients may cause falsely low HbA1c levels whereas high concentrations of carbamylated hemoglobin may cause false elevations of these levels. Thus, HbA1c levels might under- or overestimate the degree of long-term glycemic control in the dialysis population. Alternate markers have been proposed, specifically glycated albumin, which has been shown not only to better correlate with plasma glucose concentration in dialysis patients than HbA1c [18, 19] but also to be a significant predictor of cardiovascular morbidity and mortality [20, 21]. However, assays of glycated albumin are not readily available and can be affected by conditions that alter protein metabolism. Nevertheless, and despite its limitations, HbA1c is considered a reasonable marker of glycemic control in diabetic patients with ESRD [22] and is still widely used in clinical practice.

Hypoglycemic agents in ESRD

The main oral hypoglycemic agents that can be used in dialysis patients are the dipeptidyl peptidase-4 inhibitors, with appropriate dose reduction, and the sulfonylurea glypizide. Insulin is an alternative option: preferably a combination of basal insulin and rapid acting insulin analogues with adjustment of the doses based on glucose patterns.

Most oral hypoglycemic agents are contraindicated in ESRD patients [23]: (1) the biguanides pose a significant risk of lactic acidosis; (2) the sulfonylureas (with the exception of glypizide, which is metabolized mainly by the liver) are subject to extensive renal excretion and pose a significant risk of hypoglycemia; (3)

this is also applicable to the meglitinides; (4) the thiazolidinediones have a risk of fluid overload, precipitation of heart failure, and increased cardiovascular risk; (5) GLP-1 analogues undergo extensive renal excretion and can cause hypoglycemia; and (6) the alpha-glucosidase inhibitors have limited data on their use in ESRD.

Impact of glycemic control on outcomes

Glycemic control has been consistently associated with a beneficial impact on outcomes in diabetic patients, including those with early stage CKD. However, such data in ESRD patients are limited largely because of small and observational studies, which generally show that poor glycemic control is associated with higher morbidity (Table 16.2). However,

Table 16.2 Observations on the impact of glycemic control on morbidity and mortality in hemodialysis patients

Authors and year of publication	Type of study	Number and type of patients	Results
Wu et al, 1997	Retrospective observational	137 Hemodialysis	Increase in mortality and cardiovascular morbidity with poor glycemic control
Morioka et al, 2001	Prospective observational	150 hemodialysis	Better survival with good glycemic control (HbA1c <7.5%)
Oomichi et al, 2006	Prospective observational	114 hemodialysis	Decrease in mortality with lower HbA1c levels
Williams et al, 2006	Observational	24,875 hemodialysis	No correlation between HbA1c and mortality at 12 months
Kalantar-Zadeh et al. 2007	Observational	26,187 hemodialysis	Decrease in mortality with lower HgbA1c levels
Tsujimoto et al, 2009	Prospective observational	134 hemodialysis	Decrease in cardiovascular events with good glycemic control (HbA1c <7%)
Ishimura et al, 2009	Observational	122 hemodialysis	Decrease in mortality with good glycemic control (HbA1c <6.3%)
Drechsler et al, 2010	Observational	1255 hemodialysis	Poor glycemic control (HbA1c >8%) increases the risk of sudden cardiac death when compared with good glycemic control (HbA1c <6%)

taking into account their inherent design limitations, proper conclusions cannot be drawn regarding the ideal blood glucose level. Moreover, a recent observational study conducted by Miklos Molnar and his team on 54 757 diabetic patients treated with dialysis found a link between high death rates and HbA1c levels of 8% or greater [24]. Sylvia Paz Ramirez and her colleagues recently analyzed data on 8437 dialysis patients from 12 countries who had diabetes and showed that the lowest risk of death occurred when HbA1c levels were between 7% and 8% (Paz *et al.*, unpublished, 2011). Thus, while ESDN patients are treated in clinical practice according to the guidelines established for patients with normal kidney function (target HbA1c between 6% and 7%, a fasting blood glucose level <140 mg/dL, and a postprandial glucose level <200 mg/dL (level of evidence C) [25], a revision of these guidelines is needed to highlight the importance of avoiding strict glycemic control in this patient population and maybe set a new target HbA1c level between 7% and 8%.

Hypertension in diabetic patients with end-stage renal disease

Poorly controlled hypertension is a major cardiovascular risk factor in the general population and in patients with CKD. The prevalence of hypertension exceeds 50% in hemodialysis patients, and such patients do not manifest the normal nocturnal decline of blood pressure (BP) that occurs in healthy individuals, thereby predisposing them to the development of left ventricular hypertrophy, which is a strong predictor of cardiovascular disease [26]. A meta-analysis of eight randomized controlled trials showed that BP control in dialysis patients is associated with a reduction in the incidence of cardiovascular events and mortality [27].

Assessment of hypertension in ESRD patients

Unlike the general population, there are no uniform guidelines addressing evaluation of BP in patients with ESRD, particularly in the diabetic population. To date, there is no agreement concerning the optimal method and time for BP measurement. When daily home BP monitoring was compared with the 44-hour interdialytic ambulatory BP readings in chronic hemodialysis patients, an excellent correlation was found between average systolic and diastolic ambulatory BP and respective home BP readings. Moreover, prehemodialysis diastolic, but not systolic, BP was a good reflection of diastolic ambulatory BP [28]. Home BP monitoring is therefore suggested as a cost-effective way to diagnose hypertension in hemodialysis patients.

Although the optimal BP range has been determined in the general population and in patients with either diabetes or CKD, there is no consensus concerning target BP levels in hemodialysis patients whether diabetic or not. Besides, a U-curve relationship between cardiovascular mortality and BP has been shown in these patients [29]. Despite the controversial data, the NKF-K/DOQI clinical practice guidelines in dialysis patients set the predialysis and postdialysis BP goals as <140/90 mm Hg and <130/80 mmHg, respectively (level of evidence C) [25].

Mechanisms of hypertension in ESRD patients

The development of hypertension in ESRD patients has been attributed to many risk factors that also apply to the diabetic subgroups, and these include (1) extracellular fluid expansion; (2) derangements of the renin–angiotensin system; (3) Sympathetic overactivity; (4) impaired vasodilatation; (5) secondary hyperparathyroidism; and (6) use of ESAs for anemia correction.

Management of hypertension in ESRD patients

Recommendations issued for ESRD patients in general can likely be applied to the subgroup of diabetic ESRD patients [25]. In all dialysis patients, management of fluid status and adjustment of antihypertensive medications are the mainstay of hypertension therapy. Importantly, adequate BP control requires dietary sodium restriction [30] and achievement of dry weight through adequate dialysis [31]. Increased ultrafiltration, longer or more frequent dialysis and drugs that reduce salt appetite are recommended (level of evidence B). Antihypertensive medications can be used if dialysis fails to ensure adequate salt and volume removal [32]. The most commonly used agents are calcium channel blockers, beta-blockers, and inhibitors of the renin–angiotensin system. The last ones are preferred according to guidelines (level of evidence C) [25] because they reduce left ventricular hypertrophy and cardiovascular risk [33, 34]. However, since their use poses an increased risk of hyperkalemia, serum potassium should be closely monitored [35]. Beta-blockers are the preferred agents in ESRD patients with dilated cardiomyopathy, in whom they improve clinical status and left ventricular function and, most importantly, reduce mortality [36]. Calcium channel blockers do not reduce left ventricular hypertrophy but they provide significant BP lowering [37]. Antihypertensive drugs should be given preferentially at night, because they may reduce the nocturnal surge in BP and minimize intradialytic hypotension, which may occur when drugs are taken the morning before a dialysis session (level of evidence C). In patients with difficult-to-control hypertension, the dialyzability of antihypertensive medications should be considered (level of evidence C).

Dyslipdemia is considered as one of the major cardiovascular risk factors in patients with diabetes and CKD. Also the pattern of dyslipidemia in diabetic patients is similar to that commonly seen in patients with CKD, with high triglyceride levels, low high-density lipoprotein cholesterol (HDL-C) levels, and average low-density lipoprotein cholesterol (LDL-C) levels [38]. Furthermore, there is a shift in the LDL particle size to the more atherogenic small, dense LDL particles in patients with type 2 diabetes [39].

Therapy of dyslipidemia in diabetic ESRD patients

Although the use of statins in various populations was associated with substantial cardiovascular benefit, there are limited trials investigating their effect in diabetic patients with ESRD. Improvement in survival has been suggested in observational studies that addressed statin use among ESRD patients [40]. To date, two major randomized controlled trials have studied the effect of such therapy in hemodialysis patients: the 4D study used atorvastatin and showed a significant relative reduction of 18 % in all cardiac events, but counterbalanced by an increased incidence of fatal ischemic stroke, and no difference in all-cause and cardiovascular mortality [41]. The AURORA study that used rosuvastatin in dialysis patients confirmed no benefit on major cardiovascular events or death [42]. However, a subgroup analysis of diabetic patients revealed a significant relative reduction of 32% in all cardiac events [43].

The SHARP trial recently assessed the use of a combination of simvastatin and ezetimibe in CKD patients, including individuals on hemodialysis. The combination pill significantly reduced the rate of non-hemorrhagic stroke and arterial revascularization procedures without any difference in the rate of myocardial infarction. Subgroup analysis showed similar results among dialysis and non-dialysis patients [44] and further *post hoc* analysis in diabetic patients on dialysis will be needed before generalization of the results to this patient population.

Based on the limited available data, the NKF-K/DOQI guidelines for the treatment of dyslipidemia in diabetic patients with CKD recommend the following [45]: (1) target LDL-C in people with diabetes and CKD stages 1–4 should be <100 mg/dL; a level <70 mg/dL is a therapeutic option (level of evidence B); and (2) treatment with a statin should not be initiated in patients with type 2 diabetes on maintenance hemodialysis who do not have a specific cardiovascular indication for treatment (level of evidence A).

Cardiovascular disease in diabetic patients with ESRD

Diabetic patients with CKD are at a much higher risk of cardiovascular morbidity and mortality than any other at-risk population [46]. One of the discrete subtypes of the so-called "cardiorenal syndrome" encompasses how diabetes can affect both the renal and cardiovascular systems. Hence, proper identification and prevention of cardiovascular events in diabetic patients with CKD is critically important [47].

Cardiovascular risk factors

Traditional predictors of poor cardiovascular outcomes such as poor glycemic control, hypertension, dyslipidemia, and smoking are also aggravated by some others unique to the ESRD population; these include anemia, disorders in phosphate metabolism and vascular calcification, hyperparathyroidism, and intra-

dialytic hypotension [48], in addition to non-conventional risk factors such as endothelial dysfunction, oxidative stress, and the microinflammatory state of the uremic environment.

Evaluation of cardiovascular disease in ESRD

According to the NKF-K/DOQI guidelines [25], all dialysis patients, regardless of symptoms, require assessment for cardiovascular disease and screening for both traditional and non-traditional risk factors (level of evidence C), including a baseline electrocardiogram (ECG) (level of evidence C) and echocardiogram (level of evidence A). Further evaluation by exercise or pharmacological stress echocardiographic or nuclear imaging tests should be reserved for patients who are either candidates for kidney transplantation or have a history of CAD. Thus, universal CAD evaluation with stress imaging is currently not recommended for all dialysis patients (level of evidence C). Among these tests, exercise-ECG is usually not advised because of poor exercise tolerance and high incidence of left ventricular hypertrophy in this population. Both thallium scintigraphy and dobutamine stress echocardiography can be used, as they help stratify cardiac risk among diabetic and non-diabetic ESRD patients [49].

Aspirin use in ESRD

It has been hypothesized that aspirin can be useful as part of the primary prevention strategy in ESRD patients. However, there are no RCTs in this area. Data from the cohort studies DOPPS I and II showed that the use of aspirin in hemodialysis patients was associated with a higher risk of cardiac events and lower risk of cerebrovascular events without an increase in the hemorrhagic risk [50]. A subgroup analysis of the Hypertension Optimal Treatment trial investigated the use of aspirin in various stages of CKD and revealed a greater reduction in mortality and major cardiovascular events in patients with worse kidney function; the benefits appeared to outweigh bleeding risks [51]. As regards the subgroup of diabetic patients with ESRD, trials addressing the use of aspirin are lacking. Given the available limited and controversial data, the NKF-K/DOQI guidelines did not issue any specific recommendation regarding the use of aspirin but stated that "it may be useful for primary prevention of atherosclerotic disease in dialysis patients, with careful monitoring for bleeding complications," without addressing the subgroup of diabetic patients.

Management of acute coronary syndromes (ACS) in ESRD

Dialysis patients have a higher mortality rate after acute myocardial infarction and they receive less optimal treatment than patients with normal kidney function [52]. There are no RCTs investigating the medical management of ACS in either diabetic or non-diabetic patients with ESRD, but observational studies showed that the use of aspirin and beta-blockers is generally protective in ESRD [53]. Thus, in the absence of strong evidence, the NKF-K/DOQI guidelines on the evaluation and management of cardiovascular disease in dialysis patients issued the following recommendations with a level of evidence C [25]: (1) all dialysis patients presenting with ACS should be treated as in the non-dialysis population, with the exception of specific attention to drugs that have altered clearances in kidney failure (e.g., low molecular weight heparin); and (2) dialysis patients with ST-segment elevation acute myocardial infarction should receive acute reperfusion therapy. Prompt thrombolytic therapy is indicated if emergency percutaneous coronary intervention (PCI) is not readily available, but the latter is preferred because of the potential for increased hemorrhagic risk associated with thrombolytic

therapy. These guidelines can likely be extrapolated to diabetic patients on dialysis.

Coronary artery bypass graft (CABG) surgery in ESRD

There are no RCTs comparing outcomes with CABG against PCI in patients with ESRD, particularly in the diabetic population. A meta-analysis of 17 retrospective cohort studies addressing this issue in dialysis patients showed that the short-term (30 days or in-hospital) mortality was higher after CABG than PCI, whereas the long-term (>1 year) mortality was similar between groups or even lower after CABG in some studies. Furthermore, PCI was associated with considerably more cardiovascular events, and this trend could be attributed to the higher restenosis rate in the group of patients treated with this modality [54]. On the other hand, a meta-analysis of four randomized control trials comparing clinical outcomes after PCI with bare-metal stenting versus CABG in patients with multivessel CAD revealed that the former has a similar long-term safety profile than CABG. However, it is associated with a higher repeat revascularization rates and consequently more cardiovascular events [55]. Given the limited body of evidence, the NKF-K/DOQI guidelines recommend individualizing the decision to intervene with either PCI or CABG for dialysis patients with obstructive CAD (level of evidence C) with a preference toward CABG for patients with multivessel disease [25].

Comparing renal replacement therapies in diabetic patients with ESRD

Once a diabetic patient reaches ESRD, several options for renal replacement become available: hemodialysis, peritoneal dialysis (PD), and kidney transplantation (which is addressed in

Chapter 17). It has been established that survival with either modality of dialysis is generally worse for diabetic patients than their non-diabetic counterparts [56].

Hemodialysis versus peritoneal dialysis

Despite several advantages of PD over hemodialysis, its use progressively decreased over the last decade while that of hemodialysis increased [57], because of some observational studies showing either similar or even worse outcomes in diabetic patients treated with PD compared with hemodialysis (Table 16.3). Furthermore, a meta-analysis of six large-scale registry studies

and three prospective cohort studies comparing outcomes among ESRD patients receiving hemodialysis or PD revealed the following results [58]: (1) PD is associated with better survival than hemodialysis among non-diabetic and younger diabetic patients; (2) PD is generally associated with equivalent or even better survival during the first year or two of dialysis; and (3) conflicting results were encountered in older diabetic patients such that studies conducted in Canada and Denmark showed no difference in survival between the two dialysis modalities while others carried out in the USA showed a better survival with hemodialysis in diabetic patients more than 45 years of age.

Table 16.3 Observational studies comparing outcomes between peritoneal dialysis and hemodialysis

Authors and year of publication	Type of study	Number and type of patients	Results
Nelson et al, 1992	Observational	1,458 diabetics 2,830 non-diabetics	PD: lower mortality than hemodialysis in young diabetic patients (age 20 to 52)
Held et al, 1994	Prospective observational	1,725 diabetics 2411 non-diabetics	1. Non-diabetic patients: similar outcomes. 2. Diabetic patients: similar outcomes in patients <58 years of age. Higher mortality with PD in patients >58 years of age. 3. First year of treatment: similar outcome. After 12 months: PD associated with higher mortality
Fenton et al, 1997	Observational	2707 diabetics 9263 non-diabetics	PD: lower mortality during the first 2 years of treatment; effect less pronounced in diabetics >65 years of age
Vonesh et al, 1999	Observational	55,668 diabetics 147,930 non-diabetics	1. Older (age >50) and female diabetics: higher mortality on PD 2. Younger diabetics (age <50): lower mortality on PD 3. Male diabetics: similar outcomes
Collins et al, 1999	Observational	117,158 patients	1. PD: lower mortality in non-diabetics and diabetics <55 years of age, especially during the first 2 years of treatment 2. PD: higher mortality in female diabetics >55 years of age

Potential benefits of PD in diabetes

Hemodialysis is frequently associated with recurrent episodes of hypotension, repetitive coronary ischemia, and consequently myocardial stunning and arrhythmias [59]. Thus, the better hemodynamic profile associated with PD makes it an advantageous modality in diabetic patients who are at increased risk of cardiovascular complications [60]. Furthermore, the lack of a need to create an arteriovenous fistula, which increases cardiac overload and can precipitate heart failure, may also be a potential benefit of PD in such patients. Superior preservation of residual renal function, with a significant impact on patient outcome, has been associated with PD [61]. Finally, the avoidance of anticoagulation and the lack of need for vascular access with subsequently fewer episodes of bloodborne diseases are additional advantages that favor this dialysis modality in diabetic patients [57].

Potential disadvantages of PD in diabetes

The conventional PD modality relies mainly on D-glucose to achieve better ultrafiltration. Indeed, since 50–80% of the intraperitoneal glucose is absorbed into the systemic circulation, excessive glucose exposure not only worsens hyperglycemia but is associated also with an increased incidence of dyslipidemia [62]. Thus, glucose-sparing solutions have been developed, the most widely available being icodextrin. A meta-analysis of nine randomized controlled trials comparing icodextrin to glucose showed that the former had significant advantages over glucose in small solute clearance and plasma total cholesterol. However, no differences in plasma triglycerides, fasting plasma glucose, and body weight were observed [63]. Hence, larger and longer randomized controlled trials are needed to definitively assess the effect of glucose-sparing solutions not only

on the metabolic profile but more importantly on the survival of PD patients.

Where does the use of PD stand in diabetic patients?

Given the available body of evidence, PD is suggested as the initial modality of dialysis in all ESRD patients. Non-diabetic patients and older patients with diabetes may switch modality to hemodialysis or undergo kidney transplantation after 1–2 years while younger diabetic patients may stay longer on PD [64].

1. El-Achkar TM, Ohmit SE, McCullough PA, et al. Higher prevalence of anemia with diabetes mellitus in moderate kidney insufficiency: The Kidney Early Evaluation Program. Kidney Int 2005; **67**:1483–88.
2. Weiner DE, Tighiouart H, Vlagopoulos PT, et al. Effects of anemia and left ventricular hypertrophy on cardiovascular disease in patients with chronic kidney disease. J Am Soc Nephrol 2005;**16**: 1803–10.
3. Vlagopoulos PT, Tighiouart H, Weiner DE, et al. Anemia is a risk factor for cardiovascular disease and all-cause mortality in diabetes: the impact of chronic kidney disease. J Am Soc Nephrol 2005;**16**:3403–10.
4. Foley RN, Parfrey PS, Harnett JD, et al. The impact of anemia on cardiomyopathy, morbidity, and mortality in end-stage renal disease. Am J Kidney Dis 1996;**28**:53–61.
5. Pisoni RL, Bragg-Gresham JL, Young EW, et al. Anemia management and outcomes from 12 countries in the Dialysis Outcomes and Practice Patterns Study (DOPPS). Am J Kidney Dis 2004; **44**:94–111.

6. Jones M, Ibels L, Schenkel B, Zagari M, et al. Impact of epoetin alfa on clinical end points in patients with chronic renal failure: a meta-analysis. *Kidney Int* 2004; **65**:757–67.

7. Singh AK. The controversy surrounding hemoglobin and erythropoiesis-stimulating agents: what should we do now? *Am J Kidney Dis* 2008; **52**(Suppl 1):S5–S13.

8. K/DOQI Clinical Practice Guideline and Clinical Practice Recommendations for anemia in chronic kidney disease: 2007 update of hemoglobin target. *Am J Kidney Dis* 2007;**50**:471–530.

9. Robbins J, Aragaki AK, Kooperberg C, et al. Factors associated with 5-year risk of hip fracture in postmenopausal women. *JAMA* 2007;**298**:2389–98.

10. Rigalleau V, Lasseur C, Raffaitin C, et al. Bone loss in diabetic patients with chronic kidney disease. *Diabet Med* 2007;**24**:91–3.

11. Pei Y, Hercz G, Greenwood C, et al. Renal osteodystrophy in diabetic patients. *Kidney Int* 1993; **44**:159–64.

12. Schwartz AV, Sellmeyer DE, Vittinghoff E, et al. Thiazolidinedione use and bone loss in older diabetic adults. *J Clin Endocrinol Metab* 2006; **91**:3349–54.

13. Mehrotra R, Kermah D, Budoff M, et al. Hypovitaminosis D in chronic kidney disease. *Clin J Am Soc Nephrol* 2008; **3**:1144–51.

14. K/DOQI Clinical Practice Guidelines for bone metabolism and disease in chronic kidney disease. *Am J Kidney Dis* 2003;**42** Suppl 3:S2.

15. Agarwal R, Acharya M, Tian J, et al. Antiproteinuric effect of oral paricalcitol in chronic kidney disease. *Kidney Int* 2005;**68**:2823–8.

16. Lambers Heerspink HJ, Agarwal R, Coyne DW, et al. The selective vitamin D receptor activator for albuminuria lowering (VITAL) study: study design and baseline characteristics. *Am J Nephrol* 2009;**30**:280–6.

17. Mak RH. Impact of end-stage renal disease and dialysis on glycemic control. *Semin Dial* 2000;**13**:4–8.

18. Peacock TP, Shihabi ZK, Bleyer AJ, et al. Comparison of glycated albumin and hemoglobin A(1c) levels in diabetic subjects on hemodialysis. *Kidney Int* 2008;**73**:1062–68.

19. Inaba M, Okuno S, Kumeda Y, et al. Glycated albumin is a better glycemic indicator than glycated hemoglobin values in hemodialysis patients with diabetes: effect of anemia and erythropoietin injection. *J Am Soc Nephrol* 2007;**18**:896–903.

20. Okada T, Nakao T, Matsumoto H, et al. Association between markers of glycemic control, cardiovascular complications and survival in type 2 diabetic patients with end-stage renal disease. *Intern Med* 2007;**46**:807–14.

21. Fukuoka K, Nakao K, Morimoto H, et al. Glycated albumin levels predict long-term survival in diabetic patients undergoing haemodialysis. *Nephrology (Carlton)* 2008;**13**:278–83.

22. Joy MS, Cefalu WT, Hogan SL, Nachman PH. Long-term glycemic control measurements in diabetic patients receiving hemodialysis. *Am J Kidney Dis* 2002;**39**:297–307.

23. Shrishrimal K, Hart P, Michota F. Managing diabetes in hemodialysis patients: observations and recommendations. *Cleve Clin J Med* 2009;**76**:649–55.

24. Ricks J, Molnar MZ, Kovesdy CP, et al. Glycemic control and cardiovascular mortality in hemodialysis patients with diabetes: a 6-year cohort study. *Diabetes* 2012;**61**:708–15.

25. K/DOQI Clinical Practice Guidelines for cardiovascular disease in dialysis patients. *Am J Kidney Dis* 2005;**45**(Suppl 3): S1–S153.

26. Hörl MP, Hörl WH. Hemodialysis associated hypertension: pathophysiology and therapy. *Am J Kidney Dis* 2002;**39**: 227–44.

27. Heerspink HJ, Ninomiya T, Zounga S, *et al*. Effect of lowering blood pressure on cardiovascular events and mortality in patients on dialysis: a systematic review and meta-analysis of randomised controlled trials. *Lancet* 2009;**373**: 1009–15.

28. Agarwal R. Role of home blood pressure monitoring in hemodialysis patients. *Am J Kidney Dis* 1999;**33**:682–7.

29. Zager PG, Nikolic J, Brown RH, *et al*. "U" curve association of blood pressure and mortality in hemodialysis patients. *Kidney Int* 1998;**54**:561–9.

30. Mailloux LU. The overlooked role of salt restriction in dialysis patients. *Semin Dial* 2000;**13**:150–1.

31. Agarwal R, Alborzi P, Satyan S, Light RP. Dry-weight reduction in hypertensive hemodialysis patients (DRIP): a randomized, controlled trial. *Hypertension* 2009;**53**:500–7.

32. Scribner BH. Can antihypertensive medications control BP in haemodialysis patients: yes or no? *Nephrol Dial Transplant* 1999;**14**:2599–601.

33. Zannad F, Kessler M, Lehert P, *et al*. Prevention of cardiovascular events in end-stage renal disease: results of a randomized trial of fosinopril and implications for future studies. *Kidney Int* 2006;**70**:1318–24.

34. Suzuki H, Kanno Y, Sugahara S, *et al*. Effect of angiotensin receptor blockers on cardiovascular events in patients undergoing hemodialysis: an open-label randomized controlled trial. *Am J Kidney Dis* 2008;**52**:501–6.

35. Knoll GA, Sahgal A, Nair RC, *et al*. Renin-angiotensin system blockade and the risk of hyperkalemia in chronic hemodialysis patients. *Am J Med* 2002; **112**:110–4.

36. Cice G, Ferrara L, D'Andrea A, *et al*. Carvedilol increases two-year survival in dialysis patients with dilated cardiomyopathy: a prospective, placebo-controlled trial. *J Am Coll Cardiol* 2003;**41**:1438–44.

37. London GM, Pannier B, Guerin AP, *et al*. Cardiac hypertrophy, aortic compliance, peripheral resistance, and wave reflection in end-stage renal disease. Comparative effects of ACE inhibition and calcium channel blockade. *Circulation* 1994; **90**:2786–96.

38. Molitch ME. Management of dyslipidemias in patients with diabetes and chronic kidney disease. *Clin J Am Soc Nephrol* 2006;**1**:1090–9.

39. Feingold KR, Grunfeld C, Pang M, *et al*. LDL subclass phenotypes and triglyceride metabolism in non-insulin-dependent diabetes. *Arterioscler Thromb* 1992;**12**: 1496–502.

40. Mason NA, Baillie GR, Satayathum S, *et al*. HMG-CoA reductase inhibitor use is associated with mortality reduction in hemodialysis patients. *Am J Kidney Dis* 2005; **45**:119–26.

41. Wanner C, Krane V, Marz W, *et al*. Atorvastatin in patients with type 2 diabetes mellitus undergoing hemodialysis. *N Engl J Med* 2005;**353**: 238–48.

42. Fellstrom BC, Jardine AG, Schmieder RE, *et al*. Rosuvastatin and cardiovascular events in patients undergoing hemodialysis. *N Engl J Med* 2009;**360**: 1395–407.

43. Holdaas H, Holme I, Schmieder RE, *et al.* Rosuvastatin in diabetic hemodialysis patients. *J Am Soc Nephrol* 2011;**22**: 1335–41.

44. Baigent C, Landray MJ, Reith C, *et al.* The effects of lowering LDL cholesterol with simvastatin plus ezetimibe in patients with chronic kidney disease (Study of Heart and Renal Protection): a randomised placebo-controlled trial. *Lancet* 2011;**377**:2181–92.

45. K/DOQI Clinical Practice Guidelines and Clinical Practice Recommendations for diabetes and chronic kidney disease. *Am J Kidney Dis* 2007;**49** Suppl 2: S12-S154.

46. Foley R. Cardiac disease in diabetic patients with renal disease. *Acta Diabetol* 2002;**39**(Suppl 1):S9–S14

47. Karnib HH, Ziyadeh FN. The cardiorenal syndrome in diabetes mellitus. *Diabetes Res Clin Pract* 2010;**89**:201–8.

48. Schömig M, Ritz E. Cardiovascular problems in diabetic patients on renal replacement therapy. *Nephrol Dial Transplant* 2000;**15**(Suppl 5):S111–6.

49. Rabbat CG, Treleaven DJ, Russell JD, Ludwin D, Cook DJ. Prognostic value of myocardial perfusion studies in patients with end-stage renal disease assessed for kidney or kidney-pancreas transplantation: a meta-analysis. *J Am Soc Nephrol* 2003;**14**:431–9.

50. Ethier J, Bragg-Gresham JL, Piera L, *et al.* Aspirin prescription and outcomes in hemodialysis patients: the Dialysis Outcomes and Practice Patterns Study (DOPPS). *Am J Kidney Dis* 2007;**50**: 602–11.

51. Jardine MJ, Ninomiya T, Perkovic V, *et al.* Aspirin is beneficial in hypertensive patients with chronic kidney disease: a post-hoc subgroup analysis of a randomized controlled trial. *J Am Coll Cardiol* 2010;**56**:956–65.

52. Wright RS, Reeder GS, Herzog CA, *et al.* Acute myocardial infarction and renal dysfunction: a high-risk combination. Ann *Intern Med* 2002;**137**: 563–70.

53. McCullough PA, Sandberg KR, Borzak S, Hudson MP, Garg M, Manley HJ. Benefits of aspirin and beta-blockade after myocardial infarction in patients with chronic kidney disease. *Am Heart J* 2002; **144**:226–32.

54. Nevis IF, Mathew A, Novick RJ, *et al.* Optimal method of coronary revascularization in patients receiving dialysis: systematic review. *Clin J Am Soc Nephrol* 2009;**4**:369–78.

55. Daemen J, Boersma E, Flather M, *et al.* Long-term safety and efficacy of percutaneous coronary intervention with stenting and coronary artery bypass surgery for multivessel coronary artery disease: a meta-analysis with 5-year patient-level data from the ARTS, ERACI-II, MASS-II, and SoS trials. *Circulation* 2008;**118**:1146–54.

56. McMillan MA, Briggs JD, Junor BJ. Outcome of renal replacement treatment in patients with diabetes mellitus. *BMJ* 1990;**301**:540–4.

57. Passadakis PS, Oreopoulos DG. Diabetic patients on peritoneal dialysis. *Semin Dial* 2010;**23**:191–7.

58. Vonesh EF, Snyder JJ, Foley RN, Collins AJ. Mortality studies comparing peritoneal dialysis and hemodialysis: what do they tell us? *Kidney Int Suppl* 2006;**103**:S3–11.

59. McIntyre CW. Haemodialysis-induced myocardial stunning in chronic kidney disease—a new aspect of cardiovascular disease. *Blood Purif* 2010; **29**:105–10.

60. Selby NM, McIntyre CW. Peritoneal dialysis is not associated with myocardial stunning. *Perit Dial Int* 2011;**31**:27–33.

61. Tam P. Peritoneal dialysis and preservation of residual renal function. *Perit Dial Int* 2009;**29**(Suppl 2):S108–10.

62. Holmes CJ. Reducing cardiometabolic risk in peritoneal dialysis patients: role of the dialysis solution. *J Diabetes Sci Technol* 2009;**3**:1472–80.

63. He Q, Zhang W, Chen J. A meta-analysis of icodextrin versus glucose containing peritoneal dialysis in metabolic management of peritoneal dialysis patients. *Ren Fail* 2011;**33**: 943–8.

64. Chung SH, Noh H, Ha H, Lee HB. Optimal use of peritoneal dialysis in patients with diabetes. *Perit Dial Int* 2009;**29**(Suppl 2):S132–4.

Chapter 17

Combined pancreas and kidney transplantation or kidney alone transplantation for patients with diabetic nephropathy

Hermann J. Kissler, Christiane Rüster and Utz Settmacher

Jena University Hospital, Jena, Germany

Key points

- Multidisciplinary pretransplant evaluation is mandatory to optimize graft and patient survival.
- Cardiovascular evaluation and screening for chronic conditions, i.e., infections and malignancy, allow for appropriate management before transplantation.
- Preoperative preparation of the pancreas kidney transplant recipient is vital, with special emphasis on hydration status, cytomegalovirus prophylaxis, and immunosuppressive therapy.
- Complications after renal transplantation are delayed graft function, hemorrhage, acute rejection, and adverse effects of immunosuppressive drugs.
- Proteinuria is common after kidney transplantation and is a significant marker of graft injury.

- Urinary tract infection is the most common infection after renal transplantation.
- Chronic allograft nephropathy is the most common cause of chronic renal transplant dysfunction and managed by reducing or discontinuing calcineurin inhibitor treatment.
- Acute and chronic complications after pancreas transplantation.
- Adding a pancreas transplant to a kidney transplant not only improves diabetes and quality of life, but increases patient survival.
- Complications occur more often in pancreas than in kidney transplantation and considerably account for early pancreas transplant loss.

Rationale of pancreas kidney transplantation for patients with diabetic nephropathy

Diabetic nephropathy is the most common cause of end-stage renal disease (ESRD), followed by glomerulonephritis, polycystic kidney disease, hypertensive nephropathy, lupus nephropathy, and interstitial nephritis. Owing to the enormous advances in immunosuppressive therapy and surgical technique, kidney transplantation is now considered the best treatment for the majority of patients with ESRD. Renal transplantation clearly benefits the

Diabetes and Kidney Disease, First Edition. Edited by Gunter Wolf.
© 2013 John Wiley & Sons, Ltd. Published 2013 by John Wiley & Sons, Ltd.

recipients by being superior to dialysis in terms of quality of life, control of comorbidities, cost-effectiveness, and survival [1]. In the case of type 1 diabetes mellitus, simultaneous pancreas and kidney (SPK) or pancreas after kidney (PAK) transplantation is clearly an option to significantly improve kidney graft function and survival in selected patients [2]. This is due to pancreas transplantation being more effective in achieving glycemic control with a greater impact on secondary diabetic complications than intensive insulin therapy.

Indications and contraindications to pancreas kidney transplantation

Patients with diabetic nephropathy eligible for kidney transplantation must be on or about to go on dialysis, and have ESRD. In this case, patients should be listed for transplantation once their estimated glomerular filtration rate (eGFR) is below $20\,mL/min/1.73\,m^2$. As survival after transplantation has been shown to be better the shorter the patient is on dialysis, patients should be transferred for timely evaluation when the eGFR is below $30\,mL/min/1.73\,m^2$ [3].

Patients with ESRD and type 1 diabetes with other diabetic complications are candidates for a simultaneous pancreas and kidney transplant from the same donor because immunosuppression requirements are similar to those for a kidney transplant alone, and rejection episodes are more easily detected by monitoring kidney function. This also applies for patients with type 1 diabetes and failure of a previous renal transplant. Furthermore, pre-emptive SPK transplantation is possible in patients with ESRD before the onset of chronic dialysis. The second indication for pancreas transplantation is patients with type 1 diabetes with a well-functioning kidney transplant from either a living or cadaveric donor. These patients benefit from better control of metabolism than

achieved by exogenous insulin therapy, thereby accounting for the risk of major surgery. According to the International Pancreas Transplant Registry (IPTR), 75% of pancreas transplants were SPK and 18% PAK [4]. In 2010, 7% of patients receiving a pancreas transplant were categorized as type 2 diabetes, based on detectable serum C-peptide levels, and represented 8% of SPK and 5% of PAK [4]. According to the new US pancreas allocation system that was approved by the United Network for Organ Sharing Board in November 2010, qualifying criteria for SPK include either being on insulin with serum C-peptide $\leq 2\,ng/mL$, or being on insulin for glycemic intolerance with a body mass index (BMI) $\leq 28\,kg/m^2$ with a C-peptide $>2\,ng/mL$ [5].

Before recommending transplantation of any type, criteria precluding a successful transplant outcome must be excluded as outlined in Box 17.1. Thus, active or chronic untreated infection and recent malignancy needs to be ruled out. Patients must be compliant, without active addiction to alcohol or substance abuse, and active uncontrolled psychiatric disorder or psychologic instability. Life expectancy after transplantation must be reasonable. As diabetes and ESRD puts patients at high risk to develop complications of arteriosclerosis, i.e., cardiovascular disease and stroke, insufficient cardiovascular reserve needs to be ruled out. Patients must be able to tolerate the transplant surgery and immunosuppressive therapy. High levels of sensitization to donor tissue precludes transplantation because of a high incidence of hyperacute rejection and transplant loss, and may only be feasible with specific desensitization protocols [6].

Evaluation of candidates for pancreas kidney transplantation

The aim of the evaluation is to identify relevant comorbidities requiring treatment or

---

Box 17.1 Contraindications to pancreas and kidney transplantation

1. Reversible renal disease
2. Insufficient cardiovascular reserve
   coronary angiography indicating non-correctable coronary artery disease
   ejection fraction below 50%
   recent myocardial infarction
3. Recent malignancy
4. Active or chronic untreated infection
5. Life expectancy < 1 year
6. Sensitization to donor tissue
7. Ongoing alcohol or substance abuse
8. Uncontrolled major psychiatric illness or psychologic instability
9. History of noncompliance with medical treatment

---

constituting a contraindication for transplantation, to unmask psychosocial problems endangering the transplant outcome, and to determine the immunologic status for correct organ matching. Thus, the evaluation of the potential kidney and combined kidney–pancreas transplant candidate follow the same general guidelines [7].

The evaluation begins with a detailed history and physical examination, and the renal and urologic diseases are evaluated first. It is important to record the progression of the renal disease, time period and clinical course on dialysis, including complications, and amount of urine production. As the kidney transplant drains into the lower urinary tract, it is crucial to detect urologic problems that can affect the transplant outcome. Therefore, patients with a history of obstructive uropathy, nephrolithiasis, recurrent urinary tract infections, bladder dysfunction, and previous urologic malignancy need to be evaluated by an urologist. This allows for pretransplant medical or operative management of any urologic condition, and eventually planning of an alternate urinary drainage of the kidney transplant. All medications are recorded and medical therapy adjusted to optimize glycemic and metabolic control of diabetes in order to account for the increased risk of cardiovascular and infectious complications in this group of patients after transplantation. The review of systems should identify any extrarenal organ system issues which need to be specifically addressed by more detailed studies and specialist consultation. Extensive laboratory, radiologic, and specialty testing with special emphasis on cardiovascular and immunologic evaluation are required, as described below and detailed in Box 17.2. After completion of the evaluation, acceptance of the patient for candidacy for transplantation is decided. If accepted, the patient is placed on the waiting list.

Cardiovascular, cerebrovascular, and peripheral vascular evaluation

Diabetic patients with ESRD have considerable comorbidities, with advanced vascular disease being the most important. These patients have an increased rate of myocardial infarction, stroke, and limb amputations due to atherosclerosis of the cardiovascular, cerebrovascular, and peripheral vascular systems. Mortality from cardiovascular disease is thought to be 10–20 times that of the general population and the leading cause of death in diabetic ESRD patients. Because of diabetes-related neuropathy, patients do not experience ischemia-induced angina pectoris. Diabetic ESRD patients have a high

Evaluation of pancreas and kidney transplant recipients

Laboratory studies

General

Complete blood count, blood chemistries (creatinine, urea, uric acid, electrolytes, calcium, phosphorus, osmolarity, total protein, albumin, amylase, lipase), liver function tests (aspartate aminotransferase, alanine aminotransferase, γ-glutamyl transferase, alkaline phosphatase, bilirubin total + direct), coagulation profile (prothrombin time, partial thromboplastin time, thrombin time, fibrinogen, angiotensin III, protein C and S, activated protein C resistance), diabetes related (insulin, C-peptide, α1-antitrypsin, HbA1c, glucose day profile), bone related (vitamin D metabolites, intact parathyroid hormone, osteocalcin, bone specific alkaline phosphatase), thyroid hormones (fT3, fT4, TSH), triglycerides, total cholesterol, LDL-cholesterol, HDL-cholesterol, tumor markers (CEA, CA 19-9, PSA)

Urine: urinalysis, urine sediment, urea/creatinine clearance, urine crosslinks, urine culture

Heme occult test 3×

Infectious profile

Hepatitis B and C serologies, HIV, herpes simplex, varicella zoster serologies, CMV and Epstein–Barr virus serologies (IgM/IgG), RPR (syphilis), PPD (tuberculosis skin test)

Immunologic profile

Blood type (ABO), HLA typing, panel reactive antibody (PRA)

Auto-antibodies: islet-ab, insulin-ab, sm-ab, antinuclear ab, ds-DNA-ab, cardiolipin-ab (IgM/IgG), antibasal membrane ab, c-ANCA, p-ANCA, including anti-PR3- and anti-MPO-auto-ab

Cardiac and vascular evaluation

Electrocardiogram, echocardiography with Doppler, exercise/dipyridamole thallium scintigraphy, coronary angiogram (>40 years, positive scintigraphy)

Peripheral arterial duplex studies, carotid duplex study, duplex of iliac and lower extremity vessels, angiography (if no triphasic pattern in duplex)

Pulmonary evaluation

Chest radiograph, pulmonary function tests

Urologic evaluation

Voiding cystourethrogram, urodynamic studies, renal ultrasound, cystoscopy

Gastrointestinal evaluation

Upper gastrointestinal endoscopy, colonoscopy, gallbladder ultrasound

Specialist consultation

Ophthalmology
Neurology
Psychiatry
Otolaryngology
Dentistry
Dermatology
Gynecology: gynecology examination with Papanicolaou smear, mammography (women >35 years)

prevalence of cardiovascular disease, left ventricular hypertrophy, and congestive heart failure. Thus, they are at high risk of cardiovascular events after transplantation. Therefore, a thorough cardiac work-up is mandatory. The minimum evaluation entails ECG, echocardiography with Doppler, and a dipyridamole thallium stress test. Patients with a positive stress test need to undergo a coronary angiography. If cardiovascular disease is detected and amenable to angioplasty or coronary artery bypass grafting, these procedures need to be carried out before transplantation.

Cerebrovascular and peripheral vascular diseases are also significant in this patient group, and routine evaluation thus requires duplex studies of the carotids, iliac, and lower extremity vessels. Angiography is indicated if the duplex studies detect any pathology potentially requiring angioplasty or vascular surgery. Magnetic resonance imaging (MRI) or computed tomography (CT) scan of the head are mandatory studies after transitory ischemic attacks or stroke.

Immunologic evaluation

The aim of extensive immunologic evaluation is to assess the variables that predispose a patient to antibody-mediated hyperacute rejection. The evaluation comprises four components: ABO blood group determination, human leukocyte antigen (HLA) typing, serum screening for antibody to HLA phenotypes, and cross-matching.

Histocompatibility testing includes blood typing (ABO), and HLA typing (A, B, DR, DQ). This allows identification of potential matches and avoidance of incompatible recipient–donor pairings that would result in transplant rejection.

In addition, the serum is screened for antibody to HLA phenotypes to determine the degree of humoral sensitization to HLA antigens. This is called the panel-reactive antibody (PRA). It is expressed as the percentage of potential donor antigens against which the recipient's serum may react, and thus predispose a sensitized recipient to develop a hyperacute antibody-mediated rejection. Higher PRA levels result in fewer matches and longer waiting time. Therefore, these patients receive priority in organ allocation.

Before transplantation, donor/recipient cross-matching is required. This assay determines whether a potential transplant recipient has preformed anti-HLA Class I antibody against those of the donor. A negative cross-match is absolutely necessary before accepting organs for transplantation.

Transplantation surgery

Evaluation of pancreas kidney donor

Living kidney donor evaluation

Living kidney donation is an essential part of transplantation practice, especially in the face of the shortage of deceased donor kidneys and the growing waiting list of potential recipients, but also in the view of an optimum for patient and graft survival and in concepts of pre-emptive transplantation. On the basis of the underlying ethical principal of "doing no harm," the donor evaluation process aims to ensure the suitability of the donor and to minimize the risk of donation. This involves the identification of contraindications to donation and the presence of unreasonable medical risks. Therefore, a comprehensive and standardized medical and psychosocial routine evaluation for the potential donor has been suggested based on a consensus of the "Amsterdam Forum on the Care of the Live Kidney Donor" (Table 17.1) [8].

Limitations in living kidney donation have to be identified and to be outweighed carefully in the individual situation. A gradual donor evaluation including the testing of blood

Table 17.1 Medical evaluation of the potential live kidney donor

Routine screening for the potential living kidney donor	
Urinalysis	Dipstick for protein, blood and glucose
	Microscopy, culture and sensitivity
	Measurement of protein excretion rate
Assessment of renal function	Estimation/measurement of GFR
Blood tests	Hematologic profile
	Complete blood count
	Hemoglobinopathy (where indicated)
	Coagulation screen (PT and APTT)
	G6PD deficiency (where indicated)
	Biochemical profile
	Creatinine, urea, and electrolytes
	Liver tests
	Urate
	Fasting plasma glucose
	Bone profile
	Glucose tolerance test (if fasting plasma glucose >6–7 mmol/L)
	Blood lipids
	Thyroid function tests (if indicated)
	Pregnancy test (if indicated)
	PSA (if indicated)
Virology and infection screen	Hepatitis B and C
	Toxoplasma
	Syphilis
	HIV and HTLV 1/2
	Malaria (where indicated)
	Cytomegalovirus
	Trypanozome cruzi (where indicated)
	Epstein–Barr virus
	Schistosomiasis (where indicated)
	HHV8 and HSV (where indicated)
	Strongyloides (where indicated)
	Typhoid (where indicated)
	Brucellosis (where indicated)
Cardiorespiratory system	Chest radiograph
	Electrocardiogram
	Stress test
	Echocardiography (where indicated)
Assessment of renal anatomy	Appropriate imaging investigations should allow confirmation of the presence of two kidneys of normal size and enable abnormalities of the collecting system and calcification or stone disease in the renal tract to be detected. They must also delineate the anatomy of the renal vasculature

PSA, prostate-specific antigen; HIV, human immunodeficiency virus; HTLV, human T-lymphotropic virus; HHV, human herpes virus; HSV, herpes simplex virus.

Modified from Delmonico F. A Report of the Amsterdam Forum On the Care of the Live Kidney Donor: Data and Medical Guidelines. *Transplantation* 2005;**79**(6 Suppl):S53–66.

group compatibility, cross-match, HLA sensitization (if indicated), and primary contraindication in the donor's previous medical history as well as routine urine and blood analysis help to triage unacceptable donors at an early point of time and to identify ABO/HLA incompatibility issues [9]. The Amsterdam Forum Guidelines provide a general recommendation how to proceed with pathologic diagnostic findings according relative or absolute contraindications for living kidney donation (Table 17.2) [8].

Cadaver donor evaluation

Upon notification of the organ procurement organization (OPO) of potential organ donors, it decides upon tentative medical suitability and correct documentation of brain death. An OPO transplant coordinator then personally obtains the consent of the family for organ donation and contacts transplant programs that have patients on the waiting list for organ transplantation. Although each transplant center has its own acceptance criteria, commonly accepted contraindications are outlined in Box 17.3.

Thus, absolute contraindications for transplantation are malignancy, positive HIV status, and sepsis with multiorgan failure. Septicemia is considered a relative contraindication, based on reports of comparable transplant and graft survival between bacteremic and nonbacteremic donors [10].

The major contraindication specific for kidney transplantation is pre-existing renal disease, which can be substantiated by serum creatinine, creatinine clearance, and renal biopsy. In order to better address the shortage of cadaver kidneys, the use of kidneys from so called "expanded criteria" or "marginal" donors has been widely accepted. Therefore, scoring systems for assessment of cadaver kidneys have been developed to quantify critical donor variables for prediction of transplant

outcome, i.e., age, hypertension, creatinine clearance, cause of death, and HLA mismatch [11]. As glomerulosclerosis of 15–50% and creatinine clearance of 50–90 mL/min are considered contraindications for single kidney transplantation, another approach to expand the donor pool is to transplant a single recipient with two renal allografts [12].

Criteria for selection of pancreas donors are tighter than for kidney donors, because of the unique anatomical and physiologic properties of the pancreas with increased risk of graft failure. Major fatty infiltration of the pancreas and a predisposition to type 2 diabetes mellitus generally disqualify obese donors with a BMI above 30kg/m^2. More pancreatic fibrosis and calcification in older donors precludes their pancreas from transplantation. Hyperglycemia and hyperamylasemia are common after brain death. However, hyperglycemia is not a contraindication to pancreas procurement of donors who have no history of diabetes mellitus and normal glycosylated hemoglobin (HbA1c) levels. Hyperamylasemia is more alarming, but does not affect graft function unless pancreatitis and pancreatic damage are macroscopically detected. Thus, pancreatic assessment during procurement is of paramount importance to characterize pathologic changes of the pancreatic parenchyma and to check the vascular supply for a replaced or accessory right hepatic artery with its origin from the superior mesenteric artery, which needs to stay with the liver transplant. With the increasing demand for pancreas transplantation, two scoring systems have been proposed to expand the donor pool, one from Eurotransplant data (Preprocurement Pancreas Allocation Suitability Score, P-PASS) and from Scientific Registry of Transplant Recipients data (Pancreas Donor Risk Index, PDRI) [13, 14]. Currently, the multicenter study EXPAND prospectively evaluates an extended donor pancreas program in the Eurotransplant region (Clinical Trials.gov Identifier: NCT01384006).

Amsterdam Forum Guidelines 2005

Donor evaluation	Prior to donation, the live kidney donor must receive a complete medical and psychosocial evaluation, receive appropriate informed consent, and be capable of understanding the information presented in that process to make a voluntary decision. All donors should have standard tests performed to assure donor safety
Acceptable donor renal function	All potential kidney donors should have GFR estimated. Creatinine based methods may be used to estimate the GFR; however, creatinine clearance (as calculated from 24-hour urine collections) may under or overestimate GFR in patients with normal or near normal renal function. Calculated GFR values (MDRD and Cockcroft–Gault) are not standardized in this population and may overestimate GFR A GFR <80mL/min or 2 SD below normal (based on age, gender, and BSA corrected to 1.73/m²) generally precludes donation
Hypertension	BP >140/90 by ABPM: not acceptable as donors Patients with easily controlled hypertension + defined criteria (>50 years of age, GFR >80mL/min, urinary albumin excretion <30mg/day) may represent a low-risk group for development of kidney disease after donation and may be acceptable as kidney donors Donors with hypertension should be regularly followed by a physician
Diabetes	Individuals with a history of diabetes or fasting blood glucose ≥126mg/dL (7.0nmol/L) on at least two occasions (or 2-hour glucose with OGTT ≥200mg/dL (11.1mmol/L) should not donate
Obesity	BMI >35kg/m²: not acceptable as donors Obese patients should be encouraged to lose weight prior to kidney donation and should be advised not to donate if they have other associated comorbid conditions Obese patients should be informed of both acute and long-term risks, especially when other comorbid conditions are present Healthy lifestyle education should be available to all living donors.
Dyslipidemia	Dyslipidemia included along with other risk factors Dyslipidemia alone does not exclude kidney donation
Urine analysis for protein	A 24-hour urine protein of >300mg: contraindication to donation
Urine analysis for blood	Persistent microscopic hematuria: not be considered for kidney donation unless urine cytology/a complete urologic work up are performed. If urological malignancy and stone disease are excluded, a kidney biopsy may be indicated to rule out glomerular pathology

(Continued)

Table 17.2 (*Continued*)

Urinary tract infections	Urine should be sterile prior to donation; asymptomatic bacteria should be treated per donation
	Current pyuria and hematuria: contraindication to donation
	Unexplained hematuria or pyuria necessitates evaluation (adenovirus, tuberculosis, cancer)
	Urinary tuberculosis or cancer: contraindications to donation
Stone Disease	An asymptomatic potential donor with history of a single stone may be suitable for kidney donation if:
	– no hypercalcuria, hyperuricemia, or metabolic acidosis
	– no cystinuria, or hyperoxaluria
	– no urinary tract infection
	– multiple stones or nephrocalcinosis are not evident on CT
	An asymptomatic potential donor with a current single stone may be suitable if:
	– the donor meets the criteria shown previously for single stone formers and
	– current stone <1.5 cm in size
	– or potentially removable during the transplant
	Stone formers who should not donate are those with:
	– nephrocalcinosis on x ray or bilateral stone disease
	– stone types with high recurrence rates, and are difficult to prevent
Malignancy	A prior history of the following malignancies usually excludes live kidney donation:
	melanoma, testicular cancer, renal cell carcinoma, choriocarcinoma, hematological malignancy, bronchial cancer, breast cancer and monoclonal gammopathy
	A prior history of malignancy may only be acceptable for donation if:
	– prior treatment of the malignancy does not decrease renal reserve or place the donor at increased risk for ESRD
	– prior treatment of malignancy does not increase the operative risk of nephrectomy
	A prior history of malignancy usually excludes live kidney donation but may be acceptable if:
	the specific cancer is curable and potential transmission of cancer can reasonably be excluded

Live unrelated donors	The current available data suggest no restriction of live kidney donation based upon the absence of an HLA match. An unrelated donor transplant is equally successful to the outcome achieved by a genetically related family member such as a parent, child, or sibling, who is not HLA identical to the recipient
Determination of cardiovascular risk	The clinical predictors of an increased perioperative cardiovascular risk (for non-cardiac surgery) by the American College of Cardiology/ American Hospital Association standards fall into 3 categories: major, intermediate, minor.
	All major predictors: unstable coronary syndromes, decompensated heart failure, significant arrhythmias and severe valvular disease: contraindications to live kidney donation
	Most of the intermediate predictors: mild angina, previous myocardial infarction, compensated or prior heart failure, diabetes mellitus are also contraindications to donation
	Minor predictors: older age, abnormal ECG, rhythm other than sinus, low cardiac functional capacity, history of stroke or uncontrolled hypertension warrant individual consideration
Assessment of pulmonary issues	A careful history and physical examination are the most important parts of assessing risk
	Routine preoperative pulmonary function testing (PFT) is not warranted for potential live kidney donors unless there is an associated risk factor such as chronic lung disease
Smoking cessation and alcohol abstinence	Smoking cessation at least 4 weeks prior to donation is advised based on recommendations for patients undergoing elective surgical procedures
	Cessation of alcohol abuse defined by DSM-**3**: 60 g of alcohol/day sustained over ≥6 months should be avoided for a minimum of 4 weeks to decrease the known risk of postoperative morbidity

BP, blood pressure; ABPM, ambulatory blood pressure monitoring; GFR, glomerular filtration rate; BMI, body mass index; BSA, body surface area; CT, computed tomography; ESRD, end-stage renal disease; HLA, human leukocyte antigen; MDRD, modification of diet in renal disease.
Modified from Delmonico F. A Report of the Amsterdam Forum On the Care of the Live Kidney Donor: Data and Medical Guidelines. *Transplantation* 2005;**79** (6 Suppl):S53–66.

Box 17.3 Contraindications of kidney and pancreas procurement for transplantation

General

History of malignancy (absolute), except primary brain tumor

Infectious disease: HIV (absolute), hepatitis B or C (relative, depending on recipient status), any untreated systemic bacterial, fungal or viral infection

Septicemia (relative), sepsis with multiorgan failure (absolute)

Kidney

History of chronic renal disease (glomerulosclerosis >25–50% in renal biopsy, creatinine clearance of 50–90 mL/min for single kidney transplant)

Pancreas

Age <10 years and >55 years

Body weight <30 kg and >100 kg in consideration with height

History of diabetes mellitus or elevated HbA1c

History of alcoholism

History of pancreatic surgery

Traumatic injury of the pancreas

Intraoperative macroscopy of the pancreas: significant edema, fatty infiltration, fibrosis, or calcification, tumor, injury, hematoma, insufficient vascular supply

---

Kidney alone transplant surgery

The kidney is usually transplanted heterotopically to the iliac fossa (Figure 17.1). A right or left lower quadrant curvilinear hockey-stick type incision is made in the iliac fossa, depending on plans of a future pancreas transplant, which is usually to the right. The incision is carried down through the skin, subcutaneous tissue, and external oblique aponeurosis through the oblique muscle to the peritoneum. The peritoneum is mobilized medially and cephalad to expose the retroperitoneal fossa. The location of the vascular anastomoses depends on the length of the renal vessels, size of the donor kidney, and ascent of the psoas muscle. The transplant should lie flat in the iliac fossa avoiding greater tipping up of the lower kidney pole. The renal vein is anastomosed end-to-side to the iliac vein using 5-0 monofilament non-absorbable sutures. The iliac artery is anastomosed end-to-side with 6.0 monofilament non-absorbable sutures proximally relative to the venous anastomosis. Either the external or the common iliac artery may be

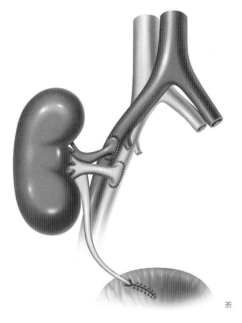

Figure 17.1 Kidney transplant in right iliac fossa with anterior ureteroneocystostomy.

used. Alternatively, an end-to-end anastomosis with the internal iliac artery is possible.

For ureteroneocystostomy, sterile saline is infused into the bladder via a Foley catheter, which is then clamped to keep the bladder distended. The ureter is properly aligned, the correct length measured, and the ureteral artery ligated. The ureter is then cut, spatulated, and slipped under the spermatic cord in males. Placement of a 6F double-J silastic ureteral stent is optional, but may prevent early urine leaks or ureteral stenosis. The stent is removed about 4 weeks after transplant via flexible cystoscopy. In the modified Lich–Gregoir procedure, the spatulated ureter is directly sutured to the bladder mucosa. The bladder musculature is incised down to the bladder mucosa. A cystostomy (2 cm) is constructed with 5-0 monofilament absorbable suture. The muscle layer is then approximated with 4-0 monofilament absorbable sutures as interrupted stitches for creation of an antireflux tunnel over the distal aspect of the ureter. Alternatively, in the Ledbetter–Politano procedure, a cystotomy is done and the ureter is tunneled posteriorly near the trigone. After positioning of the transplanted kidney without tension on the vessels and ureter to lie flat, the incision is closed by approximating the oblique musculature and external oblique aponeurosis in a single layer.

Pancreas transplant surgery

In SPK transplantation, the pancreas is transplanted first. The kidney is then transplanted to the left iliac fossa as described above.

Benchwork preparation

The pancreaticoduodenosplenic graft is transferred in a basin with chilled preservation solution. The spleen is separated from the pancreas, which is cleaned of fibrotic and adipose tissue The ampulla of Vater is identified to ensure its

center position, and the proximal and distal duodenum are trimmed to an adequate length to allow for safe anastomosis of about 6–8 cm. The superior mesenteric and splenic arteries are reconstructed using the donor iliac artery as a Y-graft. The end-to-end anastomoses are carried out with 6-0 monofilament non-absorbable sutures. This allows for one arterial anastomosis of the graft. The portal vein is carefully mobilized to gain an appropriate length for anastomosis. If the vein is too short, it is elongated using the donor external iliac vein.

Implantation surgery

Although surgical techniques differ in respect to handling the exocrine pancreatic secretions and venous outflow, there is a clear trend. Figures 17.2–17.4 illustrate all three alternative techniques. The surgical technique for duct management changed from urinary bladder drainage to enteric drainage. The latter is more physiologic in delivering pancreatic enzymes and bicarbonate to the intestines for reabsorption. Thus, urinary tract infections and

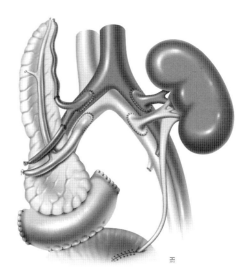

Figure 17.2 Simultaneous pancreas and kidney transplant with systemic venous and bladder drainage.

243

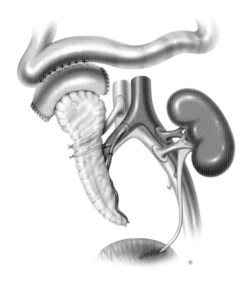

Figure 17.3 Simultaneous pancreas and kidney transplant with systemic venous and enteric drainage.

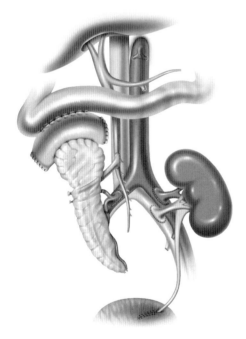

Figure 17.4 Simultaneous pancreas and kidney transplant with portal venous and enteric drainage.

metabolic acidosis, common in bladder drainage, are avoided. As there has been no real advantage of the more physiologic venous drainage of the pancreas transplant in the superior mesenteric vein with preservation of the first-pass effect of insulin, the technically easier systemic venous drainage in the iliac vein or infrarenal inferior vena cava is used in the majority of transplants. Thus, description of the surgical technique is restricted to the now favored procedure.

The abdomen is entered by a midline incision form 6–8 cm below the xiphoid to the pubis. The retroperitoneal tissue is opened medial to the ascending colon to expose the common iliac vessels. The portal vein of the pancreas graft is anastomosed end-to-side to the inferior vena cava using 5-0 monofilament non-absorbable sutures. The common iliac artery portion of the extension Y-graft that was previously anastomosed to the donor splenic and superior mesenteric arteries is sutured end-to-side to the recipient common iliac artery distal to the position of the venous anastomosis using 6.0 monofilament non-absorbable sutures.

The donor-to-recipient duodenoenterostomy is done after reperfusion of the pancreas to the terminal ileum 80 cm cephalad from Bauhin's valve. It is performed as a two-layer anastomosis using 4-0 absorbable monofilament running sutures. The length of the anastomosis is about 6–8 cm. Alternatively, a duodeno-duodenostomy can be performed. The pancreas transplant is then placed with the pancreatic head cephalad and the tail in the retrocystic pouch of Douglas.

Perioperative management

Pre- and postoperative management of pancreas kidney transplantation

Preoperative management includes physical examination, routine laboratory parameters depending on the local standard protocol (e.g., blood count, C-reactive protein, liver enzymes, coagulation parameters, pancreatic enzymes, baseline creatinine and urea, virologic screening, blood sample for cross-match for erythrocyte concentrates, etc.), a chest radiograph, and an electrocardiogram. Depending on the situation, acute preoperative hemodialysis therapy needs to be performed. If the patient does not have a functional vascular access or performs peritoneal dialysis, an intraoperative Shaldon catheter implantation should be considered. Preoperative thrombosis prophylaxis, perioperative antibiotic therapy, and application of immunosuppressive therapy depend on local standards.

Because of the high prevalence of early pancreas rejection with rates of 5–25%, induction therapy is routinely included in immunosuppressive protocols for pancreas transplant recipients [15]. Induction therapy with either alemtuzumab or antithymocyte globulin in combination with a calcineurin inhibitor and mycophenolate mofetil or sirolimus appears to be safe and effective in the setting of rapid steroid withdrawal [16]. Anti-interleukin (IL)-2 receptor antibody induction and no induction in combination with a calcineurin inhibitor, mycophenolate mofetil (MMF), or sirolimus, and prednisone have demonstrated excellent graft survival rates but are associated with a higher incidence of acute rejection [17]. Mycophenolate mofetil in combination with tacrolimus or ciclosporin is more effective in the prevention of rejection than is the combination of ciclosporin and azathioprine [18]. Comparison of cyclosporine with tacrolimus in combination with mycophenolate mofetil, and steroid plus induction with antithymocyte globulin showed a reduction in the rates of severe rejection with much lower rates of pancreas graft loss at 3 years in the tacrolimus group [19]. A rapid steroid taper with induction therapy is safe and effective in simultaneous pancreas kidney transplantation, and also steroid-free regimens seem to be possible in combination with tacrolimus and antibody induction showing no significant differences in patient and graft survival and rejection rates [20].

As in general postoperative care, usually on an intensive care unit, the focus is on cardiopulmonary stabilization, monitoring of diuresis, and volume status as well as on tight blood glucose controls. In the first 7 postoperative days, in addition to standard laboratory controls daily C-peptide controls are recommended and daily color-coded duplex sonography controls.

Complications after pancreas kidney transplantation

Complications of kidney transplantation

Surgical complications after renal transplant are comparatively low with reported rates of 5–10% [21]. Bleeding is uncommon and usually from vessels not ligated at the hilum or from small retroperitoneal vessels of the recipient. Vascular complications can involve the donor vessels: renal artery thrombosis (<1%), renal artery stenosis (1–10%), renal vein thrombosis or the recipient vessels [iliac artery thrombosis, pseudoaneurysm, deep vein thrombosis (5%)] [21]. Urologic complications either present as a leak or obstruction (2–10%), often as a result of ischemia of the transplant ureter [21].

Lymphoceles are common and well-known complications that occur in 1–26% of kidney transplant recipients [22]. The cause of lymphocele formation is unclear, but it is believed to result from transection of the lymphatic vessels accompanying the external iliac vessels during transplantation surgery and subsequent lymph accumulation in a non-epithelialized cavity in the extraperitoneal plane adjacent to the transplanted kidney.

Wound complications represent the most common surgical complication after renal transplant, including wound infections (5%), fascial dehiscences, or incisional hernias (3–5%) [21].

After exclusion of surgical and other reversible complications, postoperative kidney graft failure could be the result of rejection, and a contemporary kidney graft biopsy needs to be performed. A hyperacute rejection on the basis of preformed antidonor antibodies and complement activation occurs within minutes and hours, whereas acute accelerated rejection is due to sensitized T-cells and is observed within the first days. Both early types of rejection follow a mainly humoral immunologic pattern. Acute rejection in days to weeks after transplantation, mainly mediated by primary activation of T-cells, can often be different, either in a mainly cellular or mainly humoral process. Chronic allograft rejection occurs during a span of months to years, and it appears to be unresponsive to current treatment. The most commonly reported pathologic changes are chronic interstitial fibrosis and tubular atrophy, which are accompanied by vascular changes and glomerulosclerosis implicating its multifactorial genesis

Delayed graft function is a well-known complication affecting the kidney allograft in the immediate post-transplantation period. The frequency of delayed graft function ranges from 5% to 50% in deceased-donor kidney transplants [23]. It is the result of predominant ischemic injury to the graft before and during procurement and is further aggravated by the reperfusion syndrome, a multifactorial event in which immunologic factors also play a role [23]. Delayed graft function can contribute either to acute rejection or to accelerated interstitial nephritis and tubular atrophy, reducing graft survival. It is associated with a 41% increased risk of graft loss and is also associated with a 38% increased risk of acute rejection in the first year and results in a higher serum creatinine concentration. In this regard, delayed graft function is important for the prognosis of the clinical outcome after kidney transplantation [23].

Since the introduction of calcineurin inhibitors, initially ciclosporin followed by tacrolimus, graft survival has improved significantly, but these drugs are nephrotoxic [24]. Calcineurin inhibitor nephrotoxicity is mainly expressed as progressive arteriolar hyalinosis and downstream glomerulosclerosis, and is a common secondary diagnosis in 30% of so-called troubled transplants [25]. Although isolated calcineurin inhibitor nephrotoxicity without rejection has a good outcome, early recognition and treatment is important. In high-risk recipients, as in simultaneous pancreas kidney transplantation, calcineurin inhibitor withdrawal is not recommended [25]. Therefore either calcineurin inhibitor minimization or substitution with sirolimus or everolimus can be considered under close monitoring [26].

Residual human polyomavirus 1 (BK virus) in the renal cortex or medulla transmitted within transplanted kidneys can reactivate depending on the intensity of the immunosuppressive regimen, mostly within the first year. Asymptomatic viremia can result in transplant infection and tubulointerstitial nephritis followed by progressive transplant dysfunction in severe BK virus nephropathy, clinically very often mimicking graft rejection [27]. Early identification of BK virus infection by screening of viremia with blood nucleic acid testing and cautious reduction of immunosuppressive therapy generally reduces and eliminates circulating virus, preventing destructive parenchymal infection [26]. The prognosis of once established active BK virus nephropathy is poor and therapeutic approaches often are unsatisfactory.

Glomerular diseases can recur in kidney transplants with different frequency. The risk of recurrence is particularly increased in focal segmental glomerulosclerosis, immunoglobulin A nephropathy, membranoproliferative glomerulonephritis, hemolytic uremic syndrome, oxalosis, and Fabry's disease, and, to a lesser extent, with lupus nephritis, antiglomerular basement membrane disease, and vasculitis [26]. Recurrence usually can be screened easily by determination of proteinuria, hematuria and decrease in GFR rate leading to specific therapy.

The most common medical complications during the first weeks after transplantation are infectious problems. Infectious complications, especially early urinary tract infections with a rate of up to 81.9 % during the first 3 months are highest in the early postoperative period [28]. In spite of prophylaxis with valganciclovir or co-trimoxazol, mostly applied for the first 3–6 months, cytomegalovirus infections and pneumocystis pneumonia still present a threat and strict surveillance by the clinician must be ensured.

Complications of pancreas transplantation

Pancreas transplantation has the highest rate of complications of all organ transplants. Despite declining complication rates, the overall technical failure rate is 8–9% [4]. The most frequent and severe complications, which commonly occur within the first half year of transplantation, comprise vascular thrombosis of the pancreas graft, transplant pancreatitis, and intra-abdominal infections. Exocrine drainage leaks and bleeding are rare. Graft monitoring therefore includes frequent duplex sonography, measurement of C-peptide and procalcitonin in serum, as well as amylase and lipase in drains.

Vascular thrombosis

Vascular thrombosis usually occurs within the first days after transplantation. It typically affects the portal vein of the graft and is thought to be due to its low blood flow state, which is further reduced in reperfusion pancreatitis. Arterial thrombosis is rare and has a preference at the anastomosis of atherosclerotic arteries. Heparin and an antiplatelet agent early in the postoperative period are usually given to prevent thrombosis. The risk of mild bleeding hereby outweighs the fatal risk of graft loss. Signs of acute venous graft thrombosis are abruptly elevated blood glucose, accompanied by pain and tenderness at the transplant site with a swollen ipsilateral leg if the thrombus reaches the iliac vein. The diagnosis is confirmed by duplex sonography, CT scan, or MRI, and requires immediate vascular revision with thrombectomy or graft removal.

Transplant pancreatitis

Most recipients experience some form of graft pancreatitis within the fist week of transplantation. It is usually detected by elevated serum amylase and lipase levels and related to donor hemodynamic instability or injury from procurement, perfusion, preservation, and reperfusion. Clinical signs are abdominal pain and distension. Diagnosis is confirmed by CT scan, differentiating between mild edematous and necrotizing forms. Complications comprise pancreatic abscess, necrosis, perigraft infection, and pseudocyst. The graft is usually lost when complicated by intra-abdominal infection. Mild forms can be managed conservatively, whereas severe pancreatitis requires reoperation and may result in graft removal. Reflux pancreatitis occurs late in bladder-drained transplants and is due to urinary retention. Treatment is usually by short-term Foley catheter drainage. Only in recurrent pancreatitis, may enteric conversion be necessary.

Intra-abdominal infections

Among the factors contributing to intra-abdominal infections are pancreatitis, graft necrosis, bacterial translocation, and exocrine drainage leaks. The underlying diseases, i.e., longstanding type 1 diabetes and renal failure, as well as immunosuppressive treatment, increase the risk for infection. Abdominal pain, distension, ileus, fever, and elevated inflammatory parameters in blood are usually present. An abdominal CT scan is mandatory to identify the etiology. Treatment consists of radiologic drainage or surgery with appropriate antibiotic treatment.

Leaks of the exocrine drainage

Anastomotic leaks of the enteric drained pancreas invariably cause serious abdominal infection. Clinical symptoms are abdominal pain, distension, fever, and elevated inflammatory parameters in blood. Abdominal CT scan confirms the diagnosis. Surgical revision and appropriate antibiotic treatment are always necessary. If the infection cannot be eradicated, the graft needs to be removed in order to prevent sepsis and multiorgan failure. Management of a leak after bladder drainage depends on the degree of leakage and consists of primary repair or enteric conversion.

Complications related to bladder drainage

Drainage of exocrine pancreatic secretions into the bladder is responsible for several urologic and metabolic complications. Loss of about half a liter of pancreatic juice, rich in bicarbonate and pancreatic enzymes, causes metabolic acidosis and dehydration. The latter increases the risk of cardiac arrhythmias, severe hypotension with myocardial infarction, vascular thrombosis, and graft loss. Frequent monitoring of serum electrolytes and acid–base status is therefore mandatory. Treatment consists of vigorous hydration and oral bicarbonate substitution. The higher urinary pH results in a higher rate of urinary tract infections, whereas the pancreatic enzymes affect the urinary tract mucosa leading to cystitis, urethritis, and balanitis. When conservative measures fail, enteric

conversion is indicated. Because of the high complication rate, bladder drainage has been mostly replaced by enteric drainage.

Results of pancreas kidney transplantation

Results of kidney transplantation

In deceased donation for kidney transplantation 1-year graft survival rates of more than 90% and a long-term graft loss of about 4% per year resulting in 5-year survival rates of about 70% are consistently reported [29–31]. This is accompanied by an excellent patient survival of over 95% after 1 year and about 82% after 5 years [29]. Survival rates in living kidney donation are even better, with a 1-year survival of more than 95% and a 5-year survival of more than 80% [29].

Results of pancreas transplantation

The annual reports of the International Pancreas Transplant Registry (IPTR) and United Network for Organ Sharing (UNOS) are the authoritative sources for a comprehensive up-to-date analysis of pancreas transplant outcome [4, 32, 33]. From 1966 to 2010, 37 000 pancreas transplantations have been reported to the IPTR, including 25 000 from the USA and 12 000 from outside the USA. SPK accounted for 75% and PAK for 18% of pancreas transplants. The outcome is usually given as patient and graft survival. The survival rate of patients with SPK and PAK has constantly improved over time and reached more than 95% at 1 year post transplant for those carried out in 2009. The unadjusted patient survival rate reached 87% in SPK and 83% in PAK at 5 years post transplant, and more than 70% at 10 years post transplant. The leading causes of early and late death were cardiovascular and cerebrovascular problems, and infections. The pancreas and combined kidney graft function also improved over time. In 2006–2010, 1-year primary SPK pancreas graft function was 85.5% and combined SPK kidney function 93.4%, and 1-year pancreas graft function for PAK was 79.9%. The 5-year, 10-year, and 20-year pancreas graft functions were 80%, 68%, and 45%, respectively, for SPK, and 62%, 46%, and 16%, respectively, for PAK. These improvements were due to a reduction in technical failure rates and immunologic graft loss. Although there was no difference in pancreas graft survival in bladder-drained versus enteric drained pancreases, as well as in systemic versus portal venous drainage, enteric drainage in combination with systemic venous drainage has mostly replaced the other techniques. The overall technical failure rate was 8–9% in 2009. Graft thrombosis, infections, and pancreatitis were more common than leaks and bleeding. Current immunosuppression protocols generally have antibody induction therapy with tacrolimus and MMF as maintenance therapy, and showed a trend toward steroid avoidance. The most recent 1-year immunologic graft loss rate was 1.8% in SPK and 3.7% in PAK.

Effect of pancreas transplantation on secondary complications of diabetes and quality of life

Successful pancreas transplantation restores normoglycemia and HbA1c levels for as long as the transplant functions [34]. This has a positive influence on many secondary diabetic complications. Thus, it has been shown that SPK had a positive effect on cardiac disease, as evidenced by lower rates of myocardial infarction and pulmonary edema than in diabetic patients with KTA [35]. Cardiac atherosclerosis regression has also been shown in nearly 40% of patients with a functioning pancreas transplant, and reversal of diastolic dysfunction to normal 4 years post transplant [36, 37]. Neuropathy has been reported to slightly improve

with reduction of autonomic neuropathy-related sudden death [38]. Furthermore, recurrence of diabetic nephropathy, documented after KTA, could be prevented by SPK [39]. These positive effects of a pancreas transplant may explain why patient survival in SPK far exceeds that of cadaver donor KTA [40, 41], and in one study even of living donor KTA [2].

Several studies also confirmed that the quality of life in patients with a pancreas transplant is greatly improved compared with KTA [39, 42].

1. Wolfe RA, Ashby VB, Milford EL, *et al*. Comparison of mortality in all patients on dialysis, patients on dialysis awaiting transplantation, and recipients of a first cadaveric transplant. *N Engl J Med* 1999; **341**:1725–30.

2. Sollinger HW, Odorico JS, Becker YT, D'Alessandro AM, Pirsch JD. One thousand simultaneous pancreas-kidney transplants at a single center with 22-year follow-up. *Ann Surg* 2009;**250**: 618–30.

3. Bunnapradist S, Danovitch GM. Evaluation of adult kidney transplant candidates. Am *J Kidney Dis* 2007;**50**: 890–8.

4. Gruessner AC. 2011 update on pancreas transplantation: comprehensive trend analysis of 25,000 cases followed up over the course of twenty-four years at the International Pancreas Transplant Registry (IPTR). *Rev Diabet Stud* 2011;**8**: 6–16.

5. Kaufman DB, Sutherland DE. Simultaneous pancreas-kidney transplants are appropriate in insulin-treated candidates with uremia regardless of diabetes type. *Clin J Am Soc Nephrol* 2011; **6**:957–9.

6. Jordan SC, Peng A, Vo AA. Therapeutic strategies in management of the highly HLA-sensitized and ABO-incompatible transplant recipients. *Contrib Nephrol* 2009;**162**:13–26.

7. Kasiske BL, Cangro CB, Hariharan S, *et al*. The evaluation of renal transplantation candidates: clinical practice guidelines. *Am J Transplant* 2001;**1**(Suppl 2):3–95.

8. Delmonico F. A Report of the Amsterdam Forum On the Care of the Live Kidney Donor: Data and Medical Guidelines. *Transplantation* 2005;**79**(6 Suppl): S53–66.

9. URL: Accessed at www.bts.org.uk & www.renal.org; May 2011

10. Freeman RB, Giatras I, Falagas ME, *et al*. Outcome of transplantation of organs procured from bacteremic donors. *Transplantation* 1999;**68**: 1107–11.

11. Nyberg SL, Matas AJ, Kremers WK, *et al*. Improved scoring system to assess adult donors for cadaver renal transplantation. *Am J Transplant* 2003;**3**:715–21.

12. Tullius SG, Volk HD, Neuhaus P. Transplantation of organs from marginal donors. *Transplantation* 2001; **72**:1341–9.

13. Vinkers MT, Rahmel AO, Slot MC, Smits JM, Schareck WD. How to recognize a suitable pancreas donor: a Eurotransplant study of preprocurement factors. *Transplant Proc* 2008;**40**: 1275–8.

14. Axelrod DA, Sung RS, Meyer KH, Wolfe RA, Kaufman DB. Systematic evaluation of pancreas allograft quality, outcomes and geographic variation in utilization. *Am J Transplant* 2010;**10**:837–45.

15. White SA, Shaw JA, Sutherland DE. Pancreas transplantation. *Lancet* 2009;**373**(9677):1808–17.

16. Heilman RL, Mazur MJ, Reddy KS. Immunosuppression in simultaneous pancreas-kidney transplantation: progress to date. *Drugs* 2010;**70**: 793–804.

17. Burke GW, 3rd, Kaufman DB, Millis JM, *et al*. Prospective, randomized trial of the effect of antibody induction in simultaneous pancreas and kidney transplantation: three-year results. *Transplantation* 2004;**77**:1269–75.

18. Cantarovich D, Vistoli F. Minimization protocols in pancreas transplantation. *Transpl Int* 2009;**22**:61–8.

19. Malaise J, De Roover A, Squifflet JP, *et al*. Immunosuppression in pancreas transplantation: the Euro SPK trials and beyond. *Acta Chir Belg* 2008;**108**: 673–8.

20. Axelrod D, Leventhal JR, Gallon LG, Parker MA, Kaufman DB. Reduction of CMV disease with steroid-free immunosuppresssion in simultaneous pancreas-kidney transplant recipients. *Am J Transplant* 2005;**5**:1423–9.

21. Humar A, Matas AJ. Surgical complications after kidney transplantation. *Semin Dial* 2005; **18**:505–10.

22. Lucewicz A, Wong G, Lam VW, *et al*. Management of primary symptomatic lymphocele after kidney transplantation: a systematic review. *Transplantation* 2011;**92**:663–73.

23. Yarlagadda SG, Coca SG, Formica RN, Jr., Poggio ED, Parikh CR. Association between delayed graft function and allograft and patient survival: a systematic review and meta-analysis. *Nephrol Dial Transplant* 2009;**24**: 1039–47.

24. Naesens M, Kuypers DR, Sarwal M. Calcineurin inhibitor nephrotoxicity. *Clin J Am Soc Nephrol* 2009;**4**:481–508.

25. Gourishankar S, Leduc R, Connett J, *et al*. Pathological and clinical characterization of the "troubled transplant": data from the DeKAF study. *Am J Transplant* 2010; **10**:324–30.

26. Kasiske BL, Zeier MG, Chapman JR, *et al*. KDIGO clinical practice guideline for the care of kidney transplant recipients: a summary. *Kidney Int* 2010; **77**:299–311.

27. Johnston O, Jaswal D, Gill JS, Doucette S, Fergusson DA, Knoll GA. Treatment of polyomavirus infection in kidney transplant recipients: a systematic review. *Transplantation* 2010;**89**: 1057–70.

28. Saemann M, Horl WH. Urinary tract infection in renal transplant recipients. *Eur J Clin Invest* 2008;**38**(Suppl 2):58–65.

29. Wolfe RA, Roys EC, Merion RM. Trends in organ donation and transplantation in the United States, 1999–2008. *Am J Transplant* 2010;**10**:961–72.

30. McDonald S, Russ G, Campbell S, Chadban S. Kidney transplant rejection in Australia and New Zealand: relationships between rejection and graft outcome. *Am J Transplant* 2007;**7**: 1201–8.

31. Meier-Kriesche HU, Schold JD, Kaplan B. Long-term renal allograft survival: have we made significant progress or is it time to rethink our analytic and therapeutic strategies? *Am J Transplant* 2004;**4**: 1289–95.

32. Organ Procurement and Transplantation Network (OPTN) and Scientific Registry of Transplant Recipients (SRTR). *OPTN/ SRTR 2010 Annual Data Report*. Rockville, MD: Department of Health and Human Services, Health Resources and Services Administration, Healthcare Systems Bureau, Division of Transplantation, 2011.

33. Gruessner AC, Sutherland DE, Gruessner RW. Long-term outcome after pancreas transplantation. *Curr Opin Organ Transplant* 2012;**17**:100–5.

34. Robertson RP, Sutherland DE, Kendall DM, Teuscher AU, Gruessner RW, Gruessner A. Metabolic characterization of long-term successful pancreas transplants in type I diabetes. *J Investig Med* 1996;**44**:549–55.

35. La Rocca E, Fiorina P, Astorri E, *et al*. Patient survival and cardiovascular events after kidney-pancreas transplantation: comparison with kidney transplantation alone in uremic IDDM patients. *Cell Transplant* 2000;**9**:929–32.

36. Jukema JW, Smets YF, van der Pijl JW, *et al*. Impact of simultaneous pancreas and kidney transplantation on progression of coronary atherosclerosis in patients with end-stage renal failure due to type 1 diabetes. *Diabetes Care* 2002;**25**:906–11.

37. La Rocca E, Fiorina P, di Carlo V, *et al*. Cardiovascular outcomes after kidney-pancreas and kidney-alone transplantation. *Kidney Int* 2001; **60**:1964–71.

38. Navarro X, Kennedy WR, Loewenson RB, Sutherland DE. Influence of pancreas transplantation on cardiorespiratory reflexes, nerve conduction, and mortality in diabetes mellitus. *Diabetes* 1990; **39**:802–6.

39. Hopt UT, Drognitz O. Pancreas organ transplantation. Short and long-term results in terms of diabetes control. *Langenbecks Arch Surg* 2000;**385**:379–89.

40. Tyden G, Bolinder J, Solders G, *et al*. Improved survival in patients with insulin-dependent diabetes mellitus and end-stage diabetic nephropathy 10 years after combined pancreas and kidney transplantation. *Transplantation* 1999; **67**:645–8.

41. Ojo AO, Meier-Kriesche HU, Hanson JA, *et al*. The impact of simultaneous pancreas-kidney transplantation on long-term patient survival. *Transplantation* 2001;**71**: 82–90.

42. Gross CR, Limwattananon C, Matthees B, Zehrer JL, Savik K. Impact of transplantation on quality of life in patients with diabetes and renal dysfunction. *Transplantation* 2000; **70**:1736–46.

Page numbers in *italic* refer to figures.
Page numbers in **bold** refer to tables.
Page numbers followed by 'b' refer to boxes.

Diabetes and Kidney Disease, First Edition. Edited by Gunter Wolf.
© 2013 John Wiley & Sons, Ltd. Published 2013 by John Wiley & Sons, Ltd.